THE URBAN BRAIN

The Urban Brain

Mental Health in the Vital City

Nikolas Rose and Des Fitzgerald

PRINCETON UNIVERSITY PRESS
PRINCETON AND OXFORD

Published by Princeton University Press
41 William Street, Princeton, New Jersey 08540
99 Banbury Road, Oxford OX2 6JX

press.princeton.edu

Library of Congress Cataloging-in-Publication Data

Names: Rose, Nikolas S., author. | Fitzgerald, Des, author.
Title: The urban brain : mental health in the vital city / Nikolas Rose and Des Fitzgerald.
Description: Princeton, New Jersey : Princeton University Press,
    [2022] | Includes bibliographical references and index.
Identifiers: LCCN 2021035095 (print) | LCCN 2021035096 (ebook) | ISBN 9780691231655
    (hardcover) | ISBN 9780691178608 (paperback) | ISBN 9780691231648 (ebook)
Subjects: LCSH: Cities and towns—Health aspects. | Urban health. | Urban ecology
    (Sociology)—Health aspects. | Mental health—Environmental aspects. | Stress (Psychology)
Classification: LCC HT151 .R6495 2022 (print) | LCC HT151 (ebook) | DDC 307.76—dc23
LC record available at https://lccn.loc.gov/2021035095
LC ebook record available at https://lccn.loc.gov/2021035096

British Library Cataloging-in-Publication Data is available

Editorial: Fred Appel, James Collier
Production Editorial: Terri O'Prey
Jacket/Cover Design: Karl Spurzem
Production: Erin Suydam
Publicity: Kate Hensley, Charlotte Coyne
Copyeditor: Karen Verde

This book has been composed in Adobe Text and Gotham

10 9 8 7 6 5 4 3 2 1

CONTENTS

Acknowledgments   ix

Introduction   1

Embodied Brains   7

Urban Inhabitations   9

Moving People   12

Vital Sociology   14

The Plan of the Book   18

1   Modern Cities, Migrant Cities   21

Mentalities of Migration   22

Seeing the City   26

Chicago: Proud and Vigorous   30

Philadelphia: Striving, Palpitating   39

How Do They Really Live?   45

From Migrant Biopolitics to Migration Studies   53

The Migrant City Today   60

2   Migration, the Metropolis, and Mental Disorder   62

Psychiatry Encounters Migration   64

Degeneracy, Eugenics, and Migration   66

Migration and Mental Health Today   73

Refining 'Migration'   76

Mental Health and 'the Slums'   79

Crushed Dreams or First Steps   84

3 The Metropolis and Mental Life Today—Shanghai 2018 86

Migrant Nation 87

Migrant Labor 92

China: A Mental Health Crisis? 102

'Stress' and the Psy Complex 107

Measuring and Managing Migrant Mental Health 110

4 Everyone Knows What Stress Is and No One Knows
What Stress Is 118

General Adaptation Syndrome 120

Locating Stress 124

Rat Cities, City Rats 126

The Meaning of Urban Stress 132

Stress and Beyond: Toward the Urban Brain 137

5 The Urban Brain 140

The Urbanicity Effect 141

Understanding Urbanicity—To a New Style of Thought? 145

Seeing the Urban Brain 148

The Biopolitics of Stress 155

Epigenetics: Beyond the Genetic Program 161

Neuroplasticity: The Modulated Brain 167

The Exposome: An Urban Sensorium 170

Toward a Conception of the Neurosocial City 174

6 Another Urban Biopolitics Is Possible 176

Urban Justice: The Right to the City 178

Of 'Other' Urban Spaces 180

Transcorporeal Exposures: Beyond the Binary 183

Opening Our Eyes 185

Mental Maps of the Imagined City 186

Ecological Psychology 188

Niching 192

Precarious Niching   194

A New Urban Biopolitics?   198

Conclusion: Toward a Sociology of Inhabitation   200

Notes   213

Bibliography   229

Index   259

ACKNOWLEDGMENTS

This book arises from a program of research on 'the urban brain' initially supported by a grant from the UK's Economic and Social Research Council (ESRC) under its 'Transforming Social Science' scheme for a project entitled *A New Sociology for a New Century: Transforming the Relations between Sociology and Neuroscience, through a Study of Mental Life and the City* (ES/L003074/1). The co-investigators on this grant were Nikolas Rose and Ilina Singh, and Des Fitzgerald was the named researcher. This enabled NR and DF to set up the Urban Brain Lab in the Department of Global Health and Social Medicine of King's College London and to organize a series of international workshops on the issues we discuss in this book. We would like to thank Ilina Singh for our collaboration in the early stages of this work, and for her generous permission to use material in the present book from two of the initial journal articles on which she was a joint author. Work funded by the initial grant led to a subsequent grant from the ESRC's Newton Scheme, led by Professor Nick Manning, for a project entitled *Mental Health, Migration and the Megacity* (ESRC-NSFC Award ES/N010892/1), and we express our thanks to Nick, and to Ash Amin, Li Jie, and Lisa Richaud, for their collaboration on this project, and for many discussions in Shanghai, London, and elsewhere that have had a major impact on our thoughts in this book. Two further small grants arising from the collaborative arrangement between King's College and FAPESP (Fundação de Amparo à Pesquisa do Estado de São Paulo) enabled us to undertake a scoping review of mental health, migration, and the megacity in São Paulo, followed by a project on *Mental Health in Adversity: An Ethnographic Study of the Experience of Poor Mental Health in the Favelas of São Paulo*, and we would like to acknowledge our collaborators at the Institute of Psychiatry, University of São Paulo, notably Laura Andrade. We thank the Brocher foundation for their support, which enabled us to host a workshop in January 2019 at the home of the Brocher Foundation, on the banks of Lac Léman. This workshop brought together research teams from Shanghai, São Paulo, and Toronto to work on our Mental Health, Migration, and Megacities' projects, together with key urban mental health researchers from Berlin and Lausanne, and from three of the innovative 'Thrive' partnerships who are developing policies and practices for supporting mentally healthy cities—in New York (ThriveNYC), London (ThriveLDN), and Toronto (ThriveTO)—as well as others named below. We would like to thank Brenda Roche and Kwame McKenzie from the Wellesley Institute, Toronto, and we would also like to thank Milena Bister, Patrick Biehler, and Jörg Niewöhner, from Humboldt University, and Ole Söderström from Neuchâtel. We also thank the ESRC for a grant from the ESRC's Urban Transformation program for participation in a workshop in Rio de Janeiro, and we would like to thank Michael Keith and Andreza Aruska de Souza Santos for their support. NR was partly supported, in the final stages of the preparation of the book, by the ESRC's grant to the Centre for Society and Mental Health at King's College London (ES/S012567/1). DF was also supported by a grant from the Leverhulme Trust (PLP-2017–152) and, in the later stages, the Wellcome Trust (203109/Z/16/Z). Of course, the views expressed in this book are solely those of the authors. The book has benefited greatly from comments from the reviewers for Princeton University Press, especially from Michael Keith. Thanks to our copyeditor Karen Verde for helping us to greatly improve the clarity of the text and to Terri O'Prey for supporting us through the publication process. Last but not least, we would like to thank our editor at Princeton, Fred Appel, for his patience, encouragement, and advice over the many delays that we encountered in bringing this book to a conclusion.

THE URBAN BRAIN

Introduction

Our program of research on 'the urban brain' began in an unlikely way, in a series of workshops under the rather pretentious title, "a new sociology for a new century."[1] Our objective was actually more modest than it sounded: it was to bring sociological thinking into conversation with contemporary research in the biosciences, in particular with the neurosciences, and to explore the possibilities of such a conversation in relation to just one important contemporary issue. We deliberately chose to focus on an area that had been the topic of debates in sociology, psychiatry, and politics for many decades: mental health in the city (Fitzgerald, Rose, et al., 2016b; Fitzgerald, Rose, et al., 2016a). We wanted to put together an experiment to see the possibilities, and the limits, of a collaboration that brought together leading research in the social sciences and leading research in the neurosciences. What was possible in this space, and what, if anything, could be gained for understanding the ways in which urban living and human mental life were intertwined? What was it about city life that was so bad for the mental health of many people, at the same time that it was beneficial for others? And what might be the implications of the success or failure of such an experiment for our call for a 'revitalization' of social science?

Of course, there has always been traffic between the social sciences and the life sciences. No one who has tried to understand the nature and development of living organisms could ignore that those organisms make their lives in a world beyond the borders of their bodies, even though in their research that world is so often confined to a few roughly sketched 'factors' or confined to a box termed 'environment.' In their turn, sociology, anthropology, political science, even human geography, have always depended on beliefs about the kinds of creatures that human beings are, seldom articulated, usually drawing implicitly on the particular 'lay biology' that is the common sense in their time and place. Our research, initially funded under a program for 'transforming social science,' was in part driven by dissatisfaction with this dual inheritance. We were motivated not only by our disenchantment with the current state of sociology, but also by a sense that something new was taking shape in the sciences of life, in the many sub-disciplines of biology and neurobiology, and notably in genetics. Genetics, for many social scientists, had long been the last refuge of biological determinism, whatever geneticists might have said about their interest in 'gene-environment interactions.' But now, it seemed, something basic had changed: the scientific necessity of recognizing that 'the environment' was not merely something external to the organism with which an inborn genetic program 'interacted.' As the field moved from genetics to genomics, research was showing that the expression of DNA sequences and their implications for human development, and for health and illness, was fundamentally shaped by the experiences undergone by the organism as it develops in a particular milieu and hence that the pertinent dimensions of that milieu—biographical, material, social, even semantic—needed to be characterized and somehow incorporated into investigations and interpretations.

At the same time, something was happening in the social sciences. As feminist social scientists began to insist on the imperative to take seriously what it meant for humans to be 'embodied,' some also began to recognize the need to think through exactly what it meant for human capacities and attributes to be enabled and constrained by the facts of human biology.[2] Much of this work remained—and remains—at an abstract theoretical level. But, in our view, once we recognize that humans, as living organisms, are always and inescapably biosocial beings, many of the long-standing concerns of the social sciences about the implications of poverty, inequality, and exploitation, working and living conditions, the injuries of race, gender, and class, must be cast as both sociopolitical *and* corporeo-cerebral. To take this recognition seriously requires sustained conversations between social scientists and life scientists. These conversations will not be easy. They will certainly involve conflict over questions of research, evidence, truth, justice, politics, and much more. But they are crucial, especially at a time when human beings are coming to realize just how closely their fates, individually and collectively, are braided within their capacity to survive, and to make their lives, as particular kinds of organisms adapted to a very specific set of ecological and geological conditions.[3]

This book is a contribution to such a conversation. It is not a manifesto of intentions. It is rather an attempt to think about just one node of the biosocial and biopolitical everyday: mental health. In particular, it focuses on the mental health of people who live in those complex, ever-changing, often stressful places that we call cities. Our discussion raises what might seem to be a very abstract and grandiose question: how should we understand human mental life today? Perhaps this is the kind of question best left to philosophers. Whether we wish it or not, however, mental health and mental disorder force us to consider such a question directly, precisely because the now long-standing disputes between sociologists, psychiatrists, and neuroscientists about the explanation of mental disorder are, at their root, disputes about the tangles of biological, psychological, biographical, social, and political forces that shape human mental life. While philosophers wrestle with seemingly irresolvable questions about mind-body relations, the explanations forged within the empirical sciences themselves are forcing us to go beyond the heritage of debates over dualism and the snares their binaries—mind/body, organism/environment, individual/social—set for our thought. Our focus—mental disorder in cities—may seem terribly mundane for those embroiled in these grand abstract debates. But we suggest that such 'field work in philosophy' may enable us to sidestep these snares and begin to create a path for future thought.

Perhaps it was once possible to think of questions of mental order and dis-order as somewhat marginal. Philanthropists and activists might have been concerned about conditions in asylums and mental hospitals; social historians might have drawn our attention to the therapeutic consequences of the history of ideas about lunacy, madness, and mental illness. But as for mental disorders themselves, even as recently as the 1960s it seemed perfectly plausible to think of them as afflicting only a relatively small number of people whose ailments were the remit of specialist doctors and mental health professionals. No longer. It is not only that the media is full of stories about the mental problems of younger people and students; of the deep trauma of those who have suffered abuse; of the psychological effects of war and climate change; or simply of the everyday hidden struggles of people with anxiety and depression. It has become habitual to use the term 'mental health' to talk about this widening domain, but while we use the term in this book, we also ask whether mental health is the right frame within which to understand and respond to anxious children, to young people worried about their bodies, to workers stressed by the unceasing demands of their employers, to people of color experiencing the aggressions of everyday racism, to households despairing of their future as their livelihoods are destroyed by financial insecurity, to migrants experiencing economic exploitation and social exclusion, to older people struggling with the memory lapses that are so common in later life, and so on? There is pervasive uncertainty about who is or is not a suitable case for what sort of treatment, and the distinction between 'normality' and 'pathology'—always fragile and contested in relation to psychiatry—seems increasingly hard to sustain.

These issues have implications for the specific problem that we focus on in this book: the relationship between mental distress and urban life.[4] There are many reasons for thinking that urban living might actually be good for people's well-being and life chances. There are long-standing arguments in the social sciences—exemplified, for example, by Michael Lipton's 'urban bias' theory (Lipton, 1977)—to the effect that people living in urban areas are, by and large, wealthier than people elsewhere, with better access to health facilities, more political clout, often more cultural and personal opportunities, thicker social networks, and so on. And yet since at least the middle of the nineteenth century, evidence has shown that there are consistently higher rates of mental disorder in cities, as compared, not just to 'rural' or 'village' life, but also to smaller towns and settlements. There is a long history of dispute over the causes of this difference.[5] In its classic (and much oversimplified) formulation, debate has centered on whether those who are peculiarly susceptible to mental disorder 'drift' into cities, or whether there is something about urban experience itself that actually provokes mental distress.

Until recently, one might have presented this as a debate in the *history* of sociological thought. But it has come to the fore again, today, in the context of a period of renewed urbanization and the growing view that such urbanization is one of the key transformations of our own time. For the first time in human history, so it is routinely claimed, the majority of the world's population lives in cities, especially in big cities, driven in large part by migration from rural areas to emerging megacities, especially in Africa, Asia, and Latin America. Estimates suggest that in 2016, 1.7 billion people, or 23 percent of the world's population, lived in a city with at least 1 million inhabitants. Numbers like these confer a new urgency to the question of mental distress and city life. And yet it is surprising how little we know about the mental consequences of this contemporary movement of people from villages and small towns to such vast, sprawling urban environments. We do not know very much, at least with any certainty, about how these new patterns of migration affect the mental lives of the individuals and families who migrate, or how it might relate to, or disrupt, existing logics of diagnosis and treatment of mental distress. Perhaps most pressingly: despite the fact that such migration is reshaping cities itself in many parts of the world today, we know virtually nothing about how the consequential transformations in mental life and mental distress might structure the actual experience of urban living for so many people throughout the twenty-first century.

The topic of urban mental health has certainly not been ignored by sociologists and anthropologists, or by those concerned with social policy. But it has been something of a specialist area, a concern of subdisciplines. Certainly, the issues raised have not been central to social theory, nor to the work in the social and human sciences that has focused on core issues of self and society, of power and inequality, of injustice and discrimination. And yet this relative absence of interest in urban mental health at the heart of contemporary social sciences has *not* been mirrored in the neurosciences. Researchers in the domain we will call the new brain sciences[6] have proposed new ways to think about the emergence of the problems of mental illness and mental disorder that stunt human lives, in many cases particularly focusing on the implications of urban living. In so doing, in thinking about what it is about the urban environment that might lead to such problems, they have come to recognize that human neurobiology cannot be understood by conceiving of brains as closed systems bound by the skull: thinking about the developmental trajectory of those conceived and born in cities, those whose earliest childhood experiences are in families living in urban dwellings, those whose life course is fully urban, researchers have had to come to terms with the fact that human brains are fashioned and refashioned across days, months, years, decades, by the body's internal and external environments. And not just by nutrition, exposures to pollution, or styles of parenting, however important these might be, but by social relations, by culture, by forms of life. To think of human neurobiology, today, requires us to think of a dynamic interplay in which human bodies and human environments constrain each other, mark each other, intermingle in an awkward, shuffling, embrace. The central gambit of this book is that focusing on that embrace, shuffling along with it, might offer new ways of engaging with the core questions of sociology, questions of inequality and social justice, of marginality, exclusion, and violence, of hope and solidarity and care, precisely by allowing us to understand them as *vital matters*, as matters of our emergent human capacities and human limits, as a collective of living, breathing, developing, sickening, and ultimately dying creatures.[7]

We hope it is becoming clear that this book is structured by two arguments—one general, and one specific. The general argument is about *vitality*. In using this term, we wish to raise the possibility of a critical social science in which the biological exigencies of life come to the center of analysis; an analysis in which thinking with and through those exigencies does not have to be a metaphysical reductionism or a naïve scientism; where it might in fact underpin a style of thought for which being a certain kind of *living* thing really matters—matters for how we conjure, think, contest and shape those parts of human existence we have come to hold together under the term 'social.' The more specific argument is about *inhabitation*. In using this term, we are committing in particular to the spatial consequences of the vitalist position just outlined, to think about what it means to make life as a certain kind of organism, affiliated and disaffiliated to other organisms, in a particular *place*—and specifically in the kind of place that today is rather inadequately termed 'the city.' Thinking about city life as a form of inhabitation is our attempt to mingle the corporeal, social, and ecological life of place—to think about space, justice, accumulation, and marginalization, and so on, not only as grand historical or political phenomena, but also as things that are made and experienced within localized webs of highly specific organic and biological contingencies.

Of course, the argument that the social sciences need to forge a new relationship with the life sciences, while it remains contested, is no longer novel. Each of the present authors, with their different collaborators, has made this argument in different ways for some years, and indeed this was the basis on which our original urban brain project was established.[8] In our own previous work we argued that this relationship should not only be at the level of theory or philosophy, but that a genuine conversation between researchers was required. That is to say, what was needed was the rather dull but necessary work of forging the interdisciplinary concepts and methods required to shape specific problems, and to grasp and intervene in those problems. With such work in mind, this book does not attempt to build a grand conceptual edifice and will not make any large philosophical claims. While we often deploy concepts such as inhabitation, and while we often unceremoniously sidestep hallowed philosophical disputes on issues such as dualism, our goal in what follows is not to make a case *for* our arguments, as if we were presenting them in a court of law, but rather to follow them along, as if they were fibers, strands, filaments within diffuse webs, trying to comprehend what it could mean to experience mental distress in the contemporary city.

In this sense, examining debates over the boundaries and explanations of mental distress, in the city and elsewhere, as well as understanding the multiplicity of forces, processes, and pathways that shape human mental life, is more a question of cartography than of philosophy. If what policymakers sometimes call 'the burden of mental illness' is now a major concern in many regions of the world, then we need to not just understand how to create conditions of care for people who experience mental distress, but to explain how particular conditions produce so much distress, so often, for so many. And we need to tease out the relations between the cerebral, the corporeal, the sociocultural, and the biographical, in the unfolding of these individual and collective stories. In the rest of this introduction, we start to follow some of those relations—between mental health and the city, between biology and sociology, between vitality and embodiment. And we do so by saying more about the two objects that comprise the idea of the 'urban brain' which sits at the very center of our argument—the new brain sciences, on the one hand, and our increasingly urban habitat, on the other.

Embodied Brains

At least since Montesquieu published his *Persian Letters* (Montesquieu, 1773), it has been commonplace, within a certain Euro-centric intellectual tradition, to acknowledge that human beliefs, values, and mores are not universal, but shaped by language, history, and culture. For many in the century that followed, this knotting of intellectual, environmental, and cultural conditions was the justification for creating a racialized hierarchy of peoples and civilizations. It was also—indeed often in the same breath—a space from which anthropologists, sociologists, and historians began to produce descriptions of some of ways in which human experiences and understandings are shaped by the descriptions, categorizations, and forms of judgment available at a specific place and time. What might the neurosciences, whose focus since the 1960s has mainly been on the description of neuronal processes at the molecular level, often based on laboratory experiments with small rodents bred in cages, contribute to this troubled intellectual history? It is certainly true that much research in the life sciences has been reductionist, not only in its experimental approaches—where reductionism is a powerful strategy for maintaining a focus on a specific biological process—but also on its overall style of thought (Woese, 2004). And yet, most strands of the heterogenous fields of biology have acknowledged the centrality of the 'interaction' between the organism and its environment. While some maintained that the development and activities of many organisms were merely the unfolding of an inherited and inbuilt genetic program, and some still hold to this position in relation to non-human organisms, contemporary biologists recognize that human organisms are intrinsically 'social'—that at all stages of development, from the fertilized egg onward, humans are shaped by constant transactions between biological processes and their overlapping environments, within the cell, within the organ, and within the organism itself, as it in turn develops within a physical, cultural, material, and symbolic environment.[9]

Given the long history of research on rates of mental disorder in cities, and the growing awareness of the 'urban' character of much contemporary human life, it is perhaps not surprising that neurobiologists have built on these ideas in order to understand the relationship between urban life and mental distress. Much of this research does use laboratory-based methods, which have an almost inevitable focus on isolated brains, as well as a predictable reduction of the city to a number of quantitative indicators such as density, deprivation, or socioeconomic status. But not all of it. The protean concept of 'stress,' in particular, has been one important ally for researchers trying to get a better grasp on the realities of urban living, and the impacts of ecological features of urban social life. It is one of the central claims of this book that such developments in the life sciences offer real opportunities for interdisciplinary research on how spatial inequalities and injustices can work not only as social or economic phenomena, but also as collective wounds at the psychological and biological levels.

In the midst of large-scale migrations from the countryside to the city in the late nineteenth century, intellectuals, activists, and scholars—perhaps most famously, for sociologists at least, Georg Simmel (Simmel, [1903] 2002)—were struck by how novel physical environments, new urban architectural forms, new systems of transportation, new types of consumption, new practices of everyday life that were taking shape in expanding cities were reshaping urban citizens in body and in soul. Today, in another age of migration and urbanization, it is our argument that a revitalized urban sociology, in similar vein, might bring the neurological lives of urban citizens into the center of its research program. In that spirit, we take up the opportunities and challenges offered by an emerging, open, and social neurobiology, pursuing the potential it offers for a new moment of shared thinking between life scientists and social scientists. We use the figure of 'the urban brain' to hold together this way of thinking. The 'urban brain' functions as a kind of matrix—a point of intersection between neuroscientists and social scientists, between city planners and policymakers, between architects, designers, activists, and many others. It emerges into thought as urban studies and the neurosciences have become intertwined with one another in quite concrete ways. And it underpins a style of empirical and conceptual thinking for which old dualistic notions are simply irrelevant, within which the human brain—itself not so much a single organ but a kind of assemblage—is molded not only by the long timescale of evolution, but also by the short timescale of an individual life, by changing ways of living, by novel sites and practices of human inhabitation, which often require a constant work of adaptation to very difficult circumstances of existence.[10]

Urban Inhabitations

Where do these vital matters of human life take place? It is becoming common to understand places where humans live as *habitats*—to make sense of people's physical environment through an ecological gaze, as we might do with any other animal or plant species. When news reports and documentaries visualize how humans manage in the face of drought, floods, and wildfires, how they face the tests of obtaining adequate nutrition and combatting diseases, how they, their families, and communities make their lives among the (other) animals and plants that surround them, they no longer automatically portray a world from which nature has been banished.[11] Rather it has become a media commonplace to show how the lives of human beings are adapted to, and made possible by, the ecologies of their particular environments; to show how changing ecologies introduce challenges that require them both to manage their material circumstances—as forests burn, crops fail, and water levels rise—and to adapt their modes of social life. No doubt this ecological sensibility is stimulated by the growing inescapability of what many scholars call the Anthropocene, a moment when events arising from climate change are palpably transforming human habitats, most pressingly in countries such as Bangladesh, Haiti, and the Philippines, presaging a future in which forms of inhabitation that have been taken for granted for centuries will be thrown into hazardous uncertainty.

But a habitat, for a human being, as for any living creature, is not just a material place, with its climate, its topography, its relations with other species, its habitations, its practices for obtaining food and so forth. It is rather the milieu that makes possible, and is made possible by, those daily practices of living. Most of the time—like other species—we humans carry out most of the tasks of living *habitually*, which is to say, without conscious thought. To make sense of the issues that concern us in this book, we therefore need to recognize that humans are living organisms striving, sometimes instinctively, often habitually, sometimes consciously, to make a life in a particular place and time against much that would disrupt or threaten that life, transforming their 'environment' into a milieu for living. Such a vitalist perspective thus focuses our attention on how, through what processes and with what consequences, inhabitation gets *lived* in the bodies, brains, and minds of dwelling beings.

Our starting point, then, is not just the embeddedness of the brain in the whole organism, but also the embeddedness of the organism, the human being, in its whole habitat. How should we think of this embeddedness? From a traditionally ecological point of view, each organism is embedded in its specific habitat because organism and habitat are co-evolved: different species of animals and plants have evolved characteristics in line with the affordances of their ecological niches, whether forests, river edges, salt marshes, or frozen tundra. What does it mean to think of a city, or a city neighborhood, as a habitat in this sense? At first glance there does not seem to be much about modern urban life that is grounded in our evolutionary inheritances—for humans at least (a lively literature on evolutionary changes in non-human urban animals persists). Indeed, of all the habitats that humans have created for themselves, cities would strike many as being the most obviously 'artificial.'[12]

This idea that one might look at the city as a space of inhabitation—that we may usefully take the relationship between city and citizen as an *ecological* relationship, in which 'natural' and 'social' environments are inseparably intertwined with the vital capacities and characteristics of human beings—is both new and not new. As recently as the mid-1990s, the distinguished environmental and urban historian, Martin Melosi, was able to lament that "historians interested primarily in nature—and the place of humans in it—have often shunned the city or marginalized it in their studies" (Melosi, 1993: 3). But such a turning away from the intertwining of nature and society in the city is (was) itself relatively recent, as Melosi went on to point out: in fact, the idea of the city as a kind of natural system or a set of organic relations was "the dominant paradigm among the first generation of middle-class urban investigators" in the late nineteenth century and well into the twentieth (ibid.: 5). The qualifier 'middle class' is revealing here: by the turn of the millennium, pretty much all self-identified 'critical' urban theorists were scathing in their critiques of the apparently amateurish belief of these authors that one could understand the human, cultural, and political life of cities in terms of their ecological features.

Despite such criticisms of the first wave of urban social science, we argue that at least three important issues come into view when we approach the experience of living in the city as inhabitation of a socio-material eco-system.[13] First is the substantive and empirical question of how such urban inhabitations shape the physical, mental, and sociocultural lives of people who are born in cities, who live in their ambit, or who migrate to them. In using a word like habitat, our hope is that we can get some purchase on the simultaneously neurological, psychological, and sociological experience of living in a city, including an idea of what happens when that experience is manifested in physical illness or mental distress. Second, there is the methodological and epistemological question of modes of inquiry, of how we make *sense* of the inhabitation of urban space. Here, thinking through habitats motivates us to ask how or whether the standard tools of social science—ethnography, interviews, survey data, network analysis—still work for grasping the realities of vital urban life. The idea of inhabitation thus compels us to think more carefully and critically about the trajectories of social knowledge that have formed our own ways of thinking, and hence the ones we can leave behind and the others that might be worth revisiting. And third, there is the theoretical and normative question of what kind of intellectual practice we think the sociology of the city *should* be, ideally— and perhaps even about what 'sociology' itself should be. Here, a focus on habitat directs our attention to what the organized discipline of sociology has long worked hard to render invisible—that social life, whatever else it is, is also bound by the latitudes of biology and its enactment within organic and material constraints.

Of course, there is no such thing as 'urban life' in general, not least because there is no such place as 'the city.' London is not Cardiff; Cardiff is not Shanghai; Shanghai is not São Paulo; São Paulo is not Toronto; and Toronto is not even Hamilton, or London, Ontario—still less is it Detroit or Chicago. Even more troublingly, it is completely misleading to refer to each of these in the singular.[14] Cities are not entities, they are more like accidents or events; the proper name imposes a deceptive coherence upon multiplicity and diversity (Osborne and Rose, 1999).[15] Indeed, even the cliché that ours is now a planet of cities is itself misleading. As Neil Brenner and Christian Schmid have argued, while claims about imminent and inevitable urbanization have become almost unquestioned clichés in discussions of urbanists, politicians, and journalists alike (Brenner and Schmid, 2014; Brenner and Schmid, 2015), such claims over-rely on the boundary-making practices of administrators: city boundaries on a map do not necessarily enclose a shared material, social, psychological, or experiential space. Even the notion of an urban 'periphery'—as Abdoumaliq Simone points out (Simone, 2010)—needs to be re-cast in a world where a major city like Shenzhen in the southeast of China is even now constituting and re-constituting itself through a complex series of annexations, where place and space once 'outside' the city—once a separate village or town—is rapidly incorporated into an ever expanding metropolis (on Shenzhen, see Keith, Lash, et al., 2013). The question of who or what is and isn't in 'the city' remains unresolved and likely irresolvable.

How, then, can we approach our explorations of the neurological, psychological, and sociological experience of living in a city, and the pathways through which that experience transforms the mental lives of people who inhabit urban spaces, and identify what it is that sometimes leads some of them to mental distress? We argue that, first, we need to find a way to stop thinking about 'the city' in general, and to adopt a broadly ecological style of thought, to differentiate the variety of habitats that are too often agglomerated, conceptually and methodologically, in studies of the psychological and neurobiological consequences of 'city living.' Second, we need to focus on a specific empirical domain, and what better than to choose the experience of those people who are moving in their millions from villages and small towns to the places that are now termed 'megacities'—to São Paulo, to Mumbai, to Lagos, and perhaps most famously, to the city that we will discuss in some detail in what follows: to Shanghai.

Moving People

The phenomenon usually termed 'rural-to-urban migration' creates modes of urban vitality that intensify and make visible some of the most potent consequences of urban inhabitation. While migration across international borders has become the focus of fierce—often highly toxic and racist—political agitation, less attention has been paid to the migration of millions of individuals and families from the countryside, village, or provincial town, into cities.[16] But there is more at stake than simply numbers of moving people: the question of who, in fact, is a migrant, in law, in surveys, and statistical data, in public debate, in perception by self and others, remains unsettled. As Bridget Anderson has often asked (for example in Anderson, 2019), given that everyone moves, whose movement counts as migration—where, to whom, and why?[17]

Perhaps a better approach, then, is to set aside the bare fact of rural to urban migration and focus on the experience itself: what does it actually feel like to move from a small country town or a rural farming community to a vast, sprawling megacity? How does this experience differ for those whose migrant journey ends in Mumbai, Istanbul, Kinshasa, Dhaka, or Birmingham? How does it differ for those who find work—sometimes quasi legal; often not governed by formal contracts—in light industry, on building sites, in offices, in restaurants, in households, or on the streets? Is there anything like a shared or overlapping experience across such diversity? If so, how does an urban experience of crowds and noise, of interactions with strangers, trailing transport networks, often contingent and haphazard housing—how does all of this affect the life, the social, political, physiological, and *mental* life, of the migrant city dweller?

At the cusp of the nineteenth and twentieth centuries, the figure of the migrant from the countryside became a particular focus of attention within the human sciences. Major figures like W.E.B. Du Bois, Georg Simmel, Walter Benjamin, Florence Bell, and Octavia Hill speculated on the consequences of urban environments for the 'nerves' of those who migrated there. In the 1930s and 1940s, another generation of social scientists—including those from the 'Chicago School' of sociology—notably Robert Park and Ernest Burgess—tried to chart and theorize what it was about urban experience that sometimes undoes city dwellers. The movement of people to cities, whether from the countryside or from other nations, also became a focus within the thriving subdiscipline of psychiatric epidemiology, where growing evidence seemed to suggest that migration was one of the strongest predictors of significant mental health problems.[18] As the thought-style of psychiatric epidemiology began to dominate research on these questions, the experience of migration became reframed in terms of correlations of rates of psychiatric diagnoses with different population groups, with different patterns of migration, with first- and second-generation migrants, and so on. The vital concern at the heart of earlier studies—a concern with how different groups of urban citizens lived their lives, the material and social constraints that shaped those lives, and their mental consequences—split apart. Some social psychologists, notably Stanley Milgram, and some urbanists, notably William H. Whyte, continued to explore the everyday interactions of citizens in different kinds of urban space, unpacking the psychic implications of particular urban spaces. But these were unusual forays. Most sociologists and urban theorists, seeing that neither their methods, their findings, nor their concepts had much purchase on this research, did not pursue interdisciplinary collaborations on the connections between the politics of urban life, the actual experience of cities, and the biological and cerebral life of those cities' inhabitants.

In what follows, we will return to that earlier tradition and see what, if anything, can be gained from reviving some aspects of it. We do not do this in a nostalgic or uncritical way. We will discuss, especially in the next chapter, how much of the work of the Chicago School is grimly reproductive of the racism of its own time, how much it incorporates the banal and bourgeois common sense that is the hallmark of much American sociology even today. But still we want to think across the gap between a figure like W.E.B. Du Bois—tramping the streets, sketching living conditions, annotating charts of sickness, gathering the vital statistics of Philadelphia's seventh ward—and the highly abstract and often rather provincial theoretical debates that concern so many of today's urban scholars in what is often loosely termed 'the Global North.'

Vital Sociology

This book is not only about mental life in cities. It also aims to be an intervention into contemporary social theory. We have mentioned the recent excitement in anthropology, sociology, human geography, urban studies, and the humanities about the emergence of a new, less 'reductionist' biology. While some see this as a sort of passage point to a future in which their disciplines could gain in status and recognition through providing a necessary social dimension to the 'hard sciences,' others respond with the familiar, and still somewhat compelling, argument about explanatory accounts drawing on biology: that they are inherently fatalistic, deterministic, and individualistic; that they root the trouble firmly inside the individual or their immediate family; that they neglect the social, structural, cultural, and political forces that reproduce inequity; that they ignore the economic and political system that exploits and oppresses the majority to enrich the few; that they reproduce the racism that marginalizes and stunts the life chances of people of color, of migrants, of Indigenous people, of LGBTQ+ and trans people, and of anyone else who stands outside the grinding logic of capitalist heteropatriarchy. References to the biological, such critics further remind us, usually continue to underpin technocratic strategies that blame 'dysfunctional' families and 'poor mothering' for the reproduction of disadvantage while failing to recognize what it is about our societies that forces so many into precarious and unstable forms of life.

It is no surprise—nor is it a bad thing—that there are those in the social and human sciences who are trenchantly committed to such critiques. They may believe that the lines of argument we are following in this book could re-open a path to the 'biologization' of inequality and to the individualization of the causes of disadvantage, perhaps now in the service of 'late capitalism' or 'neoliberalism.' Our argument in this book is not that this diagnosis is wrong, but to point to other biologies—other ways of recognizing that social subjects are nonetheless living creatures—that point precisely *away* from biologization, *away* from individualization, *away* from normalization, fatalization, and legitimation of the status quo. Indeed, a growing number of social scientists argue, with equal passion, that a genuine mutation is under way in the biosciences, which goes beyond mere lip service to the idea that humans, like other organisms, are constituted in and through their relations with their 'environment' (e.g., Meloni, 2014). We can see such arguments emerging with particular force in the new relations between feminist and biological theories (e.g., Roy, 2018). Social theorists have pointed to the emergence of a range of approaches—whether in neuroscience (Lederbogen, Kirsch, et al., 2011), epigenetics (Youdell, 2017), or microbiomics (Lorimer, 2016)—that are beginning to tease out the precise biosocial *mechanisms* through which the bodies and brains of the human organism are developmentally shaped from conception, if not before, by their dynamic transactions with their environments. Like us, they argue that as we come to understand these mechanisms, we will also come to a better understanding of how sociopolitical inequality, disadvantage, and injustice torque and blight the lives of so many, bringing them to ill health, disability, and early death.[19] Indeed, it is precisely *because* we care about the political economy of urban life, and all the violence that it entails, that we care about the city's vital, biological consequences.

With that said, we also have two cautions. First, the image of a century-long standoff between the social sciences and biology is simply not borne out by history. It is not the case that there have previously been two cultures, proceeding in mutual indifference if not open hostility. This story of a fundamental historical divide often begins in the closing decades of the nineteenth century, with Weismann's hereditary barrier, which suggested that information moves from genes to cells, organs, and organisms, but never the reverse, and ends some one hundred years later with Michael Meaney's experiments with rat pups which seemed to show, on the contrary, the crucial role of epigenetics, that is to say the ways that specific experiences of the developing animal shape and program the expression of DNA sequences, apparently with lifelong consequences (Weaver, Cervoni, et al., 2004). But, in fact, as we will show in much more detail below, multiple interactions have occurred between the biological and social sciences across that century, interactions that are especially well exemplified in research on the problems of urban living.[20]

Second, the picture emerging from the contemporary life sciences is not always as congenial to 'the social' as is sometimes imagined. Epigenetics means many different things, and much of the research has been done with animal models: extrapolation to humans remains fraught with conceptual difficulties. Further, it may be true that, unlike many other living creatures, 'environment' or 'culture' shapes key aspects of human life, but biologists insist that it does so on the basis of the evolved characteristics of our bodies and brains: our upright posture, our binocular vision, our ability to sense light and sound within certain specified wavelengths, our patterns of physical and neural development across the life course, and so on. It is still the case that many of the basic characteristics of organisms, including human organisms, remain largely constant despite highly variable external environments. And we need to be aware that much contemporary biological research on health is the victim of premature claims and hype: for example the implications of the microbiome for human well-being, while celebrated in popular books on health and diet that advise us to care for our gut by ingesting commercial probiotics, are only just being explored in empirical research.

What, then, would a social science look like that could take seriously what we are learning about human beings, individually and collectively, as living creatures striving to maintain themselves in often hostile situations? To what extent could such a vitalized social science impel sociologists, anthropologists, human geographers, and others to become co-producers of the biopolitical worlds that they have become so adept at describing? Could it offer those scholars intellectual resources and empirical insights to participate in the development of a new politics of life—a new way of configuring knowledge, expertise and intervention to combat the injustices that are so ingrained in the fabric of contemporary urban existence? Could it challenge them—challenge *us*—to undertake such sociopolitical engagement without losing their, our, capacity to critically evaluate the truth claims of our collaborators and interlocutors, and without seeking to efface the diversity of forms that the politics of urban life has taken and will continue to take? Our argument for a vital sociology names a messily collaborative form of thought and action in and around these kinds of questions, one that entails not the denial of differences, but an active, agonistic, but still—we hope—generative form of interdisciplinary research.

We use the term *vital sociology* to emphasize the extent that our approach draws explicitly on an inheritance of vitalist thought. This book should be read as an argument for taking the individual and collective lives of human beings, of human *living*, as the central object for sociological, anthropological, and geographical attention to the city. It takes from vitalism not the metaphysics that asserts some 'élan vital' specific to living creatures, but a more mundane recognition that being alive means actively organizing one's capacities to continue to exist within the resources and the dangers afforded by a particular milieu.[21] It thus insists on understanding the urban as an array of lively ecologies, sometimes convivial, turbulent, and joyful, but sometimes solitary, unpleasant, and demanding. It asks us to take seriously the vitalist understanding of the biosocial dynamics of inhabitation not as a 'philosophical' gesture; not as a 'reduction' to biology; not as a 'turn' against some imaginary idea of what social science actually is—but as an empirical and conceptual mesh for holding together the multiple processes that shape human life as it is lived—and for holding together the specific questions of urban life and mental health that are the focus of this book.

Despite the traditions it draws upon, we do not intend this book to be an abstract theoretical intervention. Focusing on the vital relationship between urban citizens and the spaces in which they find themselves requires us to address very mundane empirical issues: how to live in a city, how to manage a city, how to design a city, how to make people safe in a city, how to shape a healthy city, how to design inclusive cities, how to imagine age-friendly and disability-friendly cities, and so on. These questions and many more are being explored by scholars in a whole range of adjacent domains. But for us, they remain, insistently, questions of *life*. In arguing for a vital sociology we are thus responding to a demand, which may be thought of as ethical, and which is certainly normative, that we orient our intellectual projects around the question of living—as it is inhabited, experienced, and so often suffered, by us and by our fellow citizens. Such a demand requires us to return to some very basic questions of everyday ethics—of the situated ethics of how we to live. Underpinning our investigations in this book are questions of how we might live differently, which requires us to think differently about urban life, and to think differently about how we can make and remake cities as engines of livable lives. And we hope, finally, that approaching the question of urban living from this perspective will have some surprising effects beyond urban studies—that urban social science may turn out to be an unexpectedly potent site for re-thinking the biological present.

The Plan of the Book

Our argument is set out in six chapters, which do not form a single narrative but which together go some way toward answering the questions we set out in this introduction. In the first chapter, 'Modern Cities, Migrant Cities,' as a prelude to our focus on mental health, we think our way through a number of different lines of thought that have, to a greater or lesser extent, approached the analysis of urban life in terms of the bodies and souls of those who inhabit cities. Drawing on the work of Georg Simmel, Seebohm Rowntree, Charles Booth, and especially W.E.B. Du Bois, the chapter sets the scene for what follows by reinvigorating a vitalist tradition that we find in these older, classical studies of urban living. It asks: what would it mean to put that tradition back at the center of urban studies today?

In chapter 2, 'Migration, the Metropolis, and Mental Disorder,' we explore how the city has been configured as a place of stress and tumult for migrants, and especially for migrants from the countryside. The chapter argues that while migration and mental health are two of the predominant themes of modern city analysis, they are rarely brought together in contemporary urban studies. Moving from degeneration theory in the nineteenth century to the epidemiology of migrant mental health today, the chapter shows how the migrant city is always simultaneously configured as a city of mental distress. It examines the ways that those who have addressed this issue have believed that the experience of migration gets into the flesh, into the bodies, and into the brains of those who migrate—and explores the ways that sociological methods have been used to address this phenomenon.

Chapter 3, 'The Metropolis and Mental Life Today—Shanghai 2018' takes these questions to the present. It draws on our own and our colleagues' empirical work in Shanghai, perhaps the most symbolic migrant city of China, a country that has been transformed by a sustained movement of millions of people from the countryside to the city. The chapter describes the particular stresses of being a migrant in contemporary Shanghai—the lack of access to local services, separation from immediate family, hostility from city authorities—but also the very real hopes and dreams that people carry to the city from their villages, and that sustain them there. The chapter asks: what would a research practice look like that was able to grasp this life, even to help ameliorate its stresses, while recognizing that there is much more to the mental and social life of migrants than mental health problems? Could we imagine a sociology that would create space for nuanced ethnographic attention to the everyday mental lives of those who are considered migrants, and that would mesh with, and transform, the ways that the disciplines of public health and the psychological sciences have approached these questions.

The key question that remains is how—through what process and mechanisms—experiences of adversity in urban existence are inscribed in the body and the brain and with what consequences? In answering this question, much of the discussion has come to focus around one word: stress. In chapter 4, 'Everyone Knows What Stress Is and No One Knows What Stress Is,' we argue that the long debate on stress and the city demonstrates both the openness of particular experimental traditions in the life sciences to questions of sociality, *and* the relevance of such openness for contemporary studies of the city. From John Calhoun's rat utopias in the 1960s to Bruce McEwen's work on the neurobiology of stress today, the chapter explores the history and the present state of research on the stresses of city life—and on the stressful effects of migration in particular. The chapter asks: could stress be a meeting point for interdisciplinary research on the realities of migrant mental life in megacities today?

We continue this analysis in chapter 5, 'The Urban Brain,' where we bring together contemporary neurobiological research on stress with work on the neurobiosocial pathways that connect the vitality of the urban citizen to their place in the city. The chapter traces the emergence of 'the urban brain' as a new scientific object that makes city life amenable to the methods of the life sciences in general, and the sciences of the brain in particular. We argue that the thought space created by the idea of the urban brain enables conceptualization and intervention into the dynamic and transactional pathways that enmesh the human brain in its milieu—making space for productive collaborations across disciplinary boundaries in a quite new conception of the neurobiological and psychosocial city.

In chapter 6, 'Another Urban Biopolitics Is Possible,' we look up from the bodies and brains of urban inhabitants themselves and re-direct our neurobiological and vitalist arguments toward ethical and political questions of how we might then think about 'good life' in the vital city. In debate with different ethical accounts of city life—from Henri Lefebvre's 'right to the city' to Michel Foucault's 'heterotopias'—the chapter sets out our argument that a new urban biopolitics is possible. This would be a politics of everyday city life that foregrounds the relationship between the body and its environment, with particular attention to the neurobiology of that inhabitation. The chapter asks: what would be entailed by a sociological project that took caring for those relations as its central project?

In the Conclusion, 'Toward a Sociology of Inhabitation,' we channel the central arguments of the book into a final claim that the sociology of the city needs to be reconfigured around a renewed attention to *inhabitation*—the term that we have used to hold together the tendrils of vitalistic, ecological, and biopolitical concern that run through this book. Pointing to some recent attempts to put questions of inhabitation right at the heart of city life, from 'dementia-friendly' architecture to the 'Healthy New Towns' initiative of the UK's National Health Service, we close with an argument for replacing a philosophical language of justice with a biosocial language of *life*—not only in urban studies, but in urban policy and urban politics, and indeed in the wider human and social sciences as such.

1

Modern Cities, Migrant Cities

Since at least the mid-nineteenth century, intellectuals and social theorists have tried to understand the social and mental characteristics of life in cities. Over the same period, the benefits and dangers of city life became the subject of political debate as well as a target of intervention for a wide range of authorities—health visitors, medics, clerics, and bureaucrats. Urban theorists and city bureaucrats have come to share a sense of fundamental tension at the heart of the urban: the city is a space of alienation and exploitation, but it is also a place of cosmopolitan belonging and opportunity; cities are marked by division and segregation, but they also embody a rich and lively culture full of unexpected and rewarding encounters; cities are vital nodes in circuits of capital accumulation and extraction, but also they foster transformational movements experimenting with a host of alternative economic and social possibilities; the urban environment is constantly being structured and restructured by expert planners, but it is also continually shaped by the informal endeavors of those who live within its boundaries.

Migrants and migration were central to early debates about the nature of modern cities. And yet today, by contrast, migration has largely become the focus of specialist migrant studies, with an emphasis on international migration—on involuntary migration and refugees, the nature of diasporic communities, conflict and human trafficking, the effects of climate change, the contribution of migrants to economic development, and so on. We do not intend to embark on a comprehensive review of this material. In this chapter, instead, we set the scene for what follows by placing migration, or

what an earlier generation of social scientists understood as 'the migrant'—
and especially 'the rural-to-urban migrant'—at the heart of our own understanding of a certain kind of vital urban life. We are doing this because we
want to recover and reinvigorate a subterranean vitalism tradition in writing
on the nineteenth-century city. In this chapter, we ask what it would mean
to again put the vital life of rural migration, as a distinctive set of corporeal
and cerebral experiences of the city, back at the center of urban studies.

Why start from these questions? Well, open any textbook on urban sociology today, and you will see a roll call of late nineteenth-century European
intellectuals, and the centers of commerce in which they made their lives:
Georg Simmel, Friedrich Engels, Charles Baudelaire, Walter Benjamin, even
Sigmund Freud, on the one hand; Berlin, Vienna, London, Paris, even Manchester, on the other. Undergirding references to these authors is a conviction
that *something happened* in the second half of the nineteenth century: the
emergence of a particular political and economic formation called 'modernity,' centered on a particular kind of sociotechnical organization called
'the city,' requiring interpretation from a new mode of intellectual inquiry
called the 'social sciences.' We do not wish to repeat what is already well
known in these writings. Instead, we wish to draw out some themes that
have often been occluded in them, in particular a certain vitalism, a certain
conviction that to understand the urban, one needs to grasp it, in some way,
as a matter of the vital lives and the liveliness of those who inhabit it.

We are certainly not the first to argue for the importance of vitalist thinking; indeed, there has been a clear re-emergence of interest in vitalism in
the social sciences in the present century (Massumi, 2002; Fraser, Kember,
et al., 2005; Greco, 2005; Wolfe and Wong, 2014). Forms of vitalism can be
found in the work of many contemporary urban theorists, especially those
who have addressed the urban from postcolonial (Robinson, 2006), non-
representational (Amin and Thrift, 2002; Amin and Thrift, 2016), and ecological (Heynen, Kaika, et al., 2006b) perspectives. Rather than review this
work as a whole, we will follow one specific thread that concerns the vital
lives of migrants, and, more specifically, the ways that rural-to-urban migration comes to shape the mental lives and mental health of those who migrate.

Mentalities of Migration

As the sociologist Charley Tilly showed many decades ago (Tilly, 1978), in
Europe before the nineteenth-century people moved a lot, often en masse,
generally from one rural location to another, in search of agricultural work.

Thereafter, however, industrialization and urbanization were associated with a clear shift in mobility patterns (see also Moch, 1995). In Britain, as Pooley and Turnbull have shown (Pooley and Turnbull, 2005), there was very significant movement of people from the countryside to towns in the period from 1750 to 1900, as well as a rapid growth of small urban centers into large cities. Manchester, for example, went from a town of 89,000 in 1801 to a city of more than half a million by 1891—with Glasgow, Birmingham, and Bristol each also growing to more than 500,000 in the same period. In Germany, changes in the rural economy similarly led to high inward mobility as well as emigration abroad in the nineteenth century, as the rural poor found themselves transformed into a fluctuating, mobile workforce, in seasonal relationship with the growing cities (Hochstadt, 1986). Through processes of urban growth and annexation of the surrounding suburbs, Paris similarly grew from a population about 600,000 in 1801 to 1,700,000 by 1861; this created, inter alia, a massive increase in the need for food to be transported into the city, as well as an increase in the levels of nitrogen in human excrement, which was in great demand for use as a fertilizer (Barles, 2007). Such are the requirements and consequences of vital lives in a growing metropolis.

The patterns are varied: in Britain, as Pooley and Turnbull point out, much urban population growth had more to do with so-called natural increases (which is to say, from fewer people dying and more people being born) than with in-migration. Still, migration, including circular migration, remained part of the urbanization process at least up to the 1880s (Pooley and Turnbull, 2005). In Paris, by contrast, much more of the increase was due to inward migration (Moch, 2003: 131). Thus, while seasonality and cyclical migration make the larger picture hard to characterize neatly, what *is* clear is that the modern European city came into existence at least partly through the migration patterns of certain population groups. This is the first way that we want to frame our way of thinking about the city: the city of modernity has always been a city of migration, a space in which people come, go, and settle, sometimes temporarily and informally, where they have to make sense of new experiences, shape new ways of living, face various kinds of discrimination and hassle, but nonetheless settle in, form bonds, and make lives. The rural migrant, not the 'flâneur,' is the defining figure of urban modernity.

What might it have been like to arrive in one of these burgeoning, nineteenth-century migrant metropolises? We do have some vivid pictures of individuals caught up in the flows from the European countryside to the city in the nineteenth and twentieth centuries, as well as accounts of how people made their lives in the 'arrival cities' where they ended up (Saunders, 2010). We know, for example, that whatever their original intentions, few of the millions of people who moved from villages in rural France to the towns actually returned to their places of origin; instead, they spent whole lives in tiny, rented rooms in the quartiers in Paris. This was consequential: as Saunders argues, drawing on the work of George Rude, "The Paris crowds that formed on the fourteenth [of July, 1789] and stormed the Bastille and sacked the Hôtel de Ville were almost entirely the people of the arrival city" (Saunders, 2010: 138). In many parts of Europe, in Scandinavia, the Low Countries, the German States, in England and Wales, while agricultural developments greatly improved food production, it also underpinned movements for the enclosure of common land, and thus the disruption of the lives of rural laborers. Thus, as Saunders puts it, enclosure generated "a surplus population of tens of millions who abandoned the countryside—by choice or by decree—and sought work in the cities, either in their own country or across the Atlantic [thereby causing] a massive shift from rural poverty to urban poverty" (Saunders, 2010: 141). Cities like Berlin, Paris, Vienna, Warsaw, Prague, and St. Petersburg, whose spatial and architectural form had been shaped by conscious planning, were quickly transformed by mass arrivals from rural villages and small towns, as people built themselves shacks on fields at the east, west, south, or north edges of towns, or else mingled with impoverished urban dwellers in tenements and courts at the heart of the city.

Things were actually not so different for Europeans who took advantage of the forms of mobility made possible by colonialism and dispossession to travel beyond their own shores: "Between 1850 and 1913, more than 40 million people emigrated from Europe to the New World [sic.] . . . The United States absorbed nearly two thirds of the emigrants, although there were sizable flows to Canada, Australasia, and Latin America, the latter including Argentina, Brazil and Cuba" (Hatton and Williamson, 1992: 1). Once more, vitality itself was the corporeal reality at stake for many of these migrants.[1] Millions of Irish people, those not killed by disease or starvation in the famine of the 1840s, emigrated, not only to Manchester, Liverpool, or London, but to New York, Chicago, and Toronto. Others who made the journey across the Atlantic moved to places where previous generations of migrants from their home country had ended up, mixing, not always happily, with others in abandoning the violence of the countryside—especially rural African Americans—in temporary housing on the outskirts of St. Louis, Milwaukee, and Detroit.

There are three critical issues involved here. First, we need to see the 'modern city' as constitutively a migrant space, an agglomeration of people who, whether by virtue of their own biography, or through their parents, or grandparents, or cousins, or just their friends and neighbors, are also partly rooted somewhere else. And not just anywhere else, but somewhere smaller, somewhere less overtly industrialized and urban, where quite a different form of life still prevails. Second, we need to think about this new form of life as precisely that: as a form of life, as a particular situation of living, as a set of living human beings co-creating their existence in a particular space. Third, to make sense of the drivers and consequences of these movements, the social and human sciences need to develop a kind of attention often missing in conventional migration studies, one that also attends to the biological and physiological conditions for human life.

That is to say, in rethinking urban modernity through the vital lives of rural migrants, we should shift attention away from factories and arcades—the familiar scenes of urban history and sociology—and toward water, food, and bedbugs; toward malnutrition and disease, toward sanitary conditions and access to doctors and nurses; toward calorific intake and the specifics of metabolism; in short toward actual, physical bodies and the requirements and ailments that attend those bodies. This also means attending to the nature and consequences of the *subjective* experiences of this migrant encounter with the urban—alienation, confusion, depression, excitement, liberation, joy, creativity, exultation, despair. These affects and experiences take shape in what in the nineteenth century was understood as a *moral* space, a space in which conscience, consciousness, and character were fused together to shape conduct. Over the course of the twentieth century, this space of conscience, consciousness, and character shaping human conduct became the object of the emergent "psy complex" (Rose, 1985; Rose, 1989), and in our own century those dimensions of human mental life have come to be understood as, at least in part, underpinned or made possible by specific *neurobiological* processes (Rose and Abi-Rached, 2013).

What, then, if the central question for urbanists over the last hundred years or so had centered not on collective action, or on new forms of economic extraction, or on modes of cultural and political efflorescence, but had concerned rather the physiological and mental experiences of rural-to-urban migrants? In fact, as some have pointed out, such attention was never far from the surface of the 'classic' texts of urban sociology.[2] Nonetheless, a slight turn of attention allows us to draw out a shared set of concerns in the work of such figures as Walter Benjamin, Georg Simmel, Seebohm

Rowntree, and William Du Bois, to place the biological and mental life of the urban migrant, as a living being trying to habituate themselves and their nervous systems to a new environmental situation, at the center of our understanding of the modern city.

Seeing the City

When social scientists, writers, and artists tried to make sense of the burgeoning migrant metropoles in which they found themselves, what exactly did they see—and how did they see it? In his account of representations of the city between the second half of the nineteenth century and the first half of the twentieth, the geographer Richard Dennis draws together reflections from visual artists, writers, social scientists, planners, and cartographers, who tried to grasp the streets, buildings, parks, and other forms of spatial configurations that were then reconstituting the city (Dennis, 2008). Dennis argues that we can identify a shared goal among these "political and theological ideologues, [. . .] social explorers, census makers and takers, insurance and tax assessors, directory samplers, surveyors" and "photographers, artists and novelists"—the ambition to grasp urbanization, not merely as a physical process, but as a novel way of life. For David Frisby, too, while the city was not the only site from which nineteenth-century intellectuals brought modernity into focus, it was certainly one of the more important (Frisby, 2001). What was the metropolis, after all, except a synecdoche of the dislocating temporal whirl that was already teaching new kinds of citizens how to experience themselves? To be an inhabitant of the metropolis was to be a modern subject of one kind or another. By the same token—so the reasoning went—to understand that modern world, and the people and objects who composed it, one had to also understand the city. For social thinkers of the period, Frisby points out, it was precisely "the cityscapes of social theories" that "reveal the ambiguities and contradictions of modernity" (Frisby, 2001).

But whose cityscape? Paris in the nineteenth century was dominated by "streams of workers from the countryside" (Fuchs and Moch, 1990: 1008), the majority of them women. And yet, when we think of French urban modernity, it is the affectations of a single Parisian-born man that usually come to mind—viz. Charles Baudelaire, who gifted social theory, via the intercessions of Walter Benjamin, the image of the *flâneur*, that familiar ambling, dilettantish, deeply affected, and now also deeply irritating figure of urban theory (Leslie, 2006; Baudelaire, 2010). The flâneur functions as a defining figure binding modernity to the city in social theory: a kind of child-genius, in Baudelaire's terms, a bastion of aristocratic nerve, a dandy, a painter, a spectating prince, a kaleidoscopic mirror of the crowd—a lone candlewick of flickering grace, holding still, with all his powers of perception, at the tumultuous crowd's beating heart (Baudelaire, 2010). Such has been the self-perception of more than a little of the urban writing that followed in Baudelaire's wake.

But there is more to Walter Benjamin's conjoining of modernity and the city than the figure of the flâneur. Of course, Benjamin himself, in horrific circumstances, was a migrant to Paris. Throughout his writing, Benjamin's attention returned again and again to the two European capitals in which he spent most of his life—the Berlin of his childhood, and the Paris of his later life (Elland and Jennings, 2014). Indeed, it is in this peripatetic, mobile existence—willed at first; then, tragically, not willed at all—that we can specify Benjamin's attention to urban experience: Beatrice Hanssen reminds us that Benjamin was centrally concerned with "modernity's alienation as a state of no longer being *heimisch* or *at home*" (Hanssen, 2006: 2), and that we might recognize his attention to the city as an attempt to bring into view the changed urban *habitat* required of the new historical subjects who were to inhabit this *unheimlich* state. Here, as elsewhere, Benjamin's attention to space and citizen is distinctively archaeological; it is concerned to show how the past and the present live within and on top of one another.

This dwelling of the past within the present, which was both Benjamin's experience of the city and his theory of modernity, finds its ideal form in the arcade: "an ideal panorama of a barely elapsed primeval age opens up when we look through the arcades that are found in all cities," writes Benjamin: "here resides the last dinosaur of Europe, the consumer" (Benjamin, 2010: 874). The consumer, in this analysis, is the crystallization of modern urban subjectivity. Crawling underneath the layered and labyrinthine structure of the arcade can become both a mode of understanding the city as it was coming into existence and also a method for learning to see that city through the sedimented layers of its own past. Both projects find a kind of surface realization in the consumer goods with which the arcades are lined—"late model autos" and "paste-jewel figures"; stockings, kimonos, umbrellas, canes, leather goods; objects that, as "pure fetish. . . . not only revealed the works of reification, but [were] linked, in however corrupt a manner, to the utopian aspirations of a dreaming collective" (Cohen, 2004).

If Benjamin is one of the authors whose work forms the base of the canon of contemporary urban theory, Georg Simmel is certainly another. Simmel's 'The Metropolis and Mental Life,' first presented to a public audience at the

German Municipal Exhibition in Dresden in 1903, is often regarded as the classic sociological statement on modernity and the city. Yet it is striking that Simmel's central concern is less with the city as such (one gets little sense of 'the urban' from his essay at all), and more with how modernity is *made sense of*—indeed, how it is made *sensible*—in an individual psychology, or what Simmel calls "the psychological basis of the metropolitan type of individuality," which is produced by the city's relentless "intensification of nervous stimulation" (Simmel, 2010 [1903]: 103). Simmel's is thus an essay about how people come to make peace (or not) with particular sorts of environments—a question of how to make sense of a "body of culture with reference to the soul" (ibid.: 103).

As Steve Pile points out, Simmel is "attempting to understand the psychological preconditions of modernity while at the same time explaining the development of those preconditions with reference to changes in the metropolis" (Pile, 2005). Indeed, Mike Savage and Alan Warde read Simmel barely as a theorist of 'the city' at all: Simmel was interested in the city, they argue, because this is where the essential features of modernity were most plainly visible, *not* because there was some causal relationship between the two (Savage and Warde, 1993). And yet if we put the question of causality to one side, it seems hard not to recognize that, for Simmel, there certainly is something distinctive about the metropolitan form of life as it was unfolding before him. What separates the city from the countryside or small town is the experience of difference—not difference measured as change in a space over time, but rather the experience of difference as *sensation*, as "the swift and continuous shift to external and internal stimuli" (ibid.: 103). To be a modern urban subject, in Simmel's account, is precisely this psycho-sensory condition; in order to cope, the metropolitan individual adapts—they "creat[e[a protective organ for [themselves] against the profound disruption with which the fluctuations and discontinuities of the external milieu threaten it" (ibid.: 104).

Thus, in the experience of difference, a certain kind of metropolitan indifference becomes habitual. This is not an indifference borne of insensitivity but precisely the opposite: it is a protective layer pulled across the acutely sensitive nervous system of the city dweller thus to hold out *against* the rapidly changing stimuli that otherwise bombards their attention. "We are saved," says Simmel, "by antipathy which is the latent adumbration of actual antagonism since it brings about the sort of distillation and deflections without which this type of life could not be carried on at all" (Savage and Warde, 1993: 107). Simmel was as much eyewitness as theorist here. As Pile notes, he was confronted with the fact that "European cities were changing in ways that were having noticeable impacts both on the organization of society and on the ways people responded to each other . . . Berliners at this time were developing new ways of relating socially to one another" (Pile, 2005: 17). But what were they reacting to—and who, exactly, were the 'Berliners' in question? It is notable that Simmel wrote his essay more or less at the peak of Berlin's growth from internal migration: as Steve Hochstadt has shown, the period between 1880 and 1920 was "the heyday of urban growth, the epitome of German urbanization" (Hochstadt, 1986: 200). Within this period, strikingly, "the rural population remained the same, while urban population more than doubled, and cities over 100,000 [including Berlin] quadrupled their total size" (ibid.). Moreover, while migrants kept coming, they also kept leaving: the Berlin that Simmel was trying to make sense of was a city teeming with flows of temporary migrants arriving from, and returning to, the countryside.

Simmel was not alone in thinking of the city at the start of the twentieth century in terms of its psychic consequences. Michael Peter Smith argues that when Freud, for example, uses the term 'civilization,' he is actually thinking of what Simmel called 'metropolitan life' and that Louis Wirth called 'urbanism' (Smith, 1980).[3] For Smith, the economic and material surrounds of Freud's thought—"intellectual and scientific activity, cultural institutions, technological change and large-scale formal social controls"— were largely phenomena of "the cities of his day" (ibid.: 50). Thus, for Smith, Freud's attention to issues such as compulsive cleanliness should be understood in relation to the forms of regulation and order that were emerging within modern urban life, and to which, we should add, the not-yet-civilized figure of the migrant stood as an obvious counter. The art historian, Richard Williams, similarly locates, in Freud's thought, a deep intertwinement between feelings of anxiety and the experience of the city (Williams, 2004). Williams reminds us that Freud's 1919 essay, 'The Uncanny,' features a striking anecdote about getting lost in a strange town—in which the wanderer, with increasing desperation and uncanny sensation, repeatedly turns back into the same place that he is trying to avoid. Here and elsewhere, says Williams, architectural space and the experience of anxiety became intimately connected for Freud (Williams, 2004: 8).

Or consider Friedrich Engels, who, in the *Conditions of the Working-Class in England*, describes his own wandering in and out of the filthy, unventilated, covered-over and river-sodden courts that made up 'working-men's dwellings' in the Manchester of his day (Engels, 2010 [1844]). Most of the inhabitants of those dwellings were, of course, migrants from the country-side, or the children of such migrants. But note that Engels is not characterizing some generalized urban modernity; he is careful, for example, to describe specific districts very precisely, and to compare different eras in the construction of these dwellings with one another. His account of Manchester is not a generalized broadside against the living conditions of the new urban working class in England as such, but rather a careful account of life in different districts in one city. We are not arguing that 'the city' is somehow the real focus of attention for writers such as Freud and Engels. Rather our point is that two distinctive intellectual concerns of the late nineteenth century—capitalism and the psyche—were were bound up with cities, city life, city thinking, and cityism in general. The emerging social theory of this period did not *depend* on a focus on the migrant city, but it nonetheless found a strikingly amenable home in it. Perhaps most significant was one American city: Chicago.

Chicago: Proud and Vigorous

In the first three decades of the twentieth century, the population of Chicago doubled (Cressey, 1938: 59). By 1930, 25 percent of people living in the city had been born elsewhere. As Paul Frederick Cressey pointed out in a contemporaneous account of immigrant "succession" for the *American Journal of Sociology*: by that date Chicago had become the world's third largest Irish, Polish, Swedish, and Jewish city, as well as the city with the second largest African American population in the United States (ibid.: 60–61). Having earned his Ph.D. in sociology at Chicago, Cressey spent most of his career at Wheaton College in Massachusetts. Interestingly, his cousin, Paul Goalby Cressy, was also a student in sociology at Chicago, studying under Ernest Burgess and working toward a much more famous book, the canonical Chicago-School monograph, *The Taxi-Dance Hall* (Cressy, 1932). The "taxi-dance hall" was a space where, in short, women were paid to dance with men—and yet, as the historian Angela Fritz points out, one of the really noteworthy aspects of Cressey's study is its fundamental lack of interest in the taxi-dance as a phenomenon of immigration (Fritz, 2018). Indeed, while P. G. Cressy thanks his cousin for his assistance in the preface to his book, there is strangely no attention to that cousin's expertise in the actual text itself, viz. immigration. All these are minor matters of course—and yet such minor histories offer a small window onto how the 'Chicago School of Sociology,' as a collective enterprise, made sense of perhaps the most significant development transforming American cities at the turn of the nineteenth and twentieth centuries: mass immigration from Europe.

Consider for example, *The Polish Peasant in Europe and America*, a classic early Chicago text, published by W. I. Thomas and Florian Znaniecki in 1918 (Thomas and Znaniecki, 1918). Migrants from Poland amounted to about a quarter of the almost 1.5 million foreign migrants living in the United States when the book was written; Chicago was already the world's third largest Polish city (Bulmer, 1984: 50). The research that became *The Polish Peasant* was funded by a grant from Helen Culver, a Chicago businesswoman and philanthropist, via her Fund for Race Psychology (Culver also funded the famous Hull House, where Jane Addams began her career). Thomas's biographer, the sociologist Rudolf Haerle, points out that the contract between Culver and Thomas specified that the research was to be on "Race Psychology of the peoples of Europe—more particularly of the countries from which immigrants to the United States are mainly supplied . . . that is to say, Russia, Poland, Bohemia, Hungary, Servia, Bulgaria, Romania and Italy," and the volumes planned were to deal with the themes of "race-mind, race temparament [sic], race-morals, race-prejudice, race-degeneration, race development, etc. . . . to be followed by one or more volumes on comparative race psychology" (Haerle Jr., 1991: 24). However, these familiar themes of US race psychology at the time were not, in fact, to be the focus of the research. Thomas himself, in a panel discussion at a meeting appraising the contribution of this work in 1938, put it thus: "Immigration was a burning question. About a million immigrants were coming here annually, and this was mainly the newer immigration, from southern and eastern Europe. The larger group were Poles, Italians and Jews . . . Eventually I decided to study [the social attitudes] of an immigrant group in Europe and America to determine as far as possible what relation their home mores and norms had to their adjustment and maladjustment in America" (ibid.: 22).

Adjustment and maladjustment, attitudes, mores, and norms—these were to be the conceptual questions that underlay Thomas's methodological introduction to the five volumes of *The Polish Peasant in Europe and America* that were published between 1918 and 1920 (Thomas and Znaniecki, 1918). There was little of what we call vitalism here, largely because Thomas and Znaniecki "rejected entirely any element of biological reductionism and sought to explain social behaviour in terms of sociological and social psychological categories" (Bulmer, 1984: 58). The volumes amounted to more than 2,000 pages, including personal documents, life histories and autobiography, letters, diaries, newspaper articles, court records, and much more.

The work is more cited than read, and even when cited the focus tends to be on its methodological innovation rather than its substantive exploration of the lives of Polish immigrants and the process by which they became 'American.' Indeed, Thomas himself is probably remembered less for the insights from his study of Polish peasants, or for his concern with methods for the scientific control of human behavior, than for the phrase first articulated in a later book written with Dorothy Swaine Thomas: "If men define situations as real, they are real in their consequences" (Thomas and Thomas, 1928: 572).[4] However, *The Polish Peasant* was not to launch Chicago sociologists into a series of further studies of migration; Thomas was dismissed from the University of Chicago in 1918, following his arrest in a Chicago hotel where he had registered himself and a female (married) companion under a false name. His companion, who did marry W. I. Thomas in 1935 (when she was 36 and he was 74), was Dorothy Swaine Thomas, who was later to produce perhaps the first ever comprehensive review of migration studies (Thomas, 1938) as well as many further studies in population changes and migration (Thomas, 1936; Thomas, 1941; Kuznets and Thomas, 1957). But while subsequent Chicago sociologists remained faithful to W. I. Thomas in his insistence on patient, careful, and detailed empirical investigation, the organizing feature of the sociology that became known as 'the Chicago School' moved in a different direction: towards a new ecology of the city, in particular of Chicago itself.

Perhaps the best way to grasp the vexed history of Chicago 'urban ecology' is to begin with its later memorializations and repudiations. Reflecting on the School's influence in the mid-1960s, for example, R.E.L. Faris, a son of Ellsworth Faris, who was one of the School's central figures, argued that "the most distinctive and most widely known development" among the Chicago scholars, at least in this period of their shared endeavor, was "the unprecedented surge of highly original research in urban ecology," such that Chicago "acquired the reputation for almost exclusively concentrating on spatial distributions in its own city" (Faris, 1970: 51). For Mike Savage and Alan Warde, a quarter of a century later, the picture is very different: "The key themes still relevant today that can be extracted from the Chicago School," they argue, "do not concern formalised ecological theory nor early versions of ethnographic method, but are three interconnected substantive elements: sociation, its changing modes within modernity, and social reform" (Savage and Warde, 1993: 11). They go on: "The work of the Chicago School is best seen as an extended empirical inquiry into the nature of social bonding in the modern, fragmented city. The city interested [the Chicago sociologists] for empirical, rather than conceptual reasons" (ibid.: 13). Dennis Smith agrees that the city was not itself the focus of this work: "Chicago sociologists," says Smith, "were always aware of two potent influences. One consisted of the moral imperatives associated with being 'good Americans,' a phrase that could be uttered without irony. The other was the power of private capital" (Smith, 1988: 1). Martin Bulmer, writing around the same time as Smith, describes the School in terms of a shared "commitment to empirical research and to grounding broader and more general insights in the results of inquiries made into the contemporary world. The hallmark of the Chicago school of sociology was this blending of firsthand inquiry with general ideas, the integration of research and theory as part of an organized program" (Bulmer, 1984: 2–3). For Robert Sampson, reflecting from the early twenty-first century, the heart of the project was in bringing "neighbourhood-centred research to the fore of the discipline during the early twentieth century" (Sampson, 2012: 35).

Andrew Abbott, in his recent history of Chicago sociology and its impact on US sociology more generally, argues that 'the Chicago School' is itself a cultural object: it is less a coherent and unified 'School' than it is a "stance" or an "intensity" (Abbott, 1999). The authors and texts gathered under its name may lack a "single paradigm," but taken in the round, they tended toward the city, toward an interest in processes of social movement and change, to a certain kind of interactionist viewpoint, to a broadly observational empirical style, and so on (ibid.: 6). For Abbott, what holds all of this together is an attention to time and place: he argues that for Louis Wirth and Ernest Burgess, especially, it was this "location in time and space, certainly social time and social space," that was at the heart of what they had tried for two decades to defend (ibid.: 72). Later he says: "Chicago felt that no social fact makes any sense abstracted from its context in social (and often geographic) space and social time. Social facts are *located*. . . . Every social fact is situated, surrounded by other contextual facts and brought into being by a process relating it to past contexts" (ibid.: 197). Abbott is at least partly railing against the self-consciously scientific and quantitative American sociology of his own time, with its stultifying insistence on identifying the role of distinct individual variables, as if interdependence is the thing that had to be abstracted out, rather than being itself the center of inquiry. It is for this reason, Abbott suggests, that when contemporary urban sociologists think of Chicago at all, they focus on its legacy for core sociological commitments, rather than substantive questions about specific forms of human life that animate the migrant city.

We hesitate to add to this weight of commentary. But for us, two different aspects make the Chicago approach worth thinking about. The first is that their work developed at a time when their city was in the midst of mass immigration The second is the complex, descriptive, and often strikingly *biological* ways in which their knowledge of this migrant city took shape. Consider for example two key texts from the early years of the School: Robert Park's famous essay 'The City,' first published in 1915, and Ernest Burgess's 'The Growth of the City,' first published in 1925, brought together in the 1925 monograph *The City* edited by Park, Burgess, and Mackenzie (Park, Burgess, et al., 1967). Both scholars unquestionably were setting out at a propitious moment: "the ground had been cleared by able predecessors . . . the soldiers had returned from the war and were eager for study. The nation was optimistic and the city proud and vigorous" (Faris, 1970: 26). Vigorous is the word. Perhaps the most striking thing about Park's essay to the contemporary reader is the intensity of his naturalistic imagery: the city, he says, is not merely a "congeries" of people, services, and buildings; it is rather a "state of mind," a set of sentiments and customs (recall that Park studied under Georg Simmel at Heidelberg), something "involved in the vital processes of the people who compose it; it is a product of nature, and particularly of human nature" (Park, Burgess, et al., 1967: 1). The city, Park goes on, forms a "natural area," which can therefore be understood as a "human, as distinguished from plant and animal, ecology" (ibid.: 2). Social analysts, hitherto, may have been inclined to focus on buildings, street furniture, the legal and bureaucratic setup of the city, and so on. But such things, says Park, "become part of the *living* city only when, and in so far as, through use and wont they connect themselves, like a tool in the hand of man, with the *vital* forces resident in individuals and the community . . . the city is the natural habitat of civilized man" (ibid.: 2, our emphases).

Martin Bulmer argues that what Park is doing in this paper, following the influence of his German teachers—who included not only Simmel but also Wilhelm Windelband—is seeking to make the city a social laboratory (Bulmer, 1984: 92). To understand Park, in other words, it is vital to understand his view of the city as "a living entity" that gives itself up to "patient methods of observation" (Park, Burgess, et al., 1967: 3–4). A researcher might study the basic plan and organization of the city ("What are the sources of the city's population?," Park asks; "how many people own their homes?" ibid.: 6–8); they might study the division of labor (looking variously at "the shop girl, the policeman, the peddler, the cabman, the nightwatchman, the clairvoyant . . ." Park goes on for several more lines). They might study social order ("what are the mores, for example, of the shopgirl?"), or temperament and character ("do professional burglars and professional confidence men represent different mental types?") or communication ("what is news?"), and so on.

What one gets from Park's essay is not a theory—or even much of an account—of the city, but rather an efflorescence of questions and topics for investigation (Park would spend the next twenty years supervising students addressing many of these questions). Indeed, it is hard not to read in Park's essay, in the sheer tumult of questions he sets out, a mirror of the excitement, the stimulation, the 'excess' that he claims to find in the city itself. Ernest Burgess's 'The Growth of the City,' by contrast, is very different in tone, and though it is not explicitly presented as such, forms a kind of methodological counterpart to Park's essay. It is here that Burgess first sketches the famous diagram of the city that—so Abbott informs us—still dominates a seminar room at the University of Chicago today: "the typical processes of the expansion of the city," says Burgess, "can best be illustrated, perhaps, by a series of concentric circles, which may be numbered to designate both the successive zones of urban extensions and the types of areas differentiated in the process of expansion" (Park, Burgess, et al., 1967: 50). Burgess's influential diagram stretches from a small circle marked 'Loop' at the center (the Loop is the name of the downtown area of Chicago), surrounded by a larger circle marked 'zone in transition,' in turn surrounded by 'workingmen's homes,' followed by the higher-class residential areas, and finally the suburbs, way out at the edges (ibid.: 50–51). His orienting imagery is no less biological than that of his colleague: the expansion of the city through these various zones, he says, may be thought of as an "urban metabolism." For Burgess, the key questions then are: "in what way are individuals incorporated into the life of a city? By what process does a person become an organic part of his society" (ibid.: 63). This leads him to questions of mobility (people moving in, out of, and through, different areas), and, from such movement, the development of social 'organization' and 'disorganization'—how rates of expansions, influxes of newcomers, balances of generation and gender, produce shifting waves of settlement and tumult as more and more people, and especially different *kinds* of people, are incorporated into the urban body. With this methodological approach to patterns of mobility in the city, says Burgess, one can finally open up "a cross-section of the city—to put this area as it were, under the microscope" (ibid.: 62).

An ecological view of the city underpins all of this, in fact a specifically human ecology: "a study of the spatial and temporal relations of human beings as affected by the selective, distributive and accommodative forces of the environment," as Roderick McKenzie put it in 1924 (McKenzie, 1924: 288). Strikingly, as Andrew Abbott points out, amid the many book-length treatments of the School, including those specifically focused on its method, "there is almost no work on ecology" (Abbott, 1999: 17). But human ecology was indeed the centerpiece of the Chicago approach. As Robert Faris put it: "the important discovery [at Chicago] was that a complex ecology does exist, and that it operates in important ways to select populations, to control the direction of their flow, and variously to influence behavior, especially in the variety of manifestations of social disorganization" (Faris, 1970: 62). Why, then, is there such reticence in the secondary literature?

The answer may simply be that it is very difficult to get a grip on what was actually involved in, or intended by, projects organized under the sign of this human ecology. The ecological approach is ambiguous, to say the least. It is, in one sense, plainly biological; there are times when, for example, they are comparing the city to an ant farm, as Park does, or to "anabolic and katabolic processes of metabolism in the body," as Burgess does, that these scholars almost seem to be trying too hard to provoke the reader with overtly biological imagery (Park, Burgess, et al., 1967: 29, 53). There is also a rough and ready Darwinian rhetoric permeating the project: as Robert Sampson points out, Park's work in particular is littered with terms like 'competition,' 'invasion,' 'succession,' 'segregation,' 'symbiosis' and so on. "Borrowing concepts from Darwinian theory," Sampson points out, "Park and Burgess focused on the 'balance of nature' and argued that natural forces were responsible for the initial distribution, concentration, and segregation of urban populations" (Sampson, 2012: 35, 40). But the ecological approach was more complex than that. Not least, it depended on new forms of social expertise. The empirical work of Chicago sociologists intersected with, and often relied upon, the careful accounting and describing work of (mostly women) social workers in Chicago, as well as the work of criminologists and mental health specialists, who used the ecological model to locate particular forms of deviation and disorganization as characteristic of specific neighborhoods (Faris, 1970; Sampson, 2012). Andrew Abbott reminds us that Chicago was a rival to the much more rigidly inductive, quantitative approach of Franklin Giddings (Abbott, 1999: 209). And alongside all of this biological language, what Park and Burgess were actually doing was sending students out to collect sociological data, teaching courses on social pathology and map-making, linking up with other social scientists, beginning to teach field studies, and so on.

There are also important ways in which human ecology was specifically non-biological, or at least was opposed to the way that biology figured in much social thought at the time. Robert Faris makes clear that at least one of the central goals of the ecological method was to move away from a crude biologism, a view in which poverty, crime, suicide, mental abnormality, and other behavioral defects of slum dwellers were seen as "inborn legacies from their defective ancestors" (Faris, 1970: 62). Human-ecological research, by contrast, was one of the principal bulwarks against "eugenic extremism"—it is *the city*, not the individual, or their genetic inheritance, that is disorganized—individual problems were "a result of a grand and too-rapid transition from a pre-industrial folk society to a highly mechanized urban civilization" (ibid.: 62–63).

Perhaps this tension is most visible in Louis Wirth's celebrated 1938 essay, 'Urbanism as a Way of Life,' published almost 25 years after Park's landmark contribution. "Nowhere," says, Wirth, in his opening lines, "has mankind been farther removed from organic nature than under the conditions of life characteristic of great cities" (Wirth, 1938: 1–2). What is required then, he suggests, is some kind of theory of the way of life of people in cities: only through a meaningful theoretical grip on what the city *is*, on what constitutes the mode of life that operates *in* it, says Wirth, can sociologists hope to contribute anything useful to questions of poverty, crime, delinquency, and so on. The city, for Wirth, is a kind of intensity—not simply measured by the numbers of people in it, but by how it might act as a fulcrum for the more general outpourings of economic and cultural life. Size also produces differentiation and specialization, and from these, a certain kind of anonymity and rationality from density, then comes further segmentation and friction and the need for order, as the city comes "to resemble a mosaic of social worlds" (ibid.: 15).

There is no doubt that Wirth's approach to the city is more complex and sophisticated than those of earlier members of 'the Chicago School.' Yet despite his insistence on the need to focus on the very distinctive "social psychology" of the urban mode of life (Wirth, 1938: 1), Wirth nonetheless retains an interest in explicitly 'biological' questions (for example, the slightly higher death rate and significantly lower birth rate in cities), at the same time as more obviously social questions (who belongs to what civic organizations and why) and issues of personality and mentality (how the psychosocial life of the city produces "personal disorganization, mental breakdown, suicide, delinquency, crime, corruption, and disorder" ibid.: 23).

What social scientists still call 'the Chicago School' died off soon after, being sucked into the grimly quantitative orthodoxy of elite American sociology which continues to this day. The school was brought low by a combination of methodological critique of "the ecological fallacy" (Robinson, 1950),[5] and, from an entirely different direction, the challenge of the new 'political' urban sociology of authors such as David Harvey and Manuel Castells (Sampson, 2012). How, then, should we think about Chicago urban sociology today?

Certainly, for many, the biology makes it hard. Savage and Warde note that "since forms of biological reductionism are generally considered completely unsustainable, most urban sociologists have used such interpretations as grounds for dismissing Chicago's contemporary relevance" (Savage and Warde, 1993: 14). They point out, however, that seeing ecological thought as only a kind of biological reductionism is naïve—that 'human nature' can and does mean different things, not all of them fixed in time, and even that evolutionary thought is 'social theory' first, only becoming biologized much later. And yet, having opened this possibility, these authors quickly close it: the malleability and diverse inheritance of Chicago's biological thought is used only to rescue its major figures from the fatal charge of reductionism; it is not taken as an opportunity to look more expansively at these biological issues themselves. Indeed, quite the opposite. It becomes instead the ground on which references to biology can be explained away: for example, Burgess's ecological model was "of only marginal importance to the Chicago ethnographies," and anyway "was largely used metaphorically by Chicago writers" (ibid.: 16–17). For Savage and Warde, in other words, thinking with Chicago, today, means thinking beyond, indeed without, its biological urges. There were many other theoretical interests in the School, they point out, and in any event Park really only synthesized his ecological ideas in the 1930s, "well after most of the Chicago ethnographies had been written, and when he was no longer especially influential within Chicago" (ibid.: 15). At its heart, "the school's interest was always in studying patterns of social bonding in a given historical situation and in particular spatial settings—the American City in the early twentieth century" (ibid.: 17).

Andrew Abbott's view is not very different. If we want to intervene in the forms of sociology dominant in the United States, he argues, our goal should be to revive a kind Chicagoist interest in interaction and environment, in space and time, through a refocus on new "*positivist, formal* methods for contextualism" (Abbott, 1999: 217). By this Abbott means network analysis, or sequence analysis, or some more mathematized attempt to model interactive and contextualized social action, albeit without the variabilists' anxiety about causation (freedom from causal thinking is what Abbott sees as the real goal). With these new (quantitative) methods, Abbott argues, "we now have the empirical power to return social facts to their temporal and spatial contexts," drawing on the "goodly heritage of both theoretical and empirical work in the contextualist, interactionist tradition, bequeathed to us by the Chicago school" (ibid.: 222).

Well, maybe. But we end this section with two questions that point in other directions. First: why is migration so marginal both to the School itself and to its subsequent memorialization in urban theory? This is not to say that migration was ignored—indeed the 'immigrant colony' is an ever-present in Chicago style attentions to 'the neighborhood', as for example in Burgess's essay, 'Can Neighborhood Work Have a Scientific Basis?" (Burgess, 1925). But what is lacking in these commentaries is any attention to the 'Chicago' of 'the Chicago School' time as, fundamentally, a migrant city, and hence to the ways in which the experience of being a migrant was at the center of the human ecology that emerged in Chicago in the 1920s and 1930s. Second: what if the infusion of the biological language in the Chicago School was not mere metaphor? What if it was not something to be wished away? What if it was not just a barrier to 'contemporary relevance'? What if the weird, often worrying mixture of biology, ecology, sociology, and fieldwork, was actually what might enable the approach of those Chicago researchers to contribute to our understanding of the present?

Philadelphia: Striving, Palpitating

In 1896, just a year after becoming the first African American scholar to be awarded a doctorate at Harvard, W.E.B. Du Bois arrived in Philadelphia from a kind of exile (or what he experienced as exile) at Wilberforce College in Ohio. His purpose was to make an in-depth sociological study of the life of the African American population in one ward of Philadelphia—"a city within a city" as he would put it at the outset of the landmark monograph he published only three years later (Du Bois, 1899). Du Bois, along with Nina Gomer, who was married to him, arrived into a resolutely urban scene: "late nineteenth century Philadelphia," Thomas Sugrue and Michael Katz remind us, "was an industrial giant, the second largest city in the United States"; arriving from provincial Ohio, "Du Bois undoubtedly sensed the dynamism, the promise, and the deep-rooted problems of a city under-going wrenching economic changes" (Sugrue and Katz, 1998). Unlike the mostly transnational migrants who were swelling Chicago, Philadelphia "was drawing a steady flow of African Americans from Virginia, North and South Carolina, Georgia, and other southeastern states," pushed out of their homes by the "disastrous consequences of the crop lien and sharecropping systems" and seeking better economic opportunities in the North (Franklin, 1998: 198). While there was a black elite in Philadelphia, living in substantial homes, Southern migrants could generally only find residence in the Seventh Ward of the city, a place of "decrepit brick row homes," spread across "narrow alleys, courtyards and back streets," surrounded by "open sewers and waste disposal areas" (Sugrue and Katz, 1998: 4).

Du Bois had been brought to Philadelphia through a familiar late-Victorian philanthropic concern with 'improvement,' rooted in the Philadelphia Settlement, which sponsored the Seventh Ward project, to which it recruited Du Bois via the University of Pennsylvania. The Philadelphia Settlement was itself part of the broader College Settlement movement, led mostly by wealthy white women, bent toward their own idea of improving the lives and the souls of the urban poor, and greatly influenced by Toynbee Hall in East London (Franklin, 1998). The ward where these reformers were trying to intervene, says Du Bois's biographer, David Levering Lewis, "was a progressive reformer's worst nightmare" (Lewis, 1993: 186). Living a "hard, noisy and deadly life" in "miserable shotgun row houses," the residents of the area were "the bane of respectable Philadelphia," while the Pennsylvania Hospital, two blocks away, found itself "practically swamped by the grisly medical problems of black males in the grip of social pathologies" (ibid.: 186). It was the conditions of life in this scene that Du Bois was charged to describe and understand. And he did so largely on foot: "Du Bois," says Lewis, "sallied forth on quick firm steps each morning, accoutered with cane and gloves, to spend an eight-hour day knocking on the doors of his new neighbors" (ibid.: 190). Drawing on the work of Charles Booth in London, and also on the Hull House project in Chicago, Du Bois went from street to street, house to house, family to family, interviewing, observing, surveying, and mapping: according to Lewis (drawing on the work of Herbert Aptheker) this effort produced 2,500 interviews and 15,000 interview schedules in just three months. The book that Du Bois produced in 1899, *The Philadelphia Negro*, was only one of several forays he made into the African American urban experience—including, as Aldon Morris points out, further studies of "black communities in New York, Boston and Philadelphia" published in the *New York Times* in 1901 (Morris, 2015: 69). For Morris, *The Philadelphia Negro* is not only, as it is often acclaimed, "the first study of an

urban black community," but also "America's first major empirical sociological study" as such (ibid.: 45). "Du Bois," he argues, "emerged from *The
Philadelphia Negro* as the first number-crunching, surveying, interviewing,
participant-observing and field-working sociologist in America" (ibid.: 47).

It is this sense of *The Philadelphia Negro* as a pioneering—indeed *the*
pioneering—work of social science that interests us here. In its exploration
of African American urban life as it gets interwoven with white supremacy
in the industrial cities of the North, Du Bois is strikingly alive to the different bodies of thought necessary to make sense of the conditions of human
urban life: social science and social work, the biological capacities of human
bodies, and bureaucratic management of the migrant city. Yet, in notable
contrast to the Chicago work that followed him, Du Bois placed the movement of people to Philadelphia and the surrounding districts at the center
of his work. As he points out, in the century before his study, the population of the county of Philadelphia increased by 2000 percent (Anderson,
1996; Du Bois, 1996 [1899]: 46). "[T]he Negroes were bought here early,"
says Du Bois at the outset of Chapter III, and "were held as slaves along
with many white serfs" (ibid.: 10). Through the eighteenth century, he suggests, the long march to abolition coincided with mass arrival of immigrants
into the city from "the continual stream of Southern fugitives and rural
freedmen," which was then followed by the early stages of an "inpouring of
the newly emancipated blacks from the South" (ibid.). Into the nineteenth
century, Philadelphia, as a kind of "natural gateway between the North and
the South," experienced significant movements of people from the South but
even more so—and much to the detriment of the city's black population—
from Europe (ibid.: 25). It was this latter form of migration, Du Bois points
out, that predominated in the mid-nineteenth century: from 1840 to 1870,
the white population grew from fewer than 240,000 to more than 650,000,
while the black population grew from 19,833 to 22,147—and indeed the latter
only at century's end, Du Bois shows, in a *fin-de-siècle* "rush to the cities on
the part of both white and black" (ibid.: 36, 47).

At the heart of Du Bois's study of this migrant metropolis, and quite
against the presumptions, perhaps even the hopes, of his employers, is an
argument that while citizens of the Seventh Ward made and lived their
lives—worked, produced families, formed civic organizations, engaged in
politics, sometimes broke the law, such as it was—in incredibly straitened
and difficult circumstances, these circumstances were *not* the product of the
inherent deficiencies of what was termed the "black race." In fact, they were
the prosaic and predictable outcomes of a social and political environment

that, at every turn, worked to keep the black population in its place. Du Bois's argument is that, whatever the problems that were found within African American communities in Philadelphia, these were artefacts of history and the environment, *not* of character, or of biology. As Elijah Anderson puts it, for Du Bois, "the problems of black Philadelphians stemmed largely from their past condition of servitude as they tried to negotiate an effective place in a highly competitive industrial urban setting in which the legacy of white supremacy was strong and their competitors were favored because of their white skin" (Anderson, 1996: xix).

This is the pathbreaking contribution that Du Bois made to the emerging practice of social science. As Mia Bay points out, his contribution was both conceptual and empirical: through an innovative use of maps, surveys, and other techniques, "The *Philadelphia Negro* analyzed the city as a setting where spatial arrangements revealed racial dynamics . . . Du Bois documented racial configurations within city spaces as planned phenomena rather than as outgrowths of natural ecological processes" (Bay, 1998: 49). Here, as Katz and Sugrue make clear, some 800 miles east of—and a quarter of a century prior to—the founding myths of Chicago and its 'hobohemia' is a very different story of American sociology, centered on social welfare and social reform, on statistics, on the investigation of social problems and entanglements with philanthropy, based on a deep account of institutional racism, its embodiment and the vital experience of mobile life in the city (Sugrue and Katz, 1998). As Aldon Morris puts it: "Du Bois's pioneering community studies utilized scientific methodology two decades before Park and his students" (Morris, 2015: 4). It is important to remember that the discipline of sociology was at an embryonic moment as Du Bois was writing. Attempts at making a systematic study of social life were still taking place in the shadow of Herbert Spencer, Francis Galton, and even Charles Darwin, and the wider moralistic and 'reformist' milieu in which their ideas took root. But this was also an era of rapid methodological innovation: even though Du Bois was only ever admitted to the lowly level of instructor, despite his education and experience, the University of Pennsylvania sociology department was pioneering the use of statistics, and the study of population.

Mia Bay is surely right that *The Philadelphia Negro* is "a classic across the disciplines precisely because it was written before the modern disciplines of sociology, anthropology, history and economics were fully formed" (Bay, 1998: 41). As she argues, *The Philadelphia Negro* is best read through the nineteenth-century intellectual traditions in which it was written, and where "Du Bois broke ranks with the white social scientists of the 1890s, who almost invariably assumed that deficiencies characteristic of the race made Negro problems quite different from other people's problems" (ibid.: 42). Du Bois's singular achievement in *The Philadelphia Negro* was to replace the scientific racism of ethnology with dry empirics. Well in advance of Franz Boas's culture concept, Du Bois relies not on transcendental principles, but on "empirical evidence to controvert white racial theories": he had a "striking faith in the relations of science and justice" (ibid.: 51).

But Du Bois's relationship to the methods and concepts of the natural sciences was complex—not least on the context of migration. *The Philadelphia Negro*, in advancing sociological explanations for the grim conditions of life in the Seventh Ward in opposition to the eugenically inflected biological accounts then in vogue among progressive reformers, recruited science to the cause of anti-racism, and thereafter to sociology. Aldon Morris argues that the work Du Bois undertook and directed at Atlanta University, where he took up a post on completion of his work in Philadelphia, has a better claim than Chicago to be the foundation of American empirical sociology (Morris, 2015). Indeed, Morris argues, the clear evidence of Du Bois's pre-eminence was suppressed by white social scientists seeking a very different foundation for their own discipline, because Du Bois's "sociological arguments stressing that races were socially constructed and blacks were not biologically inferior flew in the face of white racial beliefs" (ibid.: 3). For Morris, it is vital to understand that the anti-racist thrust of Du Bois's work is tightly braided through his attention to empirical detail, and a commitment to sociology as a science.

Nevertheless, this call upon science was not without tension. On the one hand, those who argued for white supremacy claimed biological support for their view of the dire consequences of the migration of freed slaves to the heart of the expanding city. On the other hand, arguments that sought to make precisely the opposite case also claimed scientific methods and data. As David Levering Lewis reminds us, the progressives who established the settlement that sponsored the study "were prey to eugenic nightmares about Native Stock and the better classes being swamped by fecund dysgenic aliens. The conservative CSA [College Settlement Association, sponsors of Du Bois's project] thought of poverty in epidemiological terms, as a virus to be quarantined . . . Du Bois was expected to take responsibility for diagnosing the exact nature of the virus among Philadelphia's African-Americans" (Lewis, 1993: 188). Indeed, Du Bois himself was by no means wholly removed from the Social Darwinism of his day, and his book not infrequently shows the traces of his struggles between this ideology and the evidence he reports (Bay, 1998: 53–54). Hence there is another literature that sees, in Du Bois's undoubted elitism, a lurking biological conception of black inferiority (see Morris, 2015: 30).

While many are keen to portray Du Bois as a precursor to contemporary urban ethnography, we follow Mia Bay in drawing out the ways that he put scientific methods and biological concepts to work in his text. It is Du Bois's attention to the corporeal reality of urban life that strikes the contemporary reader. Indeed, the book is sometimes overwhelming in its catalogue of bodies and buildings, of bodies *in* buildings, exhaustive discussion of family size and conjugal life, of age and sex, of marriage, of alcoholism, of the precise layout of streets, of the condition of houses—and so on. "I made a study of the Philadelphia Negro so thorough that it has withstood the criticism of forty years," Du Bois recalled many years later, "it revealed the Negro group as a symptom, not a cause; as a striving, palpitating group, and not an inert sick body" (Du Bois quoted in Anderson, 1996: xvi). The imagery is not accidental: if Du Bois's text is the keystone of twentieth-century urban studies, then it is a foundation that refused to give up on science, on biology, on *life*.

Chapter Ten of the book, where Du Bois describes the "conditions of life in the ward" and offers an account of how "the Negroes as a class dwell in the most unhealthful parts of the city, and in the worst houses in those parts" (Du Bois, 1996[1899]: 148), is where this theme emerges most strongly. Here Du Bois shows his skill in intertwining differently sourced accounts of bodies and environments, working through tables showing the results of "bad ventilation, lack of outdoor life for women and children, [and] poor protection against dampness and cold [which] are undoubtedly the chief causes of [the ward's] excessive death rate" (ibid.: 152). Setting himself against the calumny that African Americans were more prone to consumption because of their inherently inferior physical condition, Du Bois points out that "the Irish were once thought to be doomed by that disease—but that was when Irishmen were unpopular" (ibid.: 160). The death rate, he says firmly, "is largely a matter of conditions of living" (ibid.: 156). And he identifies those conditions precisely: unsanitary homes, limited air and light, damp walls and bad sewers, raggedy clothes in a cold climate, food quality, the capacity to keep one's self clean. To all of this he adds the intergenerational burden of slavery: "many generations of unhealthy bodies have bequeathed to the present generation impaired vitality and hereditary tendency to disease" (ibid.: 162). For Du Bois, reform must begin with "a crusade for fresh air, cleanliness, healthfully located homes and proper food" (ibid.: 163).

We must not over-interpret this material. It is no surprise that a highly educated person, moving in elite intellectual circles between Europe and North America in the late nineteenth century, would have recourse to particular images of life and its requirements. And yet it also seems undeniable, not only in this chapter (Du Bois's account of housing, for example, works through a similar register), that Du Bois poses the question of racial injustice in the city specifically as a vital question, a question of life. Further, he positions white supremacy in the industrial north as a necropolitics, to use Achille Mbembe's term (Mbembe, 2019), noting how, for example, an anti-black animus is expressed, if not in precisely exterminationist terms, then at least through a willingness to tolerate the dying-off of the black population, while moralizing on "inferior species" (ibid.: 163). In Du Bois, we find an insistence on the basic vulnerability of the racially stratified body in the migrant city: an insistence that emancipatory projects must engage with those vulnerabilities, and with the shifting, mobile, migratory populations who are most exposed to them.

How Do They Really Live?

In the late 1880s, in a block of flats in the east end of London, a "Lady Resident" writes:

> At half-past eight [in the morning] I hear the eldest child of the A. family lighting the fire and dressing her two little brothers for school. With the departure of the children there is a lull. At ten, Mrs. A gets up, and at eleven she sallies out to make sundry purchases . . . In the afternoon a certain torpor falls upon the Buildings, only broken by the jingling cans and cat-calls of the afternoon milk-boys. But this is the favourite time for the women to call upon one another, and I can catch various fragments of conversation relating to the bad turn Mrs. D's illness is taking. . . . Various savoury smells begin to float out onto the landings. The favourite meal of the day, the "tea," is being prepared against the husband's return . . . The A.'s have sprats, as I have good reason to know. Mrs. A is aware of my partiality for this fish, and in a neighbourly spirit sends me in a plateful by her most careful child, from whom I learn that Mrs. D is much worse and wandering in her head, and that "mother is going to sit up with her." Mrs. D's husband is a nightwatch, so he is at hand by day to look after her, and the neighbours are taking turns to nurse her by night.

This report comes from the second edition of *Labour and Life of the People* (now more commonly known by the title of later editions: *Life and Labour of the People in London*), edited by Charles Booth, and published between 1891 and 1903 (Booth, 1891: 270–275). In the early 1880s, Booth, then a young shipping magnate, had moved from Liverpool to London to expand his business. Booth—described in this period by his wife's cousin, and his own future collaborator, Beatrice Webb, as "an attractive but distinctly queer figure of a man" (Webb, 1926: 188)—discovered not only the monumental imperial capital that he no doubt anticipated, but also a dirty, sickly, and deeply impoverished place. London at the end of the nineteenth century was a city "scarcely advanced beyond the middle ages. In the 1880s, with a population of over four million, it still lacked a water, sanitation, and public health system; it still suffered from periodic plagues of typhus and cholera; and its poor laws were as archaic and oppressive as ever" (Fried and Elman, 1969: xix). Public and political concern with what was usually termed 'the social problem' approached a high point.

Much of this the misery that gathered around this 'social problem' related to sheer numbers of people: the County of London grew from a population of less than one million to more than four and a half million over the nineteenth century—with more than seven million people in the greater London area by the beginning of the twentieth century (Ball and Sunderland, 2002: 42). As we have seen previously, the two major causes of the increase were 'natural increase' (falling death rates and improvements in infant mortality especially) and migration. If Britain's northern cities attracted the majority of migrants in the later eighteenth and early nineteenth centuries, the situation changed thereafter: "with its myriad of employment opportunities, high wages, and relative immunity from the trade cycle, London attracted immigrants like no other British city after the 1840s, as by then the expansion of the northern cities was slowing" (ibid.: 49). This did not go unremarked by Booth: in a chapter on influx of population in volume 1 of *Life and Labour*, his collaborator, Hubert Llewellyn Smith, writes: "the drain from the country is one of the greatest unsolved problems of London" (in Booth, 1889: 501). Indeed, says Llewellyn Smith, "London is to a great extent nourished by the literal consumption of bone and sinew from the country" (ibid.: 508). He points out that figures representing an influx of migrants in fact represent a much more complex pattern of ebb and flow: "all this internal movement though usually confined to short distances, indicates the existence of migratory habit among the people, which must in the long run produce a considerable admixture of population" (ibid.: 509). Many, he points out, came to London from "small rural towns" as "county industry" migrated to the bigger cities (ibid.: 516). But this is not only a question of the economics of labor:

> We cannot gauge by statistics the effect on the imagination of a country boy bred in the dull, if healthy, monotony of a sleepy rural district . . . add to all this the contagion of numbers, the sense of something going on, the theaters and the music halls, the brightly lighted streets and busy crowds:—All, in short, that makes the difference between the Mile End fair on a Saturday night, and a dark and muddy country lane, with no glimmer of gas, and with nothing to do. Who could wonder that men were drawn into such a vortex, even were the penalty heavier than it is? (ibid.: 518)

And it was often a heavy penalty indeed. In the series of campaigning articles later collected as *London Labour and The London Poor*, the journalist, Henry Mayhew, had already shocked an educated public with his in-depth account of the forms of life being produced by the "economic barbarism" of this era of widespread mobility (Rosenborg, 1968: v). Mayhew, Trollope, and Dickens all compellingly wrote of the conditions of life of these migrants, many of whom ended up in the 'back slums' like Jacob's Island—memorably described by Dickens as a place of "Crazy wooden galleries . . . with holes from which to look upon the slime beneath; windows, broken and patched . . . rooms so small, so filthy, so confined, that the air would seem too tainted even for the dirt and squalor which they shelter . . . dirt-besmeared walls and decaying foundations" (Dickens, 1838: ch. 50).[6] Others, notably the housing campaigner, Octavia Hill, published articles describing the "deplorable condition" of the dwellings of the urban poor (Hill, 1970 [1883]: 25)—writings that informed the arguments of Keir Hardie and the Independent Labour Party, among others (Briggs, 1961).

By the early 1880s, Booth had become a member of the Royal Statistical Society and was involved in 'social diagnosis'; he was convinced that the political economists of the day dealt with the social problem at far too high a level of abstraction, and that "personal investigation was necessary" (O'Day and Englander, 1993: 29–32). Indeed, as a reader of Auguste Comte, Booth was "convinced that empirically defined evidence of life as it was experienced, properly analysed, must form the basis of social action" (ibid.: 120). His method was, first, to draw on the records of school board visitors to estimate the extent of poverty within given households and streets, and then to interview the visitors themselves. This was supplemented with in-depth detailed primary observations, as Booth and his growing team gradually built up a detailed statistical map of poverty across the East End—later stretching out to other parts of London, and to wider investigations of working and religious life.

Booth "directly employed questionnaires, interviews, personal observation; collection of statistical data; collation of data; sampling; and statistical tabulation of data in his work" (O'Day and Englander, 1993: 18). But in this he was not especially motivated by sympathy—indeed, a significant motivation for what would become a 17-year, 17-volume obsession was Booth's conviction (wrong, as he would acknowledge in light of his empirical research) that the large numbers and desperate conditions of the London poor had been overstated. In fact, he *did* discover that the claim by the Social Democratic Federation that 25 percent of the working class of London was living in poverty was inaccurate; but this was not because it was an overstatement—indeed the true figure was nearer 35 percent (Fried and Elman, 1969: xxviii). As Raymond Williams (1969) points out, Booth hardly discovered urban poverty: Engels and Mayhew, to say nothing of Charles Dickens or Elizabeth Gaskell, got there well before him. Rather, his achievement was the formalization of analysis and intervention in a quasi-scientific method—"a method of impersonal inquiry," says Williams, which could allow the separation of "remedies" from "political analysis" (Williams, 1969: xi). As Booth's wife, Mary Booth (née Macauley, and a niece of the historian Thomas Babington Macauley) would later put it, Booth wished to know: "who are the people of England? How do they really live? What do they really want? Do they want what is good, and if so, how is it to be given to them?" (quoted in the memoir of her cousin Beatrice Webb, 1926: 192).

Booth's mammoth study became known—not least through its author's attention to his own legend—for its statistical dryness. In the final volume, speaking about the state of poverty in London, Booth writes: "for the treatment of [social] disease, it is first necessary to establish the facts as to its character, extent and symptoms. . . . The dry bones that lie scattered over the long valley that we have traversed together lie before my reader" (quoted in Pfautz, 1967: 43). Or elsewhere:

the materials for sensational stories lie plentifully in every book of our notes; but, even if I had the skill to use my material in this way—that gift of the imagination which is called 'realistic'—I should not wish to use it here. There is struggling poverty, there is destitution, there is hunger, drunkenness, brutality, and crime; no one doubts that it is so. My object [however] has been to attempt to show the numerical relation which poverty, misery and depravity bear to regular earnings and comparative comfort. (Booth, 1889: 6)

But there is some special pleading here. On the very next page of the same volume, we find lists of sample outputs from his house surveys—complete with side comments from the surveyors: "queer character"; "casual labourer—now gone hopping";[7] "two elder sons loaf about"; "a female of doubtful character"; "also have a loft, where the wife, the wife's mother (who also lives with them) and the elder children all work together at making fish baskets out of old mat sugar bags. Dirty and low, but not so poor"; "awfully poor—wife is subject to fits"; "all cripples—wife's mother also a cripple, lives here—an awful lot—younger children like withered up old men"; "injured leg prevents him working full time"; "wife drinks up all his earnings"; "used to be in regular work but some stone-work fell on him and he has been affected ever since"; "all the inmates have to use one small yard with one water tap, and w.c."; "scarcely a rag to cover themselves with—wife and children utterly neglected—a lazy vagabond"; "one child is physically and mentally afflicted" (ibid.: 7).

There is certainly more flesh on these "dry bones" than Booth wishes to admit. But what is striking to us is how often his in-depth attention to daily life in this migrant city alights on topics of health and illness, and on broader biopolitical concerns. It is the presence of sanitary taps, the flow of air, the sickliness of an underfed child, the neighbors sitting up with an ill woman at work—it is the body in its physical and social milieu experiencing sickness and in death that centers the study. In his 1893 account of the study for the Royal Statistical Society (Booth gave several papers on the study to the Society; by this time he was also its president), he threads his account of poverty and crowding through an explicit attention to natality and death, and the question of replacing populations. Thus, for example, he points out that "Bethnal Green and Shoreditch, lying side by side geographically, are fourth and fifth for crowding, fifth and sixth for early marriages, second and third for births, and sixth and seventh for deaths. Bethnal Green is Shoreditch intensified, or Shoreditch is Bethnal Green diluted" (Booth, 1893: 574). He notes that, in poor districts, high births and high deaths frequently go together: "If the lack of care which allows young children to die, is only another form of the recklessness that without thought for their future has brought them into the world. then we might confidently expect that a reduction in infant mortality would always be accompanied by fewer births" (ibid.: 574). While we can read Booth's engagement with wider Victorian imperialist and eugenicist anxiety about the virility of the body politic, he certainly brought novel techniques of observation and analysis to bear on this apparently sickly, barely reproducing body. If we can regard his study as one more moment of invention of urban sociology, then we can see again that such a sociology is invented, not so much as the dry recitation of statistics, but rather as an explicitly biopolitical—and indeed eugenic—concern. It was not for nothing that Beatrice Webb compared Booth to Darwin and Galton (Webb, 1926: 190).

London was not the only British city to grow in this period. The northern city of York, for example, grew from a population of just under 17,000 in 1901 to almost 80,000 by 1901. York was no great migrant metropolis, like London or Manchester. Yet, according to Seebohm Rowntree, the famous analyst of working life and poverty in that city at the close of the nineteenth century, the building of the railways had nonetheless "attracted many workmen to the city from other parts of England" in mid-century; at about the same period, large numbers of mostly rural Irish migrants, fleeing famine, arrived in Britain—and many of them, says Rowntree, coming "as far as York" (Rowntree, 1922: 9–10). P. M. Tillott, in his history of the city, points out that whereas York may have lost population to outward movement before 1841, thereafter inward migration clearly makes a significant contribution to population increase, especially in the middle decades of the century (Tillott, 1961).

Rowntree's study of life in York at the turn of the twentieth century, *Poverty: A Study of Town Life* (Rowntree, 2000 [1901]), was a self-conscious reproduction of Booth's efforts. Rowntree, a Quaker and social reformer, as well as the son of Joseph Rowntree (founder of the then rapidly expanding York cocoa industry), was keen to see if Booth's findings would hold up in a provincial setting. But Rowntree was a very different character than Booth: "Working as a chemist," says his biographer Asa Briggs, "he was concerned with studies that required the utmost precision. As early as the mid-nineties he was beginning to ponder the value of detailed measurement in the social sciences . . . keenly interested as he was in natural history, he himself laid special emphasis on 'natural growth,' comparing the development of Christian character to the blossoming of flowers and the lives of Christians to the 'glory of the garden'" (Briggs, 1961: 12).

This scientific desire was embedded in a particular kind of social conscience. Like his father, Rowntree was concerned, in a patrician Victorian way, with the conditions of the workers in his factory, as well as with the wider conditions of the poor in York. He was thus committed to an idea of moral improvement, but also to workers' education, and to social solutions to poverty such as the provision of state old age pensions, then the object of a lively debate among those who took 'the poor' as their object. As in London, a team of researchers was sent house to house in York between 1899 and 1900, completing a short schedule (how many people in each room, the number of people per tap, the presence or not of a yard, and so on). 'Visitors' were again used to gather the data, and Rowntree aggregated the classes according to Booth's 8-point scale of relative destitution (Rowntree, 2000 [1901]: 14, 28). To the published schedule is appended the familiar litany of grim side remarks from the researchers ('F. 10, consumptive; M.4, cripple.' 'Father has lost an eye. House not very dirty.' 'Disreputable old woman, ill; ought to be in Workhouse. Hawks[8] when able . . . House very dirty, probably used as a house of ill-fame'; 'Wife paralyzed. Respectable.' 'House dirty and unhealthy.' 'Had parish relief stopped for illegitimate child. . . . Query—how they live? [sic.]") (ibid.: 16–25).

But perhaps the most striking aspect of Rowntree's study is his attention to the relatively new science of metabolism. Of course, Rowntree is a chemist working in a food business—calorie intake is, literally, his concern. Indeed, the science of metabolism, Hannah Landecker (2019) points out, is largely inseparable from developments in industrial food manufacture in the nineteenth century. So perhaps we should not be surprised to see food, its presence, its adequacy, its chemical makeup, so much to the fore in Rowntree's study. Thus, of people in Class A, for example, the lowest class in the study, he writes: "The food of these poor people is totally inadequate . . . consisting largely of a dreary succession of bread, dripping, and tea; bread and butter and tea; bacon, bread, and coffee with only a little butcher's meat, with none of the extras and but little of the variety which serves to make meals interesting and appetizing" (Rowntree, 2000 [1901]: 43–44). He notes that one woman, while nursing infants, "lived chiefly upon bread and tea. Who can wonder that some of her children died during their first year?" (ibid.: 44). Indeed, his description of "primary poverty" (a concept that is invented in this study) is almost wholly an account of food and its role in the body: Rowntree goes on at some length about the presence of protein, carbohydrate, and fats in food, about their respective roles in repairing tissue and producing energy, about the production of albuminoids to build "muscle, tendon, and bone," and so on (ibid., 89). He calculates precisely the volume of food required of a family when a woman gets 90 percent of the husband's intake; a girl, 70 percent: and a child under two years old,

30 percent (ibid.: 91). Over and over again in the study, he remains deeply interested in "the quantity of food required for men doing varying amounts of muscular work' (ibid.).

Rowntree also offers the reader a scholarly review of the latest nutritional science, centered on the work of the metabolic chemist Wilbur Atwater at Wesleyan University, as well as J. C. Dunlop's experiments on prisoners in Scotland—the latter noting that when prisoners, breaking stones for eight hours a day, were limited to an intake of less than 3,500 calories, they "distinctly lost weight" and made complaints that "were pitiable and undoubtedly genuine" (Rowntree, 2000 [1901]: 95). Food—its metabolic properties, its cost and availability—takes up the first thirty pages of Rowntree's discussion of "the poverty line"; for "rent," the next biggest marker of poverty, he allots just one page (ibid.: 106–107). He even has participants keep food diaries (ibid.: 222–223), plots the total calorific value of the family's food, and then compares it to what he thinks they need for the amount of exertion they're undergoing (for example, a family with three children of different ages is equated to 3.3 working men)—working out not only that the food is inadequate, but, for example, how many grams of protein per statistical 'man' each household is short of (ibid.: 230, 234). Repeatedly, it is physical efficiency, measured as a relation of calorie intake to energy expended, that concerns Rowntree: "A horse fed upon hay does not feel hungry," he concludes, "and may indeed grow fat, but it cannot perform hard and continuous work without a proper supply of corn. Just so the labourer . . . is unable to do the work which he could easily accomplish upon a more nutritious diet" (ibid.: 303).

Asa Briggs argues that, whatever else we want to say about it, this was a wholly novel way of encountering the social problem: "for the foundations of his analysis [Rowntree] turned neither to socialists nor to social workers but to physiologists and dieticians" (Briggs, 1961: 32). Actually, Rowntree's interest is not *so* novel in principle; its essentials were described by Marx, more than thirty years before, in terms of the reproduction of labor power; while Marx's specific chemical attentions in his later work were not directed to bodily metabolism but to agricultural output, but the underpinning insight is much the same (cf. Saito, 2017). But Rowntree's microscopic attention to dietetics is nonetheless striking. W. O. Atwater, one of his key experts, was the inventor of the calorometer at the US Department of Agriculture (Atwater and Rosa, 1899). According to Briggs, Atwater was financially supported by the Russell Sage Foundation, which had itself conducted some of the first urban surveys in the United States. This was a revolutionary period for nutritional science, not least in the context of imperial expansion that brought questions of the 'fitness of the race' to the fore (Briggs, 1961: 33).[9] The poverty line, for Rowntree, becomes in this context a measure of adequate caloric intake. Those below it, in primary poverty, "cannot provide the bare necessities of physical efficiency"; those above the line, in secondary poverty, were still desperately poor, but had an income large enough to provide the requisite calories for the household. For Rowntree, the social problem had thus become a metabolic problem. And the solution to the problem of the migrants aggregating in the heart of the great cities lay, therefore, not in social reform, or social democracy, or conservative retrenchment—instead, it was to be found in the new population sciences of nutrition and diet. It was to be found in the industrial sciences of life.

From Migrant Biopolitics to Migration Studies

In 1938, in the aftermath of the Great Depression in the United States—which was widely believed to have been worsened by the migration of large numbers of rural Americans to the industrial centers—Dorothy Swaine Thomas produced the first systematic overview of migration research, focusing in particular on internal migration in the United States, Britain, and Germany (Thomas, 1938).[10] In her *Research Memorandum on Migration Differentials*, she argued that the question of internal migration had been neglected in the early decades of the century, "probably due in part to the apparently unlimited possibilities of economic and population expansion in America in the decades preceding the war" (ibid.: 2). Indeed, as eugenic arguments took hold in the United States, immigration from Europe, especially from southern and eastern Europe, became a burning political issue. As early as 1896, Francis Amasa Walker, director of the US Census, and the intellectual founder of the US immigration restriction movement, warned that:[11]

immigrants from southern Italy, Hungary, Austria, and Russia [now make up] something like forty per cent [of immigrants to the United States], and threatens soon to become fifty or sixty per cent, or even more. The entrance into our political, social, and industrial life of such vast masses of peasantry, degraded below our utmost conceptions, is a matter which no intelligent patriot can look upon without the gravest apprehension and alarm. These people . . . have none of the inherited instincts and tendencies which made it comparatively easy to deal with the immigration of the olden time. They are beaten men from beaten races; representing the worst failures in the struggle for existence. . . .

The problems which so sternly confront us to-day are serious enough without being complicated and aggravated by the addition of some millions of Hungarians, Bohemians, Poles, south Italians, and Russian Jews. (Walker, 2004[1896]: 752, 754)

Walker differentiated these new immigrants from those sturdier characters who he considered to have constituted the America of the first half of the nineteenth century. To support his case, he compiled maps of population density showing the prevalence of those immigrants in particular areas where he thought the "problems which so sternly confront us" were most concentrated. Such arguments played a key role in the passage of The National Origins Act of 1924, which established quotas limiting "the number of inhabitants in the continental United States in 1920 whose origin by birth or ancestry is attributable to [each] geographical area"—legislation that was warmly regarded by German racial hygienists.[12] Concern focused on the fact that those "beaten men from beaten races" were increasingly manifesting their pathological heredity in alcoholism, superstition, promiscuity, and so on in the cities where they were concentrated.

However, as Greenwood and Hunt argue, a number of changes after the First World War turned attention in the United States away from the apparently dysgenic consequences of international migration toward research on *internal* migration: the war itself had reduced the number of international migrants, as had the national origins quota system; at the same time, a demand for labor in the northern industrial centers stimulated an increasing flow of African Americans from the South (Greenwood and Hunt, 2003: 12). The Social Science Research Council appointed its Committee on the Scientific Aspects of Human Migration in 1924, and reports followed that mainly attempted to quantify this internal migration, as well as to consider its economic consequences, and to guide government policy (Thornthwaite and Slentz, 1934; Goodrich, 1936). But while Dorothy Swaine Thomas largely followed the lead of these studies in focusing on the economic motives for migration, and analyzing the age, sex, and family differentials of those who migrate, she also attempted to use the existing literature to form a richer picture of the rationale for migration, including, for example, stories told by migrants about the lure of cities compared with the dull life on the farm. Unsurprisingly, given her long collaboration with her husband, W. I. Thomas, she used language reminiscent of *The Polish Peasant* in her argument that statistical methods were not enough: "The behavior of the migrants must be observed before and after migration; the migrants' 'own stories' must be obtained; the environmental setting and the conditions of life in the communities of origin and destination much be described" (Thomas, 1938: 141–142).[13] But the vitalist styles of thought that we can identify in the works of those like Du Bois, Booth, and Rowntree were rare. Instead, attention, both in the United States and the United Kingdom— including in Thomas's own work—turned to formal analyses of the relation of migration to the "distribution of economic opportunities" (Kuznets and Thomas, 1957: 2, quoted in Greenwood and Hunt, 2003: 27).

After World War II, the subdiscipline of migration studies flourished. This is not the place for a detailed examination of this body of work. The questions of the 1950s and 1960s, to oversimplify, were divided between those seeking to quantify the flows of persons and to account for them in terms of economic pulls and pushes; and those who, in contrast, sought to engage with the challenges and difficulties of assimilation of migrants into their host communities. In the UK, postwar migration of people from former British colonies, particularly those in the Caribbean, meant that migration studies could not but intersect with academic attention to racism, with conflicts between those who worked on the psychosocial experiences of racial prejudice and those whose focus was rather on the systematic, structural effects of racist policy in education, housing, jobs, and much more. Studies of migration became caught up in what Caroline Knowles refers to as an emerging sociology of 'race relations' and in debates over the extent to which racial inequalities should be framed in terms of race and/or class (Knowles, 2010).

In the United States, scholarly interest in migration experienced a resurgence as mass international migration increased again in the late 1960s, with migrants moving not only to the large cities, but also to areas with little recent experience of immigration or, in some cases, with very little diversity (Kasinitz, 2012: 580). The initial responses of policymakers focused on the economic impacts, but official reports were remarkably sanguine: the effects on the economy and wage structure were found to be modest and largely positive. Indeed, Philip Kasinitz remarks on his "naïve surprise" at realizing that many Americans saw the cultural impact of mass immigration as a cost rather than as a benefit—that they ignored or discounted the economic benefits of immigration because of the social and cultural changes that it brought to American life (ibid.: 582). And while in 1993, in a much cited article, Alejandro Portes, writing with Min Zhou, argued that assimilation was now "segmented," so that "Children of nonwhite immigrants may not even have the opportunity of gaining access to middleclass white society, no matter how acculturated they become," it was nonetheless the case that "[r]emaining securely ensconced in their coethnic community, under these circumstances, may be not a symptom of escapism but the best strategy for capitalizing on otherwise unavailable material and moral resources. . . . a strategy of paced, selective assimilation may prove the best course for immigrant minorities" (Portes and Zhou, 1993: 96). Portes, probably the leading US sociologist of migration, remained optimistic about the consequences both for migrants themselves and for the cities they lived in. "Institutionally-complete enclaves [i.e., locally enclosed concentrations of migrants in particular urban regions such as the "Little Italys" and "Little Polands"] tend to last no more than two to three generations," Portes argued, "because the very success of immigrant entrepreneurs has pushed their descendants into positions of advantage in the American economic mainstream" (Portes, 2010: 1546). And while he agreed with others that "massive migration can transform the 'sight and smells' of a city or the ethnic composition of the masses riding public transport," he considered that these were only "'street-level' changes. The fundamental pillars of American society have remained unaltered" (ibid.: 1548). Assimilation clashes existed only in the minds of nativists: "the transformational potential of migration is limited, at every level, by the existing web of institutions reflecting deep cultural and power arrangements. These channel migrants to 'proper' places in the status system and educate them and their descendants in the language and cultural ways of the host society. This is what the process of assimilation is about" (ibid.). So, while scholars of migration were confident that upward mobility was the most common trajectory for most members of most migrant communities (Portes and Fernández-Kelly, 2008), it was left to researchers of race and racism to chart the daily reality of marginalization, exclusion, and structural violence experienced by so many migrants making their lives in urban America (Keith, 2005; Wacquant, 2008; Goldsmith and Blakely, 2010).

In the United Kingdom, studies of race and migration were both closely linked to urban studies, with work focusing for example on the dynamics of racism in patterns of housing. In the 1960s, John Rex and Robert Moore claimed to apply and extend Chicago-style analysis of spatial stratification to British cities, mapping an 'urban ecology' in which migrants from different regions of the (then) British Commonwealth were confined to low-quality housing in the city center, or to converted lodging houses for single men (notably in Rex and Moore, 1969). However, their studies had none of the vitalism that infused their Chicago forbears. By the 1980s these approaches, with their focus on racism and their hopes for multiculturalism, were criticized for their homogenization of racial experience. They fractured in the face of a renewed focus, by black and feminist scholars especially, on the heterogeneity of black experience, the intersections between race and gender, the reclaiming of diasporic identities, and the multiple forms of subjective subjugation produced by racism. Yet, as Caroline Knowles argues, this work, focused on representation and discourse, was often uninterested in "flesh-in-motion on the scenes of everyday life" (Knowles, 2010: 28). Today, the burgeoning literature in what is now called 'migration studies,' focusing on the mobility of persons and things across global circuits, certainly positions migration as a central dynamic of the contemporary world. As Pisarevskaya and colleagues have pointed out (Pisarevskaya, Levy, et al., 2019), the growing volume of contributions in the area of migration studies, with many research centers, diverse organizations, multiple conferences, and numerous journals, has led to a fragmentation of the field, but the main topics have remained relatively stable. Statistical questions of demographics and related problems of governance of migrant flows have waned, while issues of cultures and cultural diversity, diasporas and transnational networks, racism, stigma, and exclusion have become more prominent—now framed not so much in terms of migration, but rather in terms of mobilities.

But what about what George Engel might term the biopsychosocial lives of migrants (Engel, 1977)? Certainly, the ethnographic literature is full of stories of multiple, fluid, situational identities, shaped and reshaped in acts of movement and place-making. One learns much from accounts of migrant life that attend closely to issues of hybridity, creolization, and cosmopolitanism, as well as to the complexity of relations among different ways of thinking about origins and identities (Brettell and Hollifield, 2013; Vertovec, 2013; Prato, 2016). Yet, for us, there is something lacking in some of these accounts. We rarely find a concern with the vital embodied—let alone embrained—consequences of migration, that is to say with the concerns that, however problematically, were so significant for the earlier work that we have discussed above. It is true that some of these issues have been displaced to the subfield of migrant health, but the focus there tends to be on the health status and 'health behavior' of migrants, on the challenges for migrants with disabilities or with HIV, rights and access to healthcare, and of health in refugee camps (Thomas, 2016). Could one, then, find this concern with the biosocial challenges of inhabitation elsewhere?

Consider the genre of anthropological writing framed in terms of 'social suffering' (Kleinman, Das, et al., 1997; Povinelli, 2011; Biehl, 2013; Chua, 2014; Pinto, 2014; De Boeck and Baloji, 2016)? These ethnographers certainly provide moving accounts of how people make their lives amid conditions of profound marginality, exclusion, and violence, and how the work of living in decrepit and polluted environments does not preclude fleeting moments of pleasure. Their accounts reveal the ways that to live each day requires the activation of an ethic of survival, in the process showing us that the categories of psychology and psychiatry obscure the complexities of everyday mental life in these conditions of exclusion, marginalization, and structural violence. Terms like social suffering, affliction, and abandonment, whatever their problems, point to a way of grasping those experiences that the categories of the psy disciplines—mental disorder, anxiety, depression, PTSD, psychosis, schizophrenia—cannot.

For example, the focus on "affliction," in the work of Veena Das, is an attempt to enable a "mode of writing that would allow a world to be disclosed, a world in which life pulsates with the beats of suffering and also with the small pleasures of everyday life . . . Many people within the same environment move from one threshold of life marked by bleakness, even abjection, to some other threshold at which they seem to engage with others, laugh, eat, have sex, look after children, greet visitors (Das, 2015: 1–2). By contrast, she argues, more overtly psychological framings, using terms such as resilience, divert attention from important questions about how an "everyday ethics [has] been honed out of these experiences" (ibid.: 3). Das evokes this everyday ethics through narratives of individual experience, for example the psychiatric encounters of Swapan and his family, living in a migrant district of West Delhi. Das does not doubt the reality of Swapan's mental illness, but concludes rather that "the illness resides in the network of relations, in the movement over institutions . . . the pathology is struggling to find an environment in which it could reestablish new norms" (ibid.: 104). It seems inarguable that illness does indeed take its meaning within sets of norms and relationships—psychiatric norms of course represent only one way of construing what might be a normal mode of living in desperate circumstances. But it is not sufficient to simply imply or assert that such conditions and their causes are 'social.' This still leaves us to ask what experiences, in what ways, through what pathways, to what degree, with what effects, and do afflictions actually arise, and what shapes the ways that they are manifested. On these issues, the literature on "social suffering" is usually rather silent.

Clara Han's *Life in Debt* (Han, 2012) does pay particular attention to the role of psy professionals and technologies in managing people's lives. Her ethnography was conducted in La Pincoya, an impoverished district on the northern periphery of Santiago, the capital city of Chile. Her study is not specifically focused on the situation of migrants; nonetheless the growth of Chilean cities was largely due to migration from the countryside, and it was these migrants and their descendants who made their lives in slums, shanty towns, and impoverished and overcrowded neighborhoods (Norris, 2018). Han describes how psychiatric epidemiologists, attempting to bring to light the levels of suffering in such districts, encountered many challenges—not least conflicts within and between the various mental health professions, and with local authorities and bureaucrats. Han shows how studies using ICD-10 categories of mental disorder convinced the Ministry of Health to support a community intervention, combining pharmacological treatment with "psychoeducational group intervention" within the primary healthcare apparatus. Patients were given a somewhat atypical combination of fluoxetine, amitriptyline, or imipramine described as 'antidepressant medication' (Han, 2012: 180). While the decisions of experts to prescribe these drugs are not really interrogated, Han does explore how the psychological therapies in the interventions function only in combination with the religious, spiritual, and personal commitments of therapists and their clients. In mental health interventions into the lives of the very disadvantaged, she points out, communities become "social laboratories" for testing new techniques (ibid.: 184). Further, she shows how, whatever the reasons for prescribing these drugs, psycho-pharmaceuticals were not always consumed in the ways, and for the purposes, described on their information sheets; instead, they were used "sporadically to treat and thus mitigate bodily ailments emerging from confluences of the interpersonal and economic" (ibid.: 205). Antidepressants, she argues, were "intimately tied to the affective configurations of the home and the temporality of economic scarcity" (ibid.: 205). Indeed, she suggests that the drugs do not have their effects as a consequence of their chemical properties but rather through the ways that they, combined with the lay diagnoses that give them meaning, enter into particular "affective configurations" in the lives of individuals and their families in the daily business of managing living, ailing and sometimes dying in situations of penury, hunger, adversity, and drugs and violence.

Han here gives us some insights into the inseparability of bodies, minds, brains, affects, and meanings as they are intertwined in situations of impoverishment and conflict over the bare essentials of life. Her account starkly reveals the disjuncture between the explanations and interventions of psy professionals and the ways that those are experienced and made use of in everyday lives. This begins to illustrate what such studies of suffering and affliction might look like if they took a more committedly vitalist turn—if they reengaged, on the one hand, with the vital ecologies of place, crowds, noise, pollution, flows of affect across individual and collective bodies, and on the other hand, with the sciences of life, no longer the determinist biologies so rightly shunned today, but focused now on the biosocial consequences of inhabiting particular kinds of places. While they themselves do not travel far in this direction, and do not specifically address the experiences of those encountering the urban from lives elsewhere, they lay down crucial markers for the road upon which we wish to travel in this book.

The Migrant City Today

As we have seen, many of those who reflected on migration from the countryside from the mid-nineteenth century to the early twentieth century tried to make sense of the consequences of this dislocation by drawing on the biology and psychology of their times to understand its impact on the vitality of those who migrated. Their focus on migrant forms of life, on migrant diet, on migrant morbidity and mortality, on the 'quality' of the constitution of those from different races and its implications for their conduct, was inseparable from the intellectual world in which it was formed. This was a world of imperial expansion and racial hierarchy, where a eugenic 'common sense' underpinned the beliefs and practices of many of those in authority. These biological, psychological, vital threads run through the history of urban sociology and urban politics. We should not ignore them or pretend that they do not exist. If we address them here, it is in the conviction that the more we understand them, the less we are bound to reproduce them.

In trying to understand contemporary migration and its consequences for vital life, we therefore want to keep in mind those figures who we have discussed in this chapter—W.E.B. Du Bois, Georg Simmel, perhaps even Seebohm Rowntree—and to remind ourselves that thinking sociologically about these issues has often meant thinking biologically and psychologically about them. We may now be beyond the age of the calorimeter, but as social scientists committed to exposing and analyzing the vital consequences of inequity and injustice, we should not be too grand to consider the implications of studies of the neuroendocrine system, or analyses of samples of saliva, or even attention to scores on a standardized mood scale. In the next chapter we will chart the rise of a particular way of seeing the body and mind of the migrant, as it developed in the emerging discipline of psychiatric epidemiology, and examine the ways in which the migrant city—or the migrant in the city—has so often been viewed through the lens of mental pathology. How have these researchers tried to understand the ways that the experience of migration gets into the flesh, the bodies, the brains, the souls of those who migrate?

2

Migration, the Metropolis, and Mental Disorder

On July 10, 2014, the Population Division of the United Nations Department of Economic and Social Affairs released its 2014 revision of World Urbanization Prospects (UN Department of Economic and Social Affairs Population Division, 2014). It announced the conclusions on its website: "Today, 54 per cent of the world's population lives in urban areas, a proportion that is expected to increase to 66 per cent by 2050. Projections show that urbanization combined with the overall growth of the world's population could add another 2.5 billion people to urban populations by 2050, with close to 90 percent of the increase concentrated in Asia and Africa." The largest urban growth, it pointed out, "will take place in India, China and Nigeria. These three countries will account for 37 per cent of the projected growth of the world's urban population between 2014 and 2050. By 2050, India is projected to add 404 million urban dwellers, China 292 million and Nigeria 212 million."[1]

There is much that might be said about this kind of global population surveillance and its multiple histories—including the ways that it attends to some things and ignores others. The fact of the ubiquity of urban migration tells us little about its consequences for the mental lives and mental health of those whose migration constitutes new megacities in Africa, as well as East and South Asia. While it is true that, historically, the overall health of those who live in cities tends to be better than those living in the countryside, with better diets, easier access to healthcare facilities and so forth, migrants do not generally benefit from this 'urban bias.'[2] No doubt this has a great deal to do with the fact that although they may have migrated to Lagos, São Paulo, or Mumbai, most migrants captured by this report—with the notable exception of rural-to-urban migrants in China—actually live in informal housing, or what the policy literature calls "slums" (UN-Habitat, 2003).[3] Indeed, this report estimates that by 2030, at least half of this vast urban population—making up around two-thirds of the population of our planet— would live in such slums.[4] In some cases these are areas that were once in good shape but which have since had problems, become overcrowded, or have otherwise deteriorated. But this category is also composed of the new and "vast informal settlements that are quickly becoming the most visual expression of urban poverty. The quality of dwellings in such settlements varies from the simplest shack to permanent structures, while access to water, electricity, sanitation and other basic services and infrastructure tends to be limited" (ibid.: 8).

As Ash Amin points out, the verdict of the report was unequivocal: "slum life was, and would remain, a life of multiple deprivations, and few rights and reprieves, with inhabitants spending all resources and energies on sheer survival" (Amin, 2013: 480). The UN's Human Development Report published in 2010 also speaks of the plight of "over 1.75bn people suffering from multiple poverty," largely concentrated in the slums of the same set of megacities (United Nations Development Programme, 2010: 3). Poverty, deprivation, precarious work, insanitary housing, and many other deprivations seem to be the fate of most of those who leave their homes in small towns or villages and try to make a new life in the megacity.

But what are the implications for mental health of lives lived in slums? Introducing a special series in *The Lancet* on 'The Health of People Who Live in Slums' 2016, an international group of researchers found a paucity of data on *slum* health, as opposed to urban health or poverty and health more generally (Ezeh, Oyebode, et al., 2016). However, what data were available suggested that those living in slums were in worse physical health than people in others parts of the city, not just because of poverty, but also because of "neighborhood effects . . . such as faecal contamination of the environment, garbage mountains, stagnant ground water, overcrowding, poorly constructed homes, physical hazards (eg, floods, subsidence, and fires), and indoor and outdoor pollution." People housed in slums also experience many of the wider social determinants of poor health, such as "job insecurity, lack of tenure and title, poor transport networks, stigmatization," and although in many cases the social structures of slums are very supportive, in others they can be "highly toxic." City living can bring many advantages to some, and as we'll see later, few migrants from the countryside wish that they had stayed in the villages and towns. But when it comes to health, the 'urban bias' does not extend to most rural-to-urban migrants.

But what, then, of mental health? Ezeh and colleagues find that while the "living and working conditions in slums predispose to stress, and stress leads to psychological disorders . . . there is very little direct literature on slum mental health or how it might be affected by the social milieu in slum neighbourhoods" (Ezeh, Oyebode, et al., 2016: 554).[5] We will discuss the evidence on mental health of megacity migrants later in this chapter (apart from that on China, which we will discuss in chapter 3). But we agree with Ezeh and colleagues: there is indeed a dearth of research on the mental health of migrants living in informal settlements and 'slums' of various kinds in emergent megacities in India, Nigeria, Brazil, and other countries. This is surprising. One would have expected to find a great deal of research exploring the mental lives and mental health of the millions of individuals who have taken that journey—not least because discussion of the mental consequences of migration to cities is far from new. Indeed, as we shall see, it was one of the foundational issues in the professionalization of psychiatric research itself.

Psychiatry Encounters Migration

Medical experts in the second half of the nineteenth century repeatedly reflected on the consequences of the pace of modern urban living not just on physical health but also on the nerves. Indeed, the two were inseparable. For the middle classes and intellectuals, the predominant term for understanding this relationship was neurasthenia, or "exhaustion of the nervous system," as George Beard put it in 1869: "a condition of the system that is, perhaps, more frequently than any other, in our time at least, the cause and effect of disease . . . [that] may give rise to dyspepsia, headaches, paralysis, insomnia, anaesthesis, neuralgia, rheumatic gout, spermatorrhoea in the male and menstrual irregularities in the female," a condition "most frequently met with in civilized, intellectual communities . . . part of the compensation for our progress and refinement" (Beard, 1869: 217).

But it was not neurasthenia that afflicted the thousands of young men and women migrating from the countryside to the heart of the city. For writers of the time, those migrants, like other urban paupers, were caught in a vicious downward spiral in which physical deterioration and moral sensibilities were intertwined. Such moral deterioration encompassed the mental lives of these urban dwellers, their sense of right and wrong, their desires, their capacity for self-control, and all those forces that shaped their conduct (Driver, 1988). Both robust laborers seeking honest work and rogues coming to the towns in the hope of easy pickings were thrown together in impenetrable masses that were known, in England, as colonies and rookeries. In these aggregations, out of sight of the beneficial influences of civilization, virtuous habits were soon lost and vicious habits thrived—intemperance, prostitution, gambling, idleness, loss of religion, and all manner of immorality. Contemporary writers, thinkers, and scientists wrung their hands about this seemingly inescapable process of physical deterioration and moral decline, where vicious habits led to a weakened constitution which was then transmitted to children—and they, in their turn, were further debilitated by their upbringing in squalid and unsanitary conditions, subject to the foul moral miasma of corruption and criminality. This was not merely a repetition of the age-old problem of paupers; the 'social question' had acquired a worrying temporal and reproductive dimension: it was a downward spiral, in which the towns sucked in the healthy, dragged them down physically, morally, and mentally, and where these degraded characteristics were then transmitted to their numerous offspring, with consequences that threatened the constitution of the population, indeed the nation, as a whole. The relatively new profession of psychiatry would argue that this spiral of moral and mental decline constituted a specific medical process: degeneracy.

The language of degeneracy provided the moral categories of debauchery and excess with a physiological basis and a clinical rationale (Pick, 1989). Benedict Morel was its leading European theorist (Morel, 1857; Morel, 1860).[6] Degeneracy might be manifest in a whole number of ways, in excessive nervousness, in intemperance, in alcoholism, in idiocy, in mania, or in melancholia. Either way, its physiological basis lay in the individual's constitution—an inherited organic state, manifest in all aspects of the individual, from physiognomy to bodily makeup, to comportment, which might predispose an individual to pathology in the presence of particular circumstances. In this division between *predisposing* and *exciting* causes, it was not merely that inherited malfunctions in the brain could act as predisposing causes of insanity, but that such predispositions could be found in disorders of other bodily organs, such as the liver. Further, any individual may inherit a predisposition from the immoral conduct of their parents—if moral depravity, indulgence, excess, or intemperance were present at the time of conception, for example, or when the mother was carrying the child in utero, transmitted by her blood or her milk. Bad management of the developing child could also weaken its constitution, as could moral excesses in adolescence or adulthood. Such a weakened constitution would make the individual more liable to disease or mental breakdown in the presence of exciting causes, which could be unanticipated shocks such as bereavement, or perhaps immoral and vicious conduct, thus bringing on frank insanity. And this weakened constitution, whether acquired from the social milieu, from immoral habits, or from acquired damage, could itself be transmitted to any offspring, not in the form of a specific pathology, but through a 'diathesis,' which, in the presence of exciting causes, would manifest itself in one or another of a whole range of pathologies, physical or mental. Such degeneracy would course through the generations, getting worse at every stage: perhaps mere nervousness in the first generation, neurosis in the second, psychosis in the third, and, in the fourth, undeniable idiocy.

Degeneracy, Eugenics, and Migration

It was not simply that in Europe, by the later decades of the nineteenth century, almost every mentally unfit or insane individual was diagnosed with a condition arising from degeneracy. It was also that this medico-moral category became a way of thinking about all manner of other problems of the city: 'the social question' of pauperism, vice, and criminality was centrally, if not necessarily or exclusively, an urban question. Thus, migration became inextricably intertwined with ways of thinking about the moral, physical, and mental deterioration of those who were sucked into the vortex of the city. As reformulated in the almost ubiquitous eugenic style of thought, this kind of pessimistic urban vitalism, centering on the idea that the form of life lived by some in cities damaged their very constitution, their bodies and brains, with dire consequences not just for them and their descendants, but for the nation as a whole, would come to frame the thought of some of key figures who went on to study the lives of those in towns in the first half of the twentieth century.

While France was undoubtedly the focal point for the development and application of degeneracy theory in European medical psychology, the idea of degeneracy became a widespread way of describing and explaining anti-social behavior, from vice and debauchery, through indigence and crime, to idiocy and insanity. The problem of degeneracy, both physical and mental, was to become a central political concern. It did so via the hereditary principle, which was gradually reformulated to give absolute priority to the question of inheritance: the path from heredity to character, though it was influenced by all those experiences that bore upon an individual, was a one-way street. And while degeneracy theorists such as Morel believed that the end point of a degenerate lineage was sterility, later theorists argued that far from a degenerate lineage dying out, those with inferior constitutions who inhabited the slums and rookeries of the great cities were precisely those who bred most rapidly. Coupled with the fact that those with apparently superior constitutions were deferring marriage and finding other ways to limit the number of their children, the consequences for the quality of the nation, the race as a whole, seemed obvious.

This perception was to be the basis of eugenics, "the science which deals with all influences that improve the inborn qualities of a race; also with those that develop them to the utmost advantage" (Galton, 1904: 1). While the problem of differential breeding could be met by encouraging those of the best stock to have more children—positive eugenics—the real problem was the promiscuous breeding of those of worst stock (we are of course using the language of eugenics). And, as Roswell Johnson stressed as late as 1926, this eugenic problem was crucially a problem of the city (Johnson, 1926).[7] By the early years of the twentieth century, the spiral of urban degeneracy that particularly afflicted migrants from the countryside was redrawn in such hereditarian and eugenic terms. Charitable and philanthropic schemes had countered the beneficial effects of natural selection and allowed those with weak and tainted constitutions to flourish at the heart of the great cities, where they were easy prey for both physical diseases and moral degradation. Unless steps were taken to counter the increase of this class of persons, limiting their growth by immigration and their increase by reproduction, they would pose a threat to the fitness of the race as a whole.

Many of this problem group lived their lives outside the attention of the authorities, except when they were arraigned for begging or for committing crimes. However, the conduct of some did cause sufficient concern for them to be committed to one of the asylums that were now appearing in all large cities. In England, case records show that those who had migrated long distances were more likely to be admitted to an asylum (Walton, 1979; Scull, 2005).[8] Irish migrants were greatly over-represented in English asylums in the second half of the nineteenth century: some attributed their propensity to insanity to degeneracy, while others thought it was because the Irish were "particularly susceptible to the challenges of urban life, marked by intemperance, liability to general paralysis, turbulence and immorality, and the relative isolation that led to their long-term incarceration" (Cox, Marland, et al., 2012: 500).[9]

In the United States, those concerned about the mental and moral consequences of migration also drew on evidence from asylums.[10] As early as June 1850, M. H. Ranney, then Superintendent of the New York City Lunatic Asylum at Blackwell's Island (today, Roosevelt Island), read a paper, 'On Insane Foreigners' before the Association of Medical Superintendents of American Institutions for the Insane, at a meeting in Boston (Ranney, 1850). A significant proportion of inmates in his institution, Ranney pointed out, were foreigners: in the three years to the end of December 1849, only 500 of his patients were native Americans while 1,229 were foreigners, many of whom had been in America less than one year prior to their admission. These were patients whose madness seemed to have some cause either in their home country, or (this was Ranney's thesis) in the fact of their leaving it. "When leaving home," he pointed out, "they have high hopes of success, and fondly imagine that the only requisite to a realization of their expectations is a safe arrival" (ibid.: 45). But the voyage quickly disabuses them: bad food and general ill-health sets in, and the emigrants suddenly find themselves in an "impure atmosphere" of "disease," "ship fever," and "impaired and enfeebled companions" (ibid.: 46). On arrival, the migrant awakens to "a consciousness of the wretchedness of their situation in finding themselves destitute in a strange place" (ibid.). Despondence and anxiety quickly set in—made worse in women by an interruption in menstrual flow, a condition quickly followed by obscenity, nymphomania, and seduction. Female insanity is never far behind: "the sympathy existing between the brain and uterus," notes Ranney, "is very great" (ibid.: 47). He concludes by reading from a report produced by a visiting physician to his asylum, a Dr. Williams, who concluded that the real question was not actually a medical one but whether it was acceptable for "insane paupers [to] be sent from foreign countries to be supported in this" (ibid.: 62).

Ranney and Williams were pondering this question at a high point of Catholic immigration following the famine in Ireland (1845–1849) and the 1848 revolution in Germany. The issue of migrant insanity was a constant theme over the next four decades. The familiar themes in debates about migration and the city began to become clear: some argued that cities were magnets for degenerates, others thought that the conditions of urban life were actually the causal factor, and some suggested that, in fact, it was merely that the insane were more readily identified in the cities. Most statistical evidence that city living was associated with high rates of insanity was gathered in the United States. In 1903, in a study of all patients admitted to the Connecticut Hospital for the Insane between 1868 and 1901, R. H. Burr showed that rates of mental illness among inhabitants of cities were consistently 20–30 percent higher than those for towns or rural areas: "the urban life," argued Burr, "is more productive of insanity than the suburban or country life" (Burr, 1903: 311). Ten years later, another American survey on the "insane and feeble-minded," showed that "from rural communities . . . the ratio of admissions was 41.4 per 100,000 population; from cities . . . the ratio was more than twice as high, being 86 per 100,000." We must conclude, says the report, that "there is relatively more insanity in cities than in county districts and in large cities than in small cities" (US Bureau of the Census, 1914: 50). About ten years later, in 1925, Horatio M. Pollock, in the *American Journal of Psychiatry*, drawing on updated census data, showed again that admissions to mental hospitals were overwhelmingly dominated by people who lived in cities. "We can but regret," Pollock concluded, "the many unearned tears we have shed for the "poor, lonesome, languishing, isolated, farmer's wife" (Pollock, 1925: 222).

Gerald Grob has suggested that the emphasis that many of these psychiatric epidemiologists placed on the malign mental effects of urban ways of life arose from a specifically Protestant, bourgeois belief that contrasted the virtues of an agrarian existence to the temptations of the city (Grob, 1985: 230). Further, while the interpretation of disease in nineteenth-century psychiatry may have been essentially somatic, treatment was grounded in a religious, ethical, and social commitment to understanding the disturbing and deleterious relationship between urban life and mental health. As Horwitz and Grob put it, the goal of the psychiatrist was to "create a new environment that broke with those prior harmful environmental influences that led to insanity" (Horwitz and Grob, 2011: 631). In the United States, the question of what it was in the makeup of the city that led to these concentrations of mental pathology became the concern of researchers in a new discipline, at a relatively new university—the Sociology Department at the University of Chicago.[11]

Robert Faris and H. Warren Dunham's *Mental Disorders in Urban Areas* (Faris and Dunham, 1939) used the methods developed by Park and Burgess to chart "the relationship between community life and mental life" (Ernest Burgess, in his Preface to Faris and Dunham, 1939: xviii). As Burgess subsequently pointed out, Faris and Dunham started from the vitalist premise that "normal mentality can only develop through the participation of a healthy physiological mechanism in an adequate social organization" (ibid.: v). However, in mapping mental disorder across Chicago, the figures they used related only to the place of residence of those admitted to lunatic asylums. On this basis, they made two core claims. First, that mental illness associates with specific social problems: "cases of mental disorders, as plotted by residence of patients previous to admission," decrease from the center to the periphery of the city, in more or less the same distributive pattern as "poverty, unemployment, juvenile delinquency, adult crime, suicide, family desertion" (ibid.: ix–x). And second, that psychiatric diagnoses have predictable urban social geographies:

> paranoid schizophrenia [is correlated] with percentage of hotel residents and lodgers; catatonic schizophrenia with percentage of foreign-born and Negroes; manic-depressive psychosis with median monthly rentals; alcoholic psychoses with per cent of population on relief; dementia paralytica with distribution of vice resorts . . . senile psychoses with percentage of home ownership; senile psychoses combined with arteriosclerosis with percentage of population on relief and with per cent of population of native white parentage. (ibid.: x)

If they were writing today, it would perhaps not be misleading to describe Faris and Dunham's approach as 'biopsychosocial.' They argue that "the human mind is built on, and is never independent of, a physiological base . . . [However] the mind . . . is [also] a product of a process of social interaction. Mentality, abilities, behavior, are all achievements of the person, developed in a history of long interaction with his surroundings, both physical and social" (Faris and Dunham, 1939: 152). But what is particularly striking is their naturalistic feel for those physical surroundings, and the care with which they trace "influences from the community at large to persons, and from persons to intimate friends" as well as "paths of physiological communication, including sense organs, nerve paths connecting with centers, all supported by sufficiently normal functioning of many parts of the body, including glands, muscles, etc." (ibid.: 154–155).

It is true that there is not much to admire about the picture that Faris and Dunham paint of "slums" populated by "foreign-born individuals" forming a "chaotic background," nor their casual pathologization of "interracial and intercultural marriages" (Faris and Dunham, 1939: 159). Yet *Mental Disorders in Urban Areas* still bears reading as a text that refuses to take organic psychiatry and social life as separate domains of inquiry, insisting that the mental distress of human organisms can only be understood as a product of the social world they inhabit: the urban environment, in all its poverty and squalor and racism, was a bearer and producer of biological and physiological marks at the same time as it spatialized those who bore those marks across urban space.

Faris and Dunham's 'ecological study' received some positive attention from the mental health establishment: "the psychiatrist who is eager for the advancement of psychiatry will make this book a part of his library," noted a reviewer in the *American Journal of Psychiatry*, "and will welcome these sociologists and the discipline they represent as his allies" (Myerson, 1940: 997). In the *Journal of Abnormal and Social Psychology*, the reviewer commended this "pioneering" and "serious attempt to take the patient out of the clinic and study him in the full light of day in his natural habitat" (Mueller, 1940: 593). Some enthusiastic follow-up studies across the psychiatric-sociological literature appeared—notably, those of Schroeder in five other American cities (Schroeder, 1942), and in England, the work of Hare in Bristol (Hare, 1952; Hare, 1955). Yet the expansive and wide-ranging program that this research portended, and that reviewers of their monograph looked forward to—ecological, naturalistic, sociological, psychiatric—had already peaked. By the mid-1960s, this delicate tacking back-and-forth between the natural histories of cities and psyches appeared less pioneering than it did deeply naïve.

In part, the ecological approach fell out of fashion in sociology and urban studies because of methodological concerns about how well its ecological measures actually correlated with individual behavior (Robinson, 1950). More fundamentally, under the influence of critical theory and neo-Marxist sociology, scholars within the 'new urban sociology' began to turn away from "the functionalist image of society's tendency towards adaptation" (Smith, 1995). The developing 'critical' sociology not only made the naturalistic work of scholars like Faris and Dunham seem hopelessly old-fashioned, but it disrupted the relationship between sociology and psychiatry. If these had once been co-evolving sciences, with a free-flowing traffic of concepts, methods, and research topics, a new and mutually suspicious relationship developed in the 1960s. Indeed, arguing for a new 'sociology of psychiatry,' in *Social Forces*, in 1967, Schatzman and Strauss declared their "concern for some questionable benefits accruing to sociology from its association with, and application to, professional practice and service fields like psychiatry. Social scientists generally may well feel flattered by the demand for their skills and products. Yet . . . it would be much more fruitful for sociology if more research were done about psychiatry than in it or for it" (Schatzman and Strauss, 1966: 3–4).

There were good reasons for sociological criticisms of many psychiatric theories of that period, especially those that individualized and de-socialized mental disorder—and of the conditions in the psychiatric apparatus over which they presided. Yet, despite the persistence of certain kinds of social psychiatry, the breach between sociology and psychiatry that developed from the mid-1960s also marked a retreat from that earlier project in which an understanding of the forms of suffering named as mental illness demanded intense attention to the relations between living, vital human beings and their social, environmental milieu. The emerging disciplines of social and community psychiatry turned toward more easily quantified relations. Thus, "the distribution and determinants of undesirable social and health conditions" (Bloom, 1968: 424) was translated into a series of quantifiable and measurable "demographic characteristics" (Bahn, Chandler, et al., 1961), and dynamic features of the living city were quantified into tabulated ecological "correlation matrices," between specific urban characteristic and particular psychiatric diagnoses (Rowitz and Levy, 1968).

Those who were developing this more formalized and quantified social psychiatry later revisited Faris and Dunham's data with unflattering results (Mintz and Schwartz, 1964). Even Dunham himself was moved to re-situate his and Faris's earlier work within "the larger, general area that has been gradually emerging as social psychiatry" (Dunham, 1966). When it focused on the relationship between mental health and the city as such, this literature also became consumed with differentiating social 'causation' from social 'drift'—did urban life, and/or low socioeconomic status, 'cause' mental illness, or did the mentally ill inevitably 'drift'—drift toward the poorest quarters of the city, and drift down the employment scale as a result of their mental illness? By the 1980s, this notion of urban drift had won out: in a 1980 review of social psychiatry in the United Kingdom, John Wing, then professor of social psychiatry at the Institute of Psychiatry in London, firmly rejected a causal role for social experience in the etiology of schizophrenia, arguing that the person susceptible to schizophrenia actually sought out those living conditions that misguided researchers had taken to be causative:

British workers have put several hypotheses concerning the causation of schizophrenia to searching test. This is particularly true of theories suggesting that the condition was generated by living in conditions of poverty and isolation . . . [which are in fact] actively sought by the individual instead of being a cause of the breakdown. (Wing, 1980: 588)

But if it appeared that sociologists of urban mental illness did not in fact have much to offer to psychiatry, they were offered another role. Around the same period, writing in the *Community Mental Health Journal*, two American sociologists proclaimed the good news that sociologists might now become consultants to psychiatric practice: "the consultative function of the sociologist," they explained, "will be to interpret and evaluate computer outputs and their utilization by state mental health offices" (See and Mustian, 1976). Clearly, something had gone awry in the imagination of what a 'social' science might contribute to our understanding of psychiatric distress.

Migration and Mental Health Today

Today, psychiatric epidemiology remains the leading thought style for studies of the relationship between migration and mental health, and, once more, research focuses largely on international migration. Indeed, at the same time as Faris and Dunham were conducting their ecological work in Chicago, a series of influential studies on migration and psychosis were initiated by Ørnulv Ødegård.[12] Ødegård was a Norwegian psychiatrist, and, from 1938 to 1972, he served as director of Gaustad Hospital, Norway's first psychiatric hospital. In the context of the premises of racial hierarchy and the concerns about the quality of different races that suffused sociopolitical thought in the United States and Europe—and indeed much of the rest of the world—in the first decades of the twentieth century, Ødegård became interested in the question of whether the higher number of insane Norwegians (and other foreigners) in the United States was due to congenital or environmental factors. "America of course wants to protect the race against the admixture of a disproportionate number of psychopathic elements," Ødegård wrote in a famous 1932 paper, "which might cause something like a 'progressive degeneration' in the eugenic sense of the word . . . Sociologists as well as psychiatrists are inclined to regard the emigration from Europe to America as a unique experiment which deserves intensive study because it may throw light upon certain sides of human nature" (Ødegaard, 1932: 9–10).

Ødegård's innovation was that, unlike earlier studies, he did not compare rates of illness between native-born and foreign-born in the United States, because he considered that this split the constitutional from the environmental factors; it does not tell you whether the immigrant was already ill, that is to say, comes from 'poor stock,' or whether it is emigration itself that produces mental infirmity. To factor out 'racial differences,' Ødegård stuck to Norwegians alone, comparing those who had either emigrated or stayed in Norway. He took the case histories of all Norwegian-born patients in one psychiatric hospital (Rochester, in Minnesota, which importantly had both rural and urban catchment areas) and compared these with the same material from patients admitted to the asylum at Gaustad (Ødegård, 1932: 54–57). On that basis he concluded that "the ratio of insanity among the Norwegian-born of Minnesota is higher than in Norway. This is largely due to a very high incidence of senile and arteriosclerotic psychoses. The reason for this seems to be the physical and mental strain of immigrant life rather than constitutional psychopathic tendencies" (ibid.: 192). Migration itself, or rather the pressures of the immigrant life, apparently lay at the root of the problem.

While Ødegård examined statistics for all forms of insanity, it would be the specific diagnosis of schizophrenia that would dominate analyses of mental health and migration. In their meta-analysis of studies from 1997 to 2003, while recognizing the diversity of definitions of 'migrant,' and the great heterogeneity among studies of different migrant groups, Elizabeth Cantor-Graae and Jean-Paul Selten concluded that "a personal or family history of migration is an important risk factor for schizophrenia" (Cantor-Graae and Selten, 2005: 12). They report an effect size of 2.9 for the risk of schizophrenia among migrants—making migration the largest risk factor for the disorder, with only urbanization coming close. Cantor-Graae and Selten point out: "there can be little doubt about the existence of an association between migration and schizophrenia . . . the broad spectrum of migrant groups implicated would seem to refute the notion that any single biological or genetic factor could provide an adequate explanation . . . [whereas] between-population variation of this type does rather strongly support a causal role for aspects of the social environment (ibid.:18–20). They discount Ødegård's 'selection hypothesis'—that those liable to insanity are over-represented among those who chose to migrate—and suggest that what is involved is rather "the operation of environmental factors, albeit their exact nature remains uncertain." Discounting viral explanations and climate-based hypotheses, they argue that the most striking finding is not an association with migration per se, but with skin color, and with blackness in particular. Essentially, their claim is that racial discrimination, in particular against black people, is the common risk factor; referring to animal experiments using the 'defeated intruder paradigm,' they suggest that the elevated risk for schizophrenia may be linked to the long-term experience of 'social defeat' or "the chronic stressful experience of outsider status" (ibid.: 20–21)—although they admit that, as far as humans are concerned, this explanation is somewhat speculative.[13]

This focus on schizophrenia remains to the present, but with increasing emphasis on environmental factors that provoke the onset of the disorder in susceptible individuals. When Craig Morgan and his colleagues at the Institute of Psychiatry in London reviewed the evidence, for example, they presented a 'sociodevelopmental' model to account for the higher rates of schizophrenia among migrants, arguing that "the limited evidence is most consistent with the high rates being a consequence of greater exposure, in migrant and minority ethnic groups, to various forms of social adversity and problematic social contexts over the life course (Morgan, Charalambides, et al., 2010: 660). Indeed, after reviewing the evidence for alternative hypotheses—from genetic factors, to viral infections, to misdiagnosis and straight-up discrimination—they suggest that the elevated rates of psychosis among migrant groups is "largely social in origin" (ibid.: 661). Not just 'social defeat' but a broader set of potential inputs might, in their view, lead to a broad sociodevelopmental pathway: when exposure to adversity within migrant groups meets individual genetic risk, this has an impact on brain development which, in turn, produces vulnerability to the development of psychosis which is exacerbated by "further cumulative stressors . . . it is social experiences and contexts that make the difference" (ibid.: 661).

When it comes to what are normally referred to as 'common mental disorders,' on the other hand, research on mental health and migration is sparse, contradictory, and often hard to interpret, given the variety of reasons for migration and the variety of post-migration experience. Thus, an international group led by Jutta Lindert argued that "it is unclear whether migration leads to an increase or to a decrease in mental health burden. Significant differences in the mental health among different groups of migrants have been found. . . . Additionally, there may be significant differences between migrant groups especially between refugees and labor migrants with a higher burden of depression and posttraumatic stress disorder among refugees and a lower burden of depression among labor migrants" (Lindert, von Ehrenstein, et al., 2009). Inescapably, their meta-analysis brings together studies using a wide variety of measures and assessments of mental health status, many of which operate in terms of Euro-American diagnostic categories. Even when the migrants in question come from countries in the Global South, most of the studies focus on their mental health when they arrive in North America or other countries. Unsurprisingly, Lindert and her colleagues find that things are different for those who migrate for reasons of work and those who migrate as refugees: for example, prevalence rates for depression and anxiety among labor migrants are similar to those in the general population, while rates for refugees are twice as high.

A later meta-analysis, focusing on the experience of social mobility, showed that "international migrants who experienced downward social mobility as a result of migration were more likely to screen positive for common mental disorders than migrants who retained a stable socio-economic position or were upwardly mobile" (Das-Munshi, Leavey, et al., 2012: 17). The authors argue that when it comes to international migration: "attempting to examine migrant social mobility out of the context of discriminatory practices may present only part of the picture" (ibid.: 42). They point to a whole range of factors—perceived status loss, employment in an occupation for which they are overqualified, material deprivation and adversity—that may all play a role. But, of course, their significance may differ among different migrant groups with different experiences of migration—not to mention between international migrants and those who move from their homes in towns and villages to the 'arrival cities' that are the destination of the vast majority of those who migrate today.

Refining 'Migration'

Even those who carry out these studies recognize that it is necessary to refine the category of migration if one is to understand its mental health consequences. But how? Dinesh Bhugra points out that migration is not a simple before and after process, and that we need to think of it as a series of ongoing events, each of which may be accompanied by specific psychopathological phenomena—from simple high levels of morbidity in the country of origin during the pre-migration phase, to the loss of social networks during the migration experience itself, and then discrimination, financial difficulties, and the wider stress of adaptation in the post-migration period (Bhugra, 2004a; Bhugra, 2004b). For Bhugra, the concept of 'acculturation' is the key. In the psychological literature, 'acculturation' describes the process in which 'common knowledge, attitudes and values along with psychological states' begin to transition from one set of cultural experiences to another; for Bhugra and others, acculturation is a major part of the weft in self-hood, self-identity, and self-esteem—disruptions in which may have psychopathological consequences.

This idea of acculturation draws on a long anthropological tradition. As Robert Redfield and his colleagues put it in the 1930s, acculturation describes the process "when groups of individuals having different cultures come into continuous firsthand contact, with subsequent changes in the original cultural patterns of either or both" (Redfield, Linton, et al., 1936: 149). And among the psychological states of acculturation (which is distinct both from diffusion and assimilation) is a form of "psychic conflict resulting from attempts to reconcile differing traditions of social behavior and different sets of social sanctions" (ibid.: 152). This style of thought from the 'culture and personality' school, where boundaries between psychology and cultural anthropology were highly porous, is strikingly absent from much contemporary anthropology. Nonetheless, some non-anthropologists, for example the Canadian psychologist, John W. Berry, have extended this notion of acculturation into the study of what he and his colleagues call "acculturative stress" (Berry and Annis, 1974). In their much-cited paper of 1987, Berry and his colleagues identify both stressors and stress behaviors in the process of acculturation, including "lowered mental health status (specifically confusion, anxiety, depression), feelings of marginality and alienation, heightened psychosomatic symptom level, and identity" (Berry, Kim, et al., 1987: 492). A range of researchers have since utilized this model, seeking connections between migration, culture, stress, and psychopathology among a wide array of groups (Oh, Koeske, et al., 2002; Thoman and Surís, 2004; Knipscheer and Kleber, 2006).

Of course, migration is not a straightforwardly 'negative' experience for mental health: if there is, on the one hand, stress and alienation, there is also fulfillment, improved economic and social opportunities, the chance to cast off cultural and psychosocial restrictions, and so on. For example, in Canada, there is evidence of what is termed the 'healthy immigrant effect,' in which "the health of immigrants tends to be better than that of the general population in both the sending and receiving countries" (Kirmayer, Narasiah, et al., 2011: E60).[14] Kirmayer and his colleagues suggest that this may be related to the many filters and evaluations that migrants must pass if they are to be allowed to settle in a country like Canada (these are described in Picot and Sweetman, 2012). But after an initial period of optimism "disillusionment, demoralization and depression can occur early as a result of migration-associated losses, or later, when initial hopes and expectations are not realized and when immigrants and their families face enduring obstacles to advancement in their new home" (ibid.: E961). Moreover, for migrants who *do* experience problems, culture can become a barrier to treatment: different ways of experiencing and articulating symptoms, as well as different ways of relating to healthcare practitioners, means that clinicians can miss major mental health issues—leaving, in these authors' view, a role for the "cultural broker" whose job is "translating not language but cultural concepts or frameworks" (ibid.: E963).

The literature on mental health and migration is thus complex and varied, and confounded by enormous historical, cultural, and methodological constraints. Indeed, in their comprehensive review of epidemiological aspects of migration and mental illness, James Kirkbride and Peter Jones identify ten hypotheses that might explain the repeated finding of elevated rates of psychotic disorders among migrants (Kirkbride and Jones, 2010).[15] Perhaps psychosis actually predisposes people to migration, but this 'selection hypothesis' has been disproved in many studies. Perhaps there are simply higher rates of psychosis in the countries where many migrants come from, but studies do not confirm this. Perhaps the lower socioeconomic status of migrants explains it, but the rates remain elevated even when adjusted for this difference. Perhaps migrants are simply misdiagnosed, and psychiatrists are misinterpreting what are, in fact, culturally normal beliefs in the migrant population—an argument that remains current if controversial. Perhaps post-migratory experiences explain it, migration itself being a major 'life event' placing stress on the individual—this is a hypothesis we will explore in detail in a later chapter. Perhaps childhood events affecting neurodevelopment are important—for example, parental separation is much more prevalent for some migrants. Perhaps increased use of illicit substances by migrants explains the phenomenon, though this is unlikely for the majority of migrants. Perhaps different psychological responses are involved, for example, some migrant groups may externalize stressful events in particular ways, and thus find those events more difficult to cope with. Perhaps there is a genetic predisposition, but it is unlikely that migrants and their children have a greater genetic predisposition to psychosis. Or perhaps it arises from gene-environment interactions and epigenetic process—an interaction between individual genetic vulnerability and an interaction with neighborhood-level socioenvironmental stressors.

We set all this out at some length partly to show the sheer complexity of the picture. It seems that to grasp the relation between migration and mental health requires us to think our way through an incredibly complex swirl of life, culture, experience, and biology. Further, as McKenzie, Fearon, and Hutchinson point out, these complexities are often poorly dealt with in the epidemiological literature (McKenzie, Fearon, et al., 2008): researchers do not always distinguish between economic migrants, refugees and asylum seekers, self-consciously temporary migrants, and so on; similarly, discussions of mental health do not always attend well to differences in pathways to care—assuming, for example, that access to contact, assessment, and treatment are broadly invariable between migrants and non-migrants. At the same time, it is not always evident that what is being diagnosed as psychosis is the same in different cultural contexts (ibid.: 147–148). And there are frequent slippages between categories of 'race' and 'ethnicity' often reduced to crude dichotomies as they are 'operationalized' in the research, with categorizations being made in ways that are discrepant from those that would be used by the individuals or groups in question.

All in all, then, these studies suggest that there are differences in mental ill health between migrants and non-migrant populations, but these differ for different mental disorders, differ among migrants, and differ in relation to the factors that may be involved, which may have less to do with the fact of migration itself than with the situation in which those who migrate find themselves, and its relationship not only to their actual experiences, and the comparison with what they have left behind, but also to their hopes, beliefs, and expectations when they undertook their journey to the city. The prospects of those seeking to theorize some generally applicable set of relations between migration and mental health seem dispiriting.

Mental Health and 'the Slums'

As we saw at the start of this chapter, reports from UN Habitat suggest that most rural-to-urban migrants in the Global South are destined to live in 'slums'—a term they use to encompass so-called barrios, favelas, ghettos, shanty towns, townships, and informal settlements of all varieties. It seems obvious that the physical health of people living in slums will suffer when homes are so frequently without mains water or proper sewage, with electricity often pirated from legal supplies, sometimes without access to regular healthcare or education, and often without official citizenship. And surely mental health will also suffer for such people, often forced into precarious jobs, so the assumption goes, exploited by informal bosses, tyrannized by criminal gangs, and exploited by employers where they have them. So, what do we know from recent research about the mental health of the rural-urban migrant workers who make their lives in such settlements?

As Gunchar Firdaus points out, at the start of his study of the relationship between the social environment and the psychological well-being of migrants in the National Capital Territory of Delhi, "most of the research [on the effects of urban living on migrants] has been conducted in developed countries. This has been referred to as the 90/10 gap, where 10% of the research and funding takes place in developing countries which experience 90% of the global burden" (Firdaus, 2017: 164). In fact, as we shall see in the next chapter, in recent years there has been a rapid growth of research on this topic in China, mostly by Chinese researchers. But the Chinese experience of mass migration from the countryside is very different from that in most other countries, in that, to be fairly crude about it, whatever the difficulties experienced by those migrants in their new urban settings, they do not live in slums. So let us focus here on what research can and cannot tell us about rural-urban migrants in other megacities in the Global South.

Perhaps the largest epidemiological survey to cast some light on the mental health of rural-urban migrants in megacities of the South was conducted under the leadership of our colleague Laura Andrade in São Paulo.[16] The São Paulo Megacity Mental Health Survey was a survey of more than 5,000 adults carried out between 2005 and 2007 which "interviewed face-to-face using the WHO Composite International Diagnostic Interview (CIDI), to generate diagnoses of DSM-IV mental disorders within 12 months of interview, disorder severity, and treatment" (Andrade, Wang, et al., 2012: e3179). It revealed very high levels of diagnosable mental disorder among the host population, but the research seemed to show that non-migrants were actually more likely to have an active mood disorder than migrants. Among the other disorders studied, there was a complex pattern with differences between migrant men and women, as well as between them and non-migrants: for example, *non*-migrant women living in areas of high neighborhood deprivation were more likely to be diagnosable with an impulse control disorder than migrant women. Women were far more likely to have an active anxiety disorder than men, and for those migrants living in conditions of low neighborhood deprivation, women were much more likely than men to have active anxiety disorder as compared to migrant men living in the same conditions.

It is difficult to draw firm conclusions with regard to migrants as a whole from this research, as they were not a specific focus of the study. Indeed, while one might in some sense regard all members of families living in favelas in São Paulo as migrants—including those of the second or even third generation—the research defined migrants as those born outside the São Paulo Metropolitan Area (that is to say: those who had only recently made the journey to the city). In fact, this study gave some support to the argument that urbanicity—being born and raised in an urban area—was the factor that increased risk of a mental disorder, rather than recent migration to a megacity. Perhaps we are seeing here some evidence of the stoicism of migrants in the face of hardship and uncertainty that we found in Shanghai, and discuss in the next chapter. Or perhaps, to rehearse a theme familiar from many decades of dispute in transcultural psychiatry, one should question the applicability of diagnostic categories developed in the United States or Europe, to regions with often markedly different ways of signifying normality and pathology, and a radically different language for articulating mental distress. Ethnographic research, for example, work carried out by Dominique Béhague in the favelas in Pelotas in South-East Brazil, has shown that the utility of such international diagnostic schema is questioned, not only by some mental health professionals working in these areas, but also, and perhaps more important, by the people in the favelas themselves (Béhague, 2009).

This is not the place for a detailed review of this extensive and often antagonistic debate.[17] However, research on migrants to megacities in the Global South using methods of assessing mental distress that are less reliant on Euro-American diagnostic criteria paint a rather different picture.[18] We can begin with a brief look at a 'geoepidemiological study' of mental health in the slums of Dhaka, conducted by Oliver Gruebner and his colleagues.[19] Dhaka is of course the capital of Bangladesh, a major metropolis and one of the fastest growing global megacities in the first decade of this century, with more than 300,000 new migrants moving to Dhaka each year (Gruebner, Khan, et al., 2012). At the time of the study by Gruebner and colleagues, Dhaka had an estimated population of more than 14 million, of whom around 3.4 million lived in slums. Their study correlated data from a survey of mental health of around 2,000 residents in the nine slums of Dhaka, whose household location was geographically marked with GPS, with ecological and other exposure data from high-resolution land cover information from a Geographic Information System; the researchers found that "mental well-being" related to such socioeconomic factors as job satisfaction, ability to generate income, population density, and—and this was their particular focus—the physical environment (in other words, environmental pollution, lower flood risk, better sanitation, and quality, sufficiency, and durability of the house). Intriguingly, following up on their environmental focus, they argued that "individual level mental well-being was positively associated with environmental health knowledge, which reflects a person's awareness of environmental threats (i.e., that polluted, stagnant water and garbage near one's house could spread disease and that air pollution increases the risk of poor health)" (ibid.: n.p.).

The measure of mental health that was used in this study was the World Health Organization's Well-Being Index (WHO5)—a simple self-report questionnaire asking respondents to rate the extent to which they agree or disagree with five statements: I have felt cheerful and in good spirits; I have felt calm and relaxed; I have felt active and vigorous; I woke up feeling fresh and rested; My daily life has been filled with things that interest me.[20] A low total score—below 13—is often considered to be indicative of a common mental disorder, or at least enough to make the respondent a candidate for further screening, but, to say the least, it hardly tells us much about their interior psychological or neurobiological life. However, because of its ease of use and its availability in many languages, the WHO5 was also used by Gunchar Firdaus, who interviewed a sample of 1,230 respondents living in the slums of Delhi to see if he could identify socioeconomic factors linked to mental disorder. He found:

> Uneducated or less educated and unemployed or underemployed urban migrants were facing hardships in acquiring basic necessities for survival, for instance, inaccessibility to health care, educational facilities, piped water connection, overcrowding, poor housing condition, ambient environmental pollution, and the burden of paying for house rent, electricity, water, and waste collection. . . . were at much greater risk to experience poor mental health. On the contrary, educated households had better employment opportunities and feel better adjusted than others. They also had stronger aspirations to integrate into the host society. . . . At household level, the study demonstrates that the association became comparatively more significant after considering the individuals' house condition, including enough space for each person, separate kitchen, proper lavatory system, open space, and proper ventilation. (Firdaus, 2017: 167)

Firdaus acknowledges that the measure used was rather weak, and the cross-sectional design made it hard to untangle causality. However, his findings support the view that the effects of migration-driven urbanization in the 'developing world' on mental health are "structured by economic and social institutions . . . [Findings reiterate] the importance of contextual factors on individual and societal level and suggests more in-depth focus on specific areas of environmental stressor to understand the mechanisms involved in the development of mental ill-health" (Firdaus, 2017: 167).

These findings are supported and amplified by the study that comes closest to our own concerns: a 'mixed methods' study of about 12,000 people living in a slum called Kaula Bandar (KB) with a population of about 12,000 people situated on a wharf on Mumbai's eastern waterfront, carried out by Ramnath Subbaraman and colleagues (Subbaraman, Nolan, et al., 2014). KB is a 'non-notified' slum (that is, not government-recognized), as are about one-third of slums in India. Such non-notified slums have even worse access to piped water, electricity, functioning latrines, and material for housing construction, as well as receiving less support from government slum improvement schemes. Subbaraman and colleagues focused on what they termed "the psychological toll" on mental health of living in this insecure slum environment, in particular, the link with anxiety and depression. They used the General Health Questionnaire-12 (GHQ) to screen for common mental disorders (CMDs), the WHO Disability Assessment Schedule 2.0 (WHO DAS) to screen for functional impairment, and they created a slum adversity questionnaire which enabled them to create a composite Slum Adversity Index (SAI) score. Their basic finding, that around one-quarter of the inhabitants they surveyed had a score on the GHQ that indicated they were at high risk of a CMD, is probably less important for our purposes than the findings of their qualitative research, that is to say, the interviews that highlight what they call "the mechanisms of distress": "how specific adversities can cause severe stress . . . while also highlighting unique coping strategies used by KB residents to minimize the adverse impacts of these stressors" (ibid.: 159).

These adversities include a "massive garbage dump [of uncollected solid waste] which provides an ecosystem for rats and insects" in the ocean which borders KB: rats run out of the ditches and into the slum whenever the water level rises, eating the food, and having a disproportional effect on the women who have to fend them off; there are many biting insects; household density means that sometimes as many as nine people of different genders and ages have to try to sleep in one small space; very few homes have toilets, so people have to queue and pay to use the few 'pay for use' toilets situated in blocks outside the slum; water has to be bought from informal vendors—and so on, go the very grim accounts. All this is made more 'stressful' by the fact that the authorities stage periodic raids, cutting illegal electricity, trashing the mechanisms that distribute water, issuing threats of legal action and so forth. "Over time," say Subbaraman and colleagues, "these features that characterize [the slum's] relationship with government authorities, the criminalization of access to basic needs, the periodic acts of collective punishment, and the perception of [the slum] as a devalued and even depopulated spaced take a psychological toll by shaping an identity based on a feeling of social exclusion" (Subbaraman, Nolan, et al., 2014: 162). These vivid accounts, with data provided by the inhabitants themselves, provide a much more compelling biopsychosocial picture of the assault on the vital lives of these migrants to the city of Mumbai, especially drawing attention to the highly gendered nature of slum experiences in Mumbai and undoubtedly elsewhere (see also Parkar, Fernandes, et al., 2003).

Well-known ethnographic studies of Mumbai slum life have sought to paint a somewhat less grim picture, focusing on novel forms of community organizing and the use of tactics such as self-enumeration by residents to assert their right to recognition, secure tenure, and basic services—a process that has been called "deep democracy" (Appadurai, 2001). It is indeed critical not to reduce slum life to the 'bare life' indicators of epidemiological research. But, for many migrants, it seems hard to avoid the conclusion that living in the slums of Indian megacities requires constant navigation of a variety of deeply unpleasant environmental conditions, as well as the experience of legal and social exclusion. Hence, as Subbaraman and colleagues note, slum adversity *itself* should be the main focus of interventions seeking to improve 'common mental disorders'—for they are convinced that the key mechanism that translates adversity into poor mental health is stress or, as it is termed by one KB resident, "tension":

> There is so much tension in this community; I hope you are able to do something about it . . . Many people have died because of tension. After all, no one will admit that a person in her family died because of tension. It's common for people to silently drink poison or hang themselves. It's a big problem. (Subbaraman, Nolan, et al., 2014: 168)

Crushed Dreams or First Steps

In the light of the admittedly sparse research available, it is tempting to agree with the conclusions that Mike Davis draws in his coruscating account, *Planet of Slums* (Davis, 2006). Davis argues that we are witnessing the millions of dreams of a better life being crushed by the realities of migrant urban existence—all of it made worse, not better, by botched attempts to manage migration by effectively outlawing it. He is rightly critical of strategies that try to 'cleanse the city' by bulldozing migrant homes and rehousing people in bleak high-rise blocks often miles from any potential jobs—a strategy that destroys the limited infrastructure that migrant communities have built for themselves. Whatever beliefs those who migrate might have about the benefits of city life, the escape from the grinding poverty and stultifying atmosphere of the countryside, the opportunities of self-improvement offered in the city—these surely must slowly evaporate in the face of such grim realities. From such a perspective, it would be a surprise not to find high levels of mental disorders among rural-to-urban migrants.

And yet, perhaps not. Perhaps migrants are, in fact, the most 'entre-preneurial' individuals who wish, try, and in many cases actually succeed in their move to the city. This is the view of Doug Saunders in his account of migrant life in 'arrival cities' (Saunders, 2010). Maybe the life of the first generation is hard—so this story goes—but these first movers nonetheless use their experiences as a springboard to the slow and painful accumulation of resources that enables them to improve their situation. This enables them to find housing, however rudimentary, to save some money, to send remit-tances to those who they have left behind, often to obtain legal title to their land, sometimes aided by government reforms that grant them such title. Thus begins a process of upward mobility, as migrants pass on that initial equity, and in many cases bring their children and relatives to live with them in the city. Even if they themselves live difficult lives, their resources are directed toward supporting their children, especially through education, and it is those of the second generation who build a better life in the cities for themselves and their own children.

These seem like wholly contrasting accounts. And yet what holds Davis and Saunders together is that each makes assumptions about the mental life of the migrants in question—not just their hopes and dreams, their tra-vails and disappointments, but also assumptions about people's will, their desire, their capacities to act in the world and the consequences of that world acting upon them. The evidence cited in this chapter suggests that we must go beyond such generalizations, whether political or epidemiological, whether from the optimistic journalist or the pessimistic Marxist intellec-tual, and focus instead on the actual varieties of experience of those who have undertaken a journey to the city. Large-scale demographic variables make it difficult to account for variations in the prevalence of either 'com-mon' or 'severe' mental ill health among migrant populations. If specific adverse events or adverse experiences are what is important, then surely any attention to urban mental health in the burgeoning megacities of the Global South must explore these beliefs and experiences in the many different forms of the migrant life. This might enable us to characterize the forms of life of those who migrate in greater detail, to be more precise about the places that today's urban migrants inhabit and the mundane adversities that they encounter, and thereof to develop some conception of how—under what conditions, through what processes—the 'stress' that so many consider to be immanent in this experience of adversity gets inscribed into their bodies and their souls.

3

The Metropolis and Mental Life Today—Shanghai 2018

> When, so to speak, one examines the body of culture with reference to the soul, as I am to do concerning the metropolis today—the answer will require the investigation of the relationship which such a social structure promotes between the individual aspects of life and those which transcend the existence of single individuals. It will require the investigation of the adaptations made by the personality in its adjustment to the forces that lie outside of it.
>
> —(SIMMEL, 2010[1903]: 103)

The question that brought us and our colleagues to Shanghai at the beginning of the twenty-first century was not so different from the one that George Simmel addressed at the start of the twentieth, in his classic lecture on the metropolis and mental life. We frame it a little differently: how is subjectivity shaped, judged, enacted, constrained, and disrupted, both for and by those who today move from villages and small towns to make a different form of life for themselves in cities and megacities? What languages, techniques, forms of judgment, as well as ideas of normality and pathology, enable individuals to make sense of this experience to themselves and to others, to render its pleasures and their distress into thought, speech, and action, and with what consequences, for who? How is the migrant experience folded into the soul?

We focus here on Shanghai, a city whose population grew from 17.8 million in 2005 to 24.2 million in 2014, largely through the arrival of some 5.6 million people from the countryside.[1] Yet, despite this influx of migrants, and unlike the situation in São Paulo, Lagos, Mumbai, Delhi, or almost any other expanding megacity in the Global South, migrants in Shanghai, like those in other Chinese cities, do not live in slums or shanty towns. Some, a minority, live in apartments or rooming houses in 'the city,' that is, in the seven inner urban districts that make up what one might think of as 'old Shanghai.' However, most rural migrants live, not in the central city, but in the outer districts of Pudong, Minhang, Jiading, and Songjiang, often in dormitories owned by the factories in which they are employed or in basic apartment blocks close to their place of work. Some—far fewer than in other expanding Chinese cities such Guangzhou and Shenzhen—live in 'urban villages' (of which more below) that have arisen in areas of farmland enclosed by the expanding city. These urban villages are in the outer central districts and in the suburbs "mostly located close to the elevated highways and well-connected street networks, which allows for high levels of accessibility" (Wang and Ning, 2016: 98). It is clear that we cannot easily extrapolate to Chinese migrants from the epidemiological and ethnographic studies of slum life that we examined in the previous chapter. Further, it would be misleading to speak of 'migrants to Shanghai' as if they formed an homogenous mass of people. We must try to make sense of the multiple experiences, milieus, and modes of life, as well as the relationship of all of this to mental health, in these very different urban environments.[2] But before we do that, we need to examine three more general questions: (1) the character of rural to urban migration in China over the last two decades or so; (2) the current evidence on different forms of migrant life in China, linked in particular to different types of employment; and (3) the changing ways in which mental distress is being understood and managed in contemporary China.

Migrant Nation

For Mao Zedong, founder of the People's Republic, the life of the countryside was privileged over that of the city. And yet, in a few short decades, China has moved from being a nation in which—in Mao's famous phrase—the countryside would encircle the cities, to a country in which the ever-growing cities seem to swallow more and more of what was once a largely agrarian landscape. One of the most important engines for the growth of those cities, over a thirty-year period, has been rural-to-urban migration. Dorothy Solinger's detailed account of the dynamics shaping the movements and experiences of this 'floating population' (this somewhat derogatory term is remarkably persistent in the literature, including in Solinger's account) focuses largely on the period up to the mid-1990s. This is the period during which the process of migration was managed by the Chinese state and its bureaucracies, when China was moving toward a partially market-based economy, and in which the lives of families—in terms of food, housing, medical care, welfare, and security—were no longer secured by the *danwei* system, which had long been the locus of most forms of support for individuals and families (Solinger, 1997; Solinger, 1999: chs. 2, 3, and 4). In this first wave of migration, while the decision of a member of a family to migrate was an act of choice, such choices were undoubtedly shaped and constrained by other forces. As Solinger puts it, "theirs was an agency that was somewhat hobbled or bounded . . . mediated both by state policies and practices and by the specific ecosystems formed by native-place geography, resource endowments and locational situation" (Solinger, 1999: 13).[3]

The decision to migrate was undoubtedly shaped by local and regional characteristics, which varied from region to region and locality to locality. In many areas there were just too many people to work the available land; or the land was often unfertile and unproductive and agricultural labor hard and unrewarding; young people in particular were often surplus to agricultural requirements, and there were few alternative sources of employment in their home districts.[4] Further, it was clear to many that they were on the wrong end of a large income differential between countryside and city. But there was also the perception that prospects were brighter in the city, not just the availability of employment, but that work in the cities would lead to an improvement of their lives. Many thought that this improvement would not only be experienced when they were actually living in the city, where life was more varied and interesting, but would be sustained when they returned home. In some cases, they might use the money saved to start their own business. In others, they would send remittances home, some of which would be used to build a substantial house where the whole family would live. Sometimes, people living in rural areas were actively recruited by authorities to work in state-owned enterprises. Others were encouraged by networks of relatives and acquaintances from their own villages who had already migrated; they tempted them to move, made their journey itself relatively easy and cheap, and facilitated their access to employment. And so people moved, in the millions.[5]

The experience of working in the city was different for those with different skills: it was very different for those obtaining work in State-owned enterprises, those joining existing groups of construction workers, or those going into domestic labor. Employment possibilities were highly gendered, types of work were very different for male and female factory workers. They were also differentiated by region of origin; for example, factory workers from eastern regions of China were often considered to have finer skills and to be more capable of delicate work. But one thing was common to all migrants from the countryside: the planning system enshrined a whole series of divisions between migrants and more long-standing urban residents, with the former denied many of the rights and privileges of urban citizens. Yet despite their political and social exclusion, the presence of so many migrants, with their distinctive lifestyles, their social networks, and their informal organizations, reshaped the Chinese urban experience in many different and unpredictable ways (Solinger, 1999: chs. 6 and 7).

Migration not only transformed large cities such as Shanghai and Beijing, but also smaller cities that acquired skyscrapers, factories, ring roads and traffic jams, transport systems thronged with people, and soaring pollution levels—the whole urban experience. This process has been especially striking in the Pearl River Delta, in the southeast of the country. Lesley Chang, in *Factory Girls*, charts the influx of young women to Dongguan in the early years of this century (Chang, 2009). Dongguan is a prefecture city in Guangdong Province, whose official population at around 7 million in 2008 was widely believed to underestimate the actual population by omitting up to 2 million migrants who, at any one time, were working in, and jumping between, hundreds of factories, producing everything from parts for mobile phones to high-end trainers. The growth of Shenzhen, to the south of Dongguan, is even more remarkable; it grew from a settlement of around 30,000 people at the start of the 1980s into a city with an official population of around 13 million by the end of 2018, swelled to up to 20 million by large numbers of unregistered migrants living in the city at any one time (Zacharias and Tang, 2010; Keith, Lash, et al., 2013).[6]

Central to the experience of rural-urban migrants, from the period studied by Solinger up to the present day, is their *hukou*—China's system of household registration that also distributes state benefits according to whether a person lives in an agricultural area. Indeed, as far as official figures are concerned, migrants are defined, and governed, in terms of their *hukou*. "Under the *hukou* system, in operation from the mid-1950s, each individual was registered in one place of residence, and was categorized as a rural or urban resident on their *hukou* status" (Li and Rose, 2017: 21). Cindy Fan, in *China on the Move*, gives a detailed account of the origins, motives, and successive transformations of the *hukou* system as a means of state management of migrant labor flows as State priorities for economic development changed (Fan, 2007: ch. 3). The *hukou* system has been undergoing a gradual reform since the late 1980s, when the central government first allowed migration from rural areas to cities without the need for the migrants to transfer their *hukou*. From 2003 onward, the central government began to accord some basic rights to rural migrants, and since then "a series of policy reforms have taken place in many cities to provide some public services to them, and increasing numbers of small and medium cities have begun to grant rural migrants local *hukou* status on certain conditions" (Li and Rose, 2017: 21). Nonetheless, as in the period Solinger studied, those without an urban *hukou* are still stigmatized by local residents, they are also unable to access certain social welfare and housing services in the city, and, as we shall see, they are particularly vulnerable to changes in State economic and labor policies that modulate the need for urban migrant labor.

For many migrants from villages and small towns, the 'urban village' is where life in the city begins. Urban villages appear in rapidly growing cities in two main ways. In some cases, privately owned land that has been surrounded by the developing city and is now in a downtown area has been turned by landlords into densely populated housing blocks. In other cases, parcels of communally owned farmland in peripheral areas are engulfed by urban sprawl and are subsequently developed into blocks of cheap housing for rent to migrants. Such urban villages, often surrounded by new, modern skyscrapers, have a bad reputation, carrying much of the general stigma faced by many migrants in China. The term 'village' should not conjure up a rural scene (indeed, nor do most rural villages bear much relation to the idyllic scenes of peasant life captured by the Chinese YouTube star Li Ziqi).[7] The buildings in which migrants live provide very basic amenities, and are crowded together around shopping streets, where small shops, food stalls, restaurants, and repair shops are interspersed with closed markets for food and other essentials. Yuting Liu and her colleagues point out that, because of their "crowded and cluttered material landscape, their apparently unhealthy living environment, and the resulting security and social problems, "urban villages in Chinese cities are widely condemned by the media, the government and even academia" (Liu, He, et al., 2010: 136). Yet, amid such hostility, these villages do not merely provide shelter for those who inhabit them; they offer a space and a place to find a new mode of life, to develop new habits for the inhabitation of a radically different environment. As Yan Yuan points out in her ethnography of one such urban village, in Wuhan (the capital city of Hubei province in central China), urban villages are not simple enclaves, but places of "fluidity" within the network of migrant trajectories that constitute the Chinese megacity; in that experience of constant mobility, "life routines are readjusted, the sense of place is reconfigured, the belongingness to place is renegotiated, and mechanisms in space ordering and regulations are reinvented" (Yuan, 2014: 19–21).[8]

There are urban villages in Shanghai, but most migrants live neither in these nor in the old center of Shanghai, but rather in the ring of 'new towns' that have grown around the periphery of metropolitan Shanghai. These towns, though formally part of Shanghai, are often one- or two-hours' drive from the tourist center, with its nightlife, its colonial history, and its famous Bund; they are also often beyond the reach of the expanding Shanghai metro system. Migrants on the periphery may live in temporary accommodation in building sites, in factory dormitories, or in purpose-built blocks with relatively basic facilities. Not all live there, of course: others find rooming houses in the center of Shanghai, working in restaurants or as domestic workers. For all, however, whatever their form of employment, precarity is a constant feature of existence. This precarity intensified in the second decade of this century, as Shanghai tried to move 'up the value chain,' away from the low-wage, cheap-goods economy that has under-pinned its recent growth. Official attempts to curb low-skilled migration to the city sometimes involved sudden and drastic interventions, for example, without warning, factories making cheap goods for export that provided migrant employment were razed to the ground. As we shall see later in this chapter, drawing on our own and our colleagues' research in one such situation, many factory workers shrug their shoulders and move to find work in another area of the city. But the shops, markets, and restaurants run by other migrants are left behind, now bereft of customers, and having to seek new ways to make ends meet.

Migration in China is rarely a matter of cutting ties to the past. Most rural-to-urban migrants maintain strong connections with their home village or town throughout the years that they spend in the city, travelling home on holidays and for special occasions, sending remittances home to maintain family members in the village. In fact, through the houses they build, and the businesses that they establish on their return, they 'urbanize' their place of origin, not least though maintaining the connections that they have made while in the big city (Tang and Feng, 2015; Liu, Wang, et al., 2017). State authorities are now seeking to stem the massive tide of migrants to the major cities by making it easier for migrants to move semi-permanently to small and medium towns that can grant them *hukou* status. But most migrants to megacities such as Shanghai envisage their stay as temporary and retain their rural *hukou*. This imposes many limitations on their rights in the city. A migrant without Shanghai *hukou* may struggle to access healthcare, housing, and other services, for themselves and for their children, and indeed they often pay to place their children in private schools established specifically for migrants. The *hukou* system thus produces a particular form of social exclusion that "builds a wall between urban residents and rural migrants in their social interactions" (Li and Rose, 2017: 21). This nexus of economic, social, and 'subjective' exclusion in turn generates a set of 'stressors' that may help us to understand mental health problems among migrants in China's megacities. But we need to make matters more precise. Let us start by taking a closer look at some of the different ways of life of those we perhaps too easily group together as 'migrants.'

Migrant Labor

The urban experience of those who migrate from the countryside is significantly shaped by the kind of work they find. As Sarah Swider points out, migrants can be "porters, food preparers and servers, domestic workers, nannies, cleaners, retail and street vendors, sanitation workers," as well as factory workers and workers in construction (Swider, 2016: 2). Here we focus on three specific pathways that exemplify some of the most challenging situations encountered by rural migrants to Chinese megacities: life in the factory that is the destiny of most young women migrants, life in construction that is the destiny of many men, and last, the lives of those women and men who make their lives as local entrepreneurs.

Manufacturing Migrants

In Shenzhen, southern China, at two factories owned by the electronics manufacturer Foxconn—actually the Hon Hai Precision Industry Company—13 young workers tried to take their own lives between January and May 2010, "bringing a public relations crisis and a crisis of corporate responsibility to virtually all Foxconn's image-conscious customers, including Apple, Dell, IBM, Samsung, Nokia, Hitachi and other electronic giants" (Chan and Pun, 2010: 2).[9] As it became 'the workshop of the world' in the closing decades of the twentieth century, Chinese factory labor provided a large proportion of the electronic goods that supported a global economy of technological desire, one that many Chinese also came to participate in, of course, along with improved access to mobile and digital devices. But the labor, and sometimes the lives, of hundreds and thousands of Chinese migrants from the countryside were required to fuel this economy. According to Jenny Chan and Pun Ngai, at the time of their research in 2013, 85 percent of the 900,000 strong workforce of Foxconn were young migrants from rural areas. Like many such migrants, they mainly lived in factory dormitories—in this case, there were ten dormitory buildings within the gated compound; more than 50,000 other migrant factory workers lived outside the gates in village houses that had been turned into collective dormitories. Certainly, it is possible to over-interpret the Foxconn suicides as quasi-political acts of resistance[10]—nonetheless it seems self-evident that they were not isolated acts stemming from individual mental illness; while some may have arisen from personal troubles, most are merely the extreme manifestation of a labor regime of long hours, low pay, poor conditions, and the constant stress of just-in-time production (Chan, 2013).[11]

While a range of measures have been introduced by the Chinese government to improve the situation of migrant factory workers—minimum wage legislation, some rights for workers to obtain welfare benefits, and so forth—it is not clear how much impact they have had on the actual working conditions of most factory laborers, or if they alleviate the stress that they experience. Foxconn presented itself as a "warm family with a loving heart," and in the view of Foxconn CEO, Terry Gou, the workers who committed suicide were experiencing 'emotional problems' before they arrived at the factory gate. His response was not only to install 'suicide nets' outside all the dormitories, but to require "all job applicants to complete a psychological test with 36 questions" on the grounds that the earlier troubles had their source in "fragile spirits" with a "weak capacity to handle personal problems" (Chan, 2013: 98).[12] Jenny Chan gives us a compelling glimpse into the demands placed on the life and labor of those who work on these production lines, whose dreams turned sour, and whose education was no path to advancement toward a much-desired urban lifestyle. But not every migrant experience of factory work is the same. Each of the 'factory girls' in Dongguan whose stories are told by Leslie Chang claimed to know of at least one migrant who found her way to wealth and happiness in the city; such stories inspire many of these young women to 'jump' jobs from factory to factory, learning new skills, reading books on self-improvement, and repeating self-help mantras, in the hope and belief that by effort, diligence, and a certain amount of luck and cunning, they can become the creators of their own life story of success (Chang, 2009).

For the first generation of rural-to-urban migrants, "moving to *dagong* was not only a major trend (when a person successfully moved out to *dagong*, the whole village would follow) but also a means of realizing one's economic goals . . . These goals included building a new house, financing a sibling's education, marrying, and setting up a small business" (Pun and Lu, 2010c: 9).[13] But according to the surveys quoted by Chan and Pun, many of the next generation of migrants, those who moved in the first decade of the new millennium, were the 'left behind children' whose parents were part of the first wave of rural-to-urban migrants. The young women and men of this later generation migrated with dreams and aspirations about the possibilities of escaping the dull monotony of their rural lives and enjoying the wealth, lifestyle, and possibilities for self-advancement in the cities. In the words of Pun and Lu, this generation, born in the period of reform, were "better educated and better off materially, but spiritually disoriented" with a "structure of feeling" and a way of life characterized by less loyalty to their work, growing individualism, consumerism, the pursuit of personal development and freedom (ibid.: 3).

In a paper based on research in the 1990s, Pun recounts the case of Yan, a *dagongmei* (working girl), who left her hometown in Hunan and her job in the forestry department to follow her older sister to Dongguan. "When her sister married a local citizen there," writes Pun, "their hukou, or household registries, were transferred from their hometown to Dongguan, at a cost of five thousand renminbi for each person to the local government" (Pun, 2000: 543). But Yan left her first job as a secretary after a friendship with her boss turned into a demand for sexual relations. Subsequently, she found herself working in an electronics factory in Shenzhen, and her despair at her situation, her chronic bodily and mental pain and trauma, exacerbated by the toxic and noxious chemicals used in the production process, were expressed in the form of a nightly bout of screaming, which, for Pun, was an expression of anguish common to all the women workers in that enterprise. Yan found herself in an impasse: she did not have the *guanxi*—the networks, connections, and relationships—that would facilitate promotion in the factory, she no longer had hukou in her hometown so could not return to a job in local government, she "had no more choice. When I'm wandering about the streets of this big city, I know it is not my place, it does not belong to me. But I have to stay. I see people selling stuff at the side of the road. . . . I wonder whether my life will end up like that" (ibid.: 543).

We do not need to follow Pun's own Marxist/psychoanalytic analysis of Yan's situation to appreciate the impasse this young woman found herself in, and the ways in which it was transmuted into bodily and cerebral form. Yet, even events such as the 1993 fire in a toy factory in Shenzhen that killed more than eighty workers and seriously burned and injured over one hundred more, could not, it seemed, deter hundreds and thousands of young migrants, mainly young unmarried women, from taking the long journey by train or long-distance coach from their home villages to the industrial centers. Especially after the Chinese New Year or the Spring Festival, throngs of people arrive in Shanghai, hoping that their lives will be transformed by the opportunities offered in the city, rather than having to follow the predictable path of married life in their husband's home village. Crowds of these hopeful migrants hang around the stations, or in areas surrounding the local factories, hoping to be chosen for work, perhaps on the basis of relatives already employed, and their possession of the right documents—national identity cards, secondary school graduation certificates, certifications of unmarried status, and entry permits for the Shenzhen Special Economic Zone (Pun, 2002).

Pun and Lu argue that while the first generation of workers turned the pain and trauma of their experience inward, those of this second generation were turning it outward, finding themselves unable to access their urban dreams of upward mobility; theirs was a state of resentment, and their distress and suffering were transmuted into anger and rage, turned into multiple acts of resistance against their employers:

As new labor was needed for the use of capital, Chinese peasants were asked to transform themselves into laboring bodies, willing to spend their days in the workplace . . . Yet, as disposable labor, when they were not needed, they were asked to go back to the villages that they had been induced to forsake and to which they had failed to remain loyal . . . If transience was a dominant characteristic of the first generation of migrant workers, rupture characterizes the second generation, who now spend much more of their lives in urban areas. Transience suggests transitions, and so encourages hopes and dreams of transformation. Rupture, however, creates closure: there is no hope of either transforming oneself into an urban worker or of returning to the rural community to take up life as a peasant. (Pun and Lu, 2010a: 11)

Within that cyclical process—leave the village for the factory; leave the factory because of dissatisfaction and the recognition of exploitation; return to the village to set up some kind of farm or enterprise; return to the city on the failure of that enterprise—the migrant becomes stranger both in village and city. Pun and her colleagues argue that a process of proletarianization is thus taking place, in which these migrants, building on the collective experience that factory work has produced, turn their rage and frustration into consciousness of their exploitation, and their personal frustrations into political action. Anger at poor working conditions, low wages, and lack of rights, and the sense of profound unfairness that they experience, leads to collective action: they argue that a new Chinese working class is forming, no longer a class-in-themselves, they become a class-for-themselves, "as historical agents who have participated in making their own social change while China has evolved into the world's workshop" (Pun and Lu, 2010c: 21).

Have we witnessed the formation of a new, self-conscious, working class contesting the forces of capital and the state as Chinese migrant factory workers protest against their exploitative conditions of labor? Perhaps we should be cautious before mapping the Chinese experience in the twenty-first century onto E. P. Thompson's narrative of working-class formation in Europe in the nineteenth century (Thompson, 1963). Have "anger, frustration, and resentment" led to "the emergence of the workers' consciousness and their shared class position" (Pun and Lu, 2010c: 4)? Is it the case, as Pun predicts, that migrant workers on the factory floor and the construction site, will no longer internalize their plight in the form of mental distress and mental ill health, but will be protagonists of radical social change (Pun, 2017)? Or is it that most migrants find a way of life, and a relation to that life, which is neither that of political resistance not of mental disorder, but a somewhat stoic mode of self-management in conditions of uncertainty, underpinned by a firm belief that however difficult their life in the city might be, it offers something that is better than a monotonous existence in one's hometown.

In Pun's portrayal, migrants are treated as mere fuel in a strategy of Chinese modernization that seeks reintegration into a global capitalist economy through attracting foreign investment, and via super-exploitation of a 'reserve army of labor'—made up of migrant labor power under total control of their bosses, subjugated to disciplinary regimes, during the day in Taylorist factories and confined at night in factory dormitories.[14] But Lesley Chang, whose stories of the 'factory girls' of Dongguan we discussed earlier, is not alone in suggesting that the interior lives of migrants are more nuanced—that not all feel defeated, devastated, and overwhelmed with negativity (see also Ash, 2016). It is true that Kaxton Siu finds evidence of a pretty miserable experience of life in the letters written by factory workers in the 1990s—letters that also repeatedly spoke of loneliness, fatalism about their lives, low aspirations for their future, and the desire to return home, even if that meant being enmeshed in the rigid social roles and gender stereotypes of the countryside (Siu, 2015).[15] However, Siu suggests, things changed from around 2000 with the development of urban villages. Those locals who lived close to these factories saw ways to make profit for themselves from the influx of migrants and cleared their land in order to build multistory buildings of apartments which they could rent to migrant workers. Migrants moved to these apartments, with their rents subsidized by their employers, as the factories could not afford to build the number of dormitories necessary to accommodate them. The original villagers became rentiers. Further, their villages, and other villagers, profited from the rents that the factories paid in order to lease their sites, as part of the rent was distributed to each local who held a share in the village commune. The funds enabled new streets to be constructed, and new shops and restaurants to emerge, often themselves run by migrants, to serve the migrant population. New communal facilities and even parks were built with the funds the village received in rents.

Not that this led to harmony: now different challenges emerged, with new divisions between locals and migrants. Indeed, in the village in Southern China studied by Siu, the original villagers—now less than 2 percent or the total population—moved to newly built mansions in 'gated communities' protected by walls and security cameras (Siu, 2015: 51).[16] But for the migrants themselves, new communal relations developed, supportive social networks outside the control of the factories and their disciplinary regimes, using mobile phones to maintain connections with relatives and friends, play online games, join online communities, and share gossip. Their wages enabled them to begin to participate in Chinese consumer culture, to visit bars and department stores, and to live a certain kind of urban life. Many were also able to save, even though many factories retain some earnings to reduce the high turnover rate. Some came as married couples, sometimes with their child, and sometimes with a grandparent who cared for the child while the parents were at work; many had family responsibilities for relatives who have migrated to the same area.

The images of subjugation, domination, discipline, and super-exploitation that characterize accounts of Chinese migrant labor in the 1990s may or may not have been the general experience for that first wave that came from the countryside to work in the ever-expanding cities. But in any case, by the end of the first decade of the new millennium, Chinese migrant factory workers were increasingly authors of their own lives. While some are no doubt fatalistic, and others still seek to fulfill their dreams of achieving a life of wealth and status in the city, the majority live lives that, to quote Elizabeth Povinelli, are "ordinary, chronic and cruddy rather than catastrophic, crisis laden and sublime" (Povinelli, 2011: 132). Indeed, as the research by our colleagues Lisa Richaud and Ash Amin showed, even in circumstances that would appear objectively depressing, precarious, and full of uncertainty, Chinese migrant lives contain moments of satisfaction and even of joy.

Constructing Migrants

While much research has focused on the lives of those migrants who come from the countryside to labor in urban factories, another image of the migrant experience in China often comes to mind—that of the typically male construction worker in the informal economy, working, living, and sleeping in the scaffolding surrounding one of the hundreds of high-rise buildings—fancy apartment blocks and offices—springing up in every Chinese city. There is, as Sarah Swider has documented in her study of 'the new precariat'—as she terms those involved in construction work in contemporary China—a somewhat complex network of employment in the construction industry (Swider, 2016). While most of the senior and management positions are held by those with urban *hukou*, almost all the actual work of construction is done by teams of migrants, some of whom do have a registration permit to work in the city, but the majority of whom are unregistered. While many of those migrants who are registered for work have proper contracts and are employed in the formal sector of the industry with decent safety standards, many others are hired informally, with irregular wages, constant insecurity of employment, and difficult and dangerous working conditions (ibid.: 35). Many of these workers live on the construction sites, in dormitories made up of bare concrete, cell-like rooms, with bunk beds and few amenities for washing and cooking, seldom venturing out into the city beyond, but sending remittances back home and returning to their villages for festivals and marriage ceremonies.

In their study of Chinese construction workers, Pun and Lu found that these workers' lives were suffused with an ever-present undercurrent of violence. "The working lives of construction workers are . . . deeply affected by quarrels, individual and collective fighting, attempts to damage buildings, bodily abuse and even suicidal behaviors" (Pun and Lu, 2010a: 145). Yet, despite these seemingly dire working and living conditions, Sarah Swider paints a rather different picture: she found that "construction workers' lives were filled not only with bitterness, difficulty and struggle but also with love, laughter and companionship." All those interviewed by Swider tell versions of the same story: conditions are poor in their hometown; construction work offers the opportunity to make more money, to buy a motorcycle, to save, to marry and have a family, to pay for the education of their children, to build a new home back in their village of origin, to pay for the healthcare of their aging parents. Indeed, this is what we and our colleagues found in our own informal conversations with migrant building workers in Shanghai: we visited several sites and talked with foremen and workers, most of whom greeted us enthusiastically, and some of the construction workers willingly showed us their accommodation. These were fleeting encounters, of course, which we would not wish to over-interpret—but we did not get an impression of lives perceived as terrible by those who lived them. While accommodation was indeed spartan, as described above, no one to whom we spoke expressed any regrets about their migration and their working conditions. Some of them went back to their villages for short periods at the end of one episode of construction work, but chose to return again and again to Shanghai, to take up jobs in construction as the market for upscale apartments in fancy tower blocks boomed, especially for those luxurious properties being built along the Huangpu River.

Not all construction workers live on the sites where they work. Many of those who have come to the city through existing social ties with relatives or those from their own areas live in the kinds of urban villages that we have already discussed: in 2005, one large urban village in Beijing accommodated more than one hundred thousand migrants. In these urban villages, migrants share rooms, usually in shabby apartment blocks, not much better than the construction site dormitories, although some have tiny kitchens and washing facilities. Most apartment complexes are built around a courtyard, often with a vegetable garden as well as clothes lines and a parking area. The streets have shops, bars, restaurants, cafes, massage parlors, internet cafés, electronic shops, hairdressers, and thinly disguised prostitution services, often run by migrants, as well as street stalls where migrant vendors sell vegetables, food and drink, second-hand goods and much more. They create "an environment that supports existing social networks and fosters the development of new social networks, both of which shape the lives and work of migrants who work informally in service, retail, and construction" (Swider, 2016: 64). Many of these migrants actually settle in these urban villages for long periods, developing friendships, bringing their families, and sending their children to migrant schools where, in neat uniforms and pristine classrooms, they practiced writing and basic mathematics, learned languages (especially English), exercised in well-equipped play areas, ate their lunch and their snacks, and enjoyed afternoon naps.[17] Nonetheless, the adults remain unregistered temporary migrants, with no rights to urban citizenship and constantly under threat from government campaigns for enforcing regulations, with spot checks for permits, cleansing areas of those who do not have the right to remain, and sometimes taking individuals into detention until they pay a fine for their release. Despite the apparent hospitability of such enclaves, the lives of the construction workers who live within them are difficult and few can tolerate such working arrangements beyond middle age: as they approach this age, they must either return to their villages, find other, less demanding employment or, as Swider puts it, "end up destitute, decrepit or dead" (ibid.: 81).

Hard as lives may be for construction workers who live on site, and for those who have formed networks in urban villages, the situation is even worse for those who come to the city without a preexisting arrangement with contractors, and without family or friends. They find employment on a casual basis, waiting every morning at 'labor markets' on street corners or small parks, where contractors looking for particular kinds of work may hire a few men for a day or two to work on a specific building project, to do bricklaying, electrical work, tiling, or some other task for which they have a particular immediate need. These laborers are the worst paid, and the most exploited, the most indebted to corrupt and despotic local agents: they exist in the most precarious of situations. The consequences for the mental health of the male migrant construction workers caught in such situations are seldom discussed in the literature, but pathogenic levels of anxiety, fear, and trauma—physical and mental stress—seem to be woven through their lives.

Enterprising Migrants

Of course, most migrants work for others, in factories, building sites, in domestic labor, or in other low-status jobs. But not all. Around the apartment blocks and dormitories where migrant workers live, in the urban villages and even in some inner-city areas, enterprising migrants have set up restaurants and bars, internet cafés, flower and vegetable stalls, dumpling carts and other forms of street food, second-hand electronic goods shops, hairdressers, massage parlors and prostitution services, and much more. Migrant-run covered markets are crammed with meat, fish, and vegetable vendors who often buy their products from wholesalers or sometimes from their home villages. In other parts of the market, one can find sellers of spices, oils, knick-knacks, mobile phone accessories, and domestic goods. These markets are thronged with migrant laborers—or at least they are until their factories are destroyed, and the laborers are forced to move on.

Such, indeed, was the situation in 2016, in the Tongli Road in Jiuting in the Songjiang district on the South-West outskirts of Shanghai, where Lisa Richaud and Ash Amin carried out some of the fieldwork for our project (Richaud and Amin, 2019; Richaud and Amin, 2020).[18] When we first visited, this street, also known as "*Jinhui* shopping street," was marked off from its surroundings by elegant 'gateways' built at each end. Its construction seems to have been an initiative of the first generation of migrants, who obtained legal title to the land and whose ownership enabled them to profit from rents. For example, one first-generation migrant owns a local apartment building, rather grandly known as the Residential Centre for Floating Populations, where rooms are available for rent. The street itself is quite wide, and is flanked on either side by small buildings, two or three stories high, with small restaurants, clothes shops, DVD shops, and other shopfronts displaying their goods and services. In front of the shopfronts are stalls, many selling hot food. There was a large fresh food market, where migrants rented stalls to sell their products, and the locals came to shop, to meet, and to gossip. Behind the street, on each side, accessed by small semi-paved alleys, were dormitories where factory workers and others lived: blocks of single rooms, usually bare concrete with the minimum of decorations, each with several bunk beds and a small space for washing and cooking. Behind these dormitory blocks there was an agglomeration of small factories and workshops where many of the migrants were employed. Other migrants set up small workshops to repair tools or clothes, or worked as street sweepers and security guards. Some had their child with them, and there is a local migrant primary school, although education beyond primary school requires children to return to their home village. Many of those who live and work in and around Tongli Road have relatives who have also come to Shanghai, some living close by, some in other areas of the city.

But a few months later, when our colleagues started their intensive fieldwork, the Tongli Road had been transformed, as part of the new strategy of the Shanghai city authorities to reduce the numbers of migrant workers.

As Richaud and Amin report, "a campaign known as *Wuwei sibi* (literally, "five bans and four obligations") . . . was launched by the municipal authorities in the name of a better quality of life in the city," which aimed to "attract and develop high technology industries that will rely on educated, 'high quality' (*suzhi gao*) workers" (Richaud and Amin, 2020: 81)—and enacting this strategy meant, in the first place, bulldozing the factories that employed the workers who supported the vibrant life of Tongli Road. For many of those employed in these factories, this was by no means a new situation, and their response was to pack up and move to another area where unskilled work was still available. But in so doing, they left behind all those others who had depended upon their trade for their own living. How did they cope? What were the consequences for their mental health? We shall return to these questions later in this chapter. But at first glance, it would surely seem that people in this situation would form a part of what has often been called China's mental health crisis.

China: A Mental Health Crisis?

In the first decade of the twenty-first century, researchers, professionals, and the popular press began to suggest that China was 'in the grip of a mental health crisis' with a combination of high and increasing rates of mental ill health, shortage of psychiatric facilities and personnel, and a lack of psychotherapeutic services.[19] This perception of a mental health crisis took a further turn when the Chinese media discovered that the country was experiencing an 'epidemic of stress' focused on its rapidly growing cities—the stress of rapid social transformation, the stress of finding a way to live in a newly competitive society where the party no longer prescribes the rules for living, the stress of pressures at work, the stress on children of China's highly competitive education system . . . In 2012, under the title 'Worry and Stress Rise in China," a Gallup Poll reported that 75 percent of Chinese workers described an increase in stress over the previous year (compared with a global average of 48 percent). Stress was reported to be high, not among migrants, who were not mentioned in this Poll, but among white-collar office workers, working long hours, struggling with high costs of living in the big cities of Beijing and Shanghai, and facing rising expectations about lifestyle that are often hard to meet. Of those polled, 27 percent reported that they had worried a lot the previous day and 40 percent reported that they had felt a lot of stress, although, intriguingly, the levels of worry and negative emotions were actually higher in rural China than in the cities.[20]

Are migrants also experiencing an epidemic of stress, suffering from undiagnosed mental health problems, ground down by the combination of intense demands on them in unrelenting workplaces and the uncertainty of their living situations? Are they too 'psychologizing' their distress, even if they do not seek professional help? We have already remarked, in chapter 2, on the pitfalls that are likely to affect those who use Euro-American diagnostic systems to identify mental health problems in migrant populations living in contemporary megacities in other regions of the world. But what 'gaze' should we adopt then? What language, what criteria, what forms of judgment should we use to identify mental ill health? Should we use the diagnostic criteria developed in the United States and published in the various editions of the American Psychiatric Association's *Diagnostic and Statistical Manual of Mental Disorders*, the criteria used in the chapter on Classification of Mental and Behavioural Disorders in the ICD, the *International Statistical Classification of Diseases and Related Health Problems*, which is widely used in Europe, the indigenous language of everyday life used in China, the self-reports of individuals or their families, or their communities? From our perspective, in understanding the emergence of a therapeutic or psychological culture in China, the task is less about deciding between these options than about understanding their mutual entanglement in the ways that experts and laypersons have come to make sense of mental distress in contemporary China.

Let us take one international epidemiological category: depression. Psychiatric epidemiologists tell us that China is experiencing an upsurge in diagnoses of depression. But when can we say that the '*yali*' reported by many migrants is actually a mental disorder called 'depression'?[21] We can trace the broad outlines of the issue at stake here by focusing on a single paper. Sing Lee has argued that depression was "almost an unknown category in China until the early 1990s" and that "the term 'depression' (*youyuzheng* or *yiyuzheng*) or 'depressed' (*yiyu* or *youyu*) was rarely used" (Lee, 2011: 177). He points to the fact that national epidemiological surveys in 1982 and 1993 showed that fewer than 0.5 percent of those surveyed were diagnosed with depression when interviewed with the World Health Organization Composite International Diagnostic Interview (CIDI) to assess major depressive episode (MDE) according to *Diagnostic and Statistical Manual of Mental Disorders* (*DSM-IV*) criteria (Lee, Tsang, et al., 2009). Suffering, he suggests, was expressed in other ways, notably through physical symptoms such as headaches, insomnia, and physical pains that, in China, were termed neurasthenia or 'weakness of the nerves' (*shenjing shuairou*). As we described in chapter 2, neurasthenia was a familiar diagnosis in nineteenth-century Europe, where it was usually applied to the malaise of the wealthier classes. Lee draws on Arthur Kleinman's well-known work in Hunan in the 1980s, and Kleinman's argument that the physical symptoms of neurasthenia are actually 'idioms of distress' in a political climate in which individuals were required to repress external evidence of their emotions. On this basis, Kleinman argued that the majority of those diagnosed with neurasthenia would have been diagnosed with depression in the United States (Kleinman, 1982; Kleinman, 1986).[22] In the familiar terms of transcultural psychiatry, neurasthenia was reframed as a somatization of depression, a somatic means of expression of interpersonal distress within a culture that discouraged or prohibited the expression of feelings—where the mind dare not speak, the body became the means of communication of suffering and anguish.

It would be wrong, however, to disparage a belief in the reality of neurasthenia as merely part of Chinese 'folk psychology' or to suggest that when the migrants of Tongli Road speak of their response to their situation in corporeal terms it is because they do not think it appropriate to openly 'express their emotions.' Howard Chiang and his colleagues have argued that "Western behavioral sciences and psychological treatments [were] repudiated as 'bourgeois' in the Maoist period (1949–76)" (Chiang, 2015: 13), but Chinese experts and popular knowledges of the mind have a long and complex history, and one that has always been linked to practices of intervention and remediation. In the early years of the twentieth century, such beliefs and practices were influenced by psy experts from America and from Germany, sometimes mediated via Japan, asylums had been established in major cities, psychoanalytic ideas began to be taken up by radicals and spread into popular debate, as did ideas of mental hygiene; there was the beginning of a professionalization of medical psychiatry as well as various forms of psychology and psychotherapy (Hsuan-Ying, 2015). By the first half of the twentieth century, the reality of neurasthenia was widely accepted by most of these professionals and understood in terms of a weakening of the nervous system following excessive nervous excitement, leading to a variety of somatic symptoms. The somatic and the mental were deeply intertwined in professional expertise as well as in lay thought. Wen-ji Wang has described the ways in which, from the 1920s onward, *shenjing shuairuo* provided a fertile ground for the involvement of psy professionals in the management of malaise: "emergent Chinese neuropsychiatric and mental health professionals eagerly entered the already vibrant culture of neurasthenia and provided their explanations" (Wang, 2016: 1). There were a variety of explanations and treatments for neurasthenia, including those that focused on strengthening the nerves through diet, injections of various substances, fresh air, and exercise. Many Chinese psychiatrists and psychologists took up and reworked themes from Euro-American styles of thought about the causes and consequences of minor mental troubles. There was healthy pluralism and debate between neuropsychiatrists, sociodynamic psychiatrists and clinical psychologists, and "certain psychologically minded social elites [who] championed the cause of mental hygiene or mental health" (ibid.: 5). But most of these approaches were characterized by a familiar mix: a strong belief in a hereditary basis of the susceptibility to mental disorder, an emphasis on mental troubles as 'disorders of civilization' that could be precipitated in those susceptible by all manner of nervous excitement, or by bad conduct such as masturbation and fantasizing, together with a concern that such mental pathologies might weaken the race with dire consequences for the future of the nation.

Things started to change in the 1980s. Following the publication of Kleinman's research, a number of Chinese studies were conducted, initially with the aim of disputing this overlap between neurasthenia and depression, not least because of the bad consequences for the doctor-patient relationship that were feared to result. But 20 years later the position had reversed. The third edition of the *Chinese Classification of Mental Disorders*, published in 2001, based its descriptive definitions on the *Clinical descriptions and diagnostic guidelines* of ICD-10 and also sought to align itself with the *Research Criteria* of ICD-10, and the *DSM-IV* (Chen, 2002).[23] It stated that the diagnosis of neurasthenia was to be utilized only when all other diagnoses such as depression, anxiety, and disorders with an identifiable physical basis have been excluded. Predictably, by 2009, researchers were pointing to the heavy burden of depression in China. For example, when Michael Phillips and his colleagues conducted an epidemiological survey in order to update the data on the Global Burden of Disease through a "comprehensive country specific analyses of the perceived needs, available resources, and potential barriers for mental health care" (Phillips, Zhang, et al., 2009: 2042), they found that while 1,034 cases in their sample met the DSM diagnostic criteria for major depression and a further 404 for minor depression, there were only fifteen cases of neurasthenia in their sample of over 16,500. This is hardly surprising, given that neurasthenia could only be diagnosed after excluding cases that met the criteria for any other disorder! Nonetheless, the extrapolations that Phillips and his colleagues drew from their study made for grim reading: "Projection of our results to all of China suggests that 173 million adults in the country have a mental disorder and 158 million of these have never received any type of professional help for their condition" (ibid.: 2052).[24] Soon, one major study was claiming that depression was the second leading cause of disability in China (Yang, Wang, et al., 2013). Disputing the claim in previous research that "Along with Japan, South Korea, and Mexico, China seems to benefit from lower rates of major depression, anxiety disorders, and low back pain than do other members of the G20" (ibid.: 2013), the authors commented that "this finding, however, has been challenged; true rates might be higher."[25]

The shift in psychiatric discourse from neurasthenia to depression is intertwined with its contemporary corollary—the increasing prescription of so-called antidepressant medication—although a study in *The Lancet* claims that less than 6 percent of those with anxiety, depression, and other mental afflictions seek help due to stigma or lack of access to resources (Charlson, Baxter, et al., 2016). No wonder some market research companies see a vast untapped marked here, predicting growth in China's market for antidepressants of the order of 20 percent year on year.[26] And yet neither the rise of Euro-American diagnostic language among professional researchers, nor the increasing use of 'western' psychopharmaceuticals, tell us the whole picture—even more than elsewhere, multiple explanatory systems for one's afflictions exist side by side in China. Alongside the growth of the medically trained psychiatric profession in China, increasingly adopting Euro-American styles of thought, there has been a rapid growth of the other psy professions, of counselors more or less professionally trained and credentialed, of the entry of psychological technologies into the human resources departments of many enterprises, and of the presence of psychological help and advice on the internet, television shows—including 'confessional' shows where individuals speak of their personal problems and are offered advice, and psychology self-help literature. In what is often referred to as a 'psycho-boom' (*xinli re*) (Hsuan-Ying, 2015) we can see a rather different style of explanation and intervention, drawing on a longer Chinese tradition for understanding the ailments of everyday life, which prioritizes, not the brain, but the heart.

Thus, in her study of *ideas of* mental health in China, and the practices of mental health professionals, the Canadian trained anthropologist Jie Yang argues that "The heart is a fundamental component of being and a key precept in traditional Chinese medicine. As the seat of cognition, virtue and bodily sensation, the heart is the origin of all emotions and the grounding space for all aspects of bodily and social well-being . . . Indeed, psychology is translated in Chinese as *xinlixue* (the study of the heart's reasoning)" (Yang, 2015: 12). Some of the key elements of the idea of neurasthenia live on in much of Chinese thought, both popular and professional (Yang, 2017). Mind and body are not viewed as separate entities, and distress is understood as arising from social and intersubjective experiences, Jie Yang reminds us. The perspective of the heart (*xinli hua*) and the belief that the heart is the key organ where those experiences impact, is thus central to both explanation and treatment. The heart is where the rush to competition and self-advancement take their toll, the heart is where spiritual emptiness is felt, the heart is where the pressure (*yali*) of demands in the workplace and outside it are felt, the heart is what speaks out to the individual of their sorrows and disappointments, and depression (*yiyu*) is as much an emotion of the heart as it is a disease of the mind. The body and mind are open, permeable to outside forces, whether material, social, or interpersonal. When students complain of low spirits, exhaustion, frustration, and meaninglessness in their lives lived in endless pursuit of grades, Jie Yang tells us, University psychological counsellors do not diagnose 'depression' but *kongxin bing* (empty-heart disease), a psychological disorder caused by the collapse of one's value orientation due to the external pressure exerted by the exam-focused educational system, which is neither amenable to drugs nor psychological therapies (Yang, 2017: 70).

It is clear, then, that we cannot understand the nature and experience of mental distress in China, let alone explore questions about city effects, about the role of migration, and so on, without understanding the emergence of a very specific kind of 'psy complex' in that country in recent decades, not just in relation to serious and disabling disorders, but also in relation to the everyday, low-level, and yet pervasive ailments that often are placed under the sign of *stress*.

'Stress' and the Psy Complex

While, as we have seen, there were 'psy' precedents from the pre-1949 period to call upon, from the 1980s onward, for some Chinese citizens at least, a new 'psychological' language for shaping, organizing, understanding, and expressing one's afflictions became available: "the terms 'psychological' (*xinli*), 'stress' (*yali*), 'mood' (*xinqing*), 'feeling' (*quingxu* or *ganjue*), 'unhappiness' (*bukaixin* or *buyukuai*), 'feeling bad' (*nangua*) and 'depressed' (*youyu*)" (Lee, 2011: 186).

These new vocabularies, and modes of introspection, forms of judgment, and personal aspirations are linked to an "awakening interest in psychology books, biographical documentary films, counselling, psychological idioms of distress, psychometric methods, and training in psychotherapy . . . these big city, middle-class interests represent a set of quests for meaning in everyday life among ordinary Chinese that holds the potential to transform Chinese culture and society" (Kleinman, 2010: 1075). While some of the growth of the psy industry has resulted from traditionally trained individual psychotherapists (Chang, Tong, et al., 2005; Deng, Lin, et al., 2013) or family therapists expanding their practices and gaining more public recognition for their work (Deng, Lin et al., 2013), much has been market-driven, created by entrepreneurial individuals who, even when altruistic in their wish to ameliorate unhappiness, have also seen a market opportunity (Zhang, 2017). There has also been a remarkable rise of counseling services delivered face-to-face, by telephone, or via the internet. Psy professionals now star in television talk shows about emotional problems, marital difficulties, and parent-child relationships (Yang, 2017). Many training courses for psychological counselors have been established. Some of these are officially authorized programs delivered in universities and other educational establishments and leading to certification from the Ministry of Labor, with a license awarded on the basis of an examination. Others are of dubious provenance set up for profit and attracting gullible individuals who themselves see 'counseling' as a new and potentially profitable vocation for themselves.[27]

Some authors who have documented this trend have suggested that this amounts to the emergence of 'therapeutic governance' in China—a state-encouraged strategy to achieve political stability and economic growth, taken up enthusiastically by the growing psy professionals and incorporated into many workplaces, to manage the problems of living, not by changing material circumstances, but by defining and teaching the psychological capacities to optimize the relation between subjective states and economic requirements, transforming the consequences of sociopolitical policies into individual troubles, and hence masking and legitimating their political and social causes (Hsuan-Ying, 2015; Yang, 2015; Hizi, 2017; Yang, 2017; Zhang, 2017). Thus, Li Zhang has argued that "psychological intervention, often in the name of *guanai* (care), has gradually become a useful tool of managing the population and governing society in postsocialist China" (Zhang, 2017: 6). and that "psychological counselors and other psychological experts are becoming a new form of authority, an indispensable part of creating and managing knowable, stable, and governable subjects for the military, the police, schools, and enterprises (ibid.: 7). However, while the phenomena analyzed by these authors are real enough, it is not clear that the hidden hand of the state is directing them all—let alone the visible and invisible hands of the strong Party State of China.[28] We need more nuanced analytical tools to understand these developments in which a whole range of authorities, with different relations to the formal political apparatus, are involved in the government of conduct, drawing on regimes of knowledge and expertise and articulating novel self-technologies underpinned by beliefs about desirable forms of life and subjectivity. They may be better understood as the conse-quence of a number of interrelated events that are reshaping the subjectivity of Chinese citizens: new ways of thinking about the unease of the soul in China, new ways of acting upon it, and the emergence of a heterogeneous array of 'engineers of the human soul' (Rose, 1989; Rose, 1996). Further, as we have seen in other regions of the world, it would be misleading to regard individuals as docile recipients of these ways of thinking about and acting on themselves, far less as 'dupes' of a set of pacifying practices. If these prac-tices of the self have proliferated through the everyday lives of so many, it is because they connect with the dissatisfactions and desires of individuals, who do not merely subordinate themselves to them, but are active agents taking up and transforming these new techniques of governing themselves.

There are certainly a number of formalized and organized psy practices for managing subjectivity carried out at the behest of authorities in govern-ment agencies such as the police and the military, in state-owned enter-prises and in some non-state enterprises. Indeed, the workplace has been one key 'surface of emergence' of these new psy technologies. For it is in the workplace that human relations staff have sought to deploy the practices of psychological counseling to mitigate the stressful consequences of onerous working conditions, job insecurity, and the anger generated by poor wages. As we have seen, prior to the economic reforms, the *danwei* or work unit was the locus of most forms of support for individuals and families, from hous-ing and childcare to health and advice. In today's marketized and urbanized China, where offices and factories are the workplaces for the majority of Chi-nese adults, these support mechanisms have to be provided in other ways, and the workplace has become the site both for the appearance of many of these problems of living—experiences of sub-acute physical problems, anx-ieties, and the absenteeism and 'presenteeism' that result[29]—and for their therapeutic amelioration. As in Japan, where the increasing rates of mental ill health attributed to workplace stress have become a major public issue (Targum and Kitanaka, 2012; Kitanaka, 2016), psychotherapists and coun-selors in the workplace exist in the tension between care for the individual and maximization of productivity for the enterprise. Teaching the skills of well-being and stress management not only symbolizes an institution that cares for its employees, not only often offers some self-technologies through which individuals may be able to improve their personal lives, but also, or so it is hoped, reduces the costs to the enterprise of illness and low productivity. The genealogy of 'human relations' in China has its own characteristics and is undoubtedly distinct because of the highly politicized endeavor to create profitable market-based enterprises; nonetheless, as at an earlier moment in Europe and the United States, "psycho-social expertise has acquired a vital place in the diverse attempts to link individuals subjectively and emotionally to their productive activity" (Miller and Rose, 1995: 457).

Measuring and Managing Migrant Mental Health

Finally, let us return to migrant life. Are migrant workers among those being diagnosed with depression or anxiety and prescribed psychiatric drugs? Are they consumers of psy expertise, either in person or via their smartphones? Is their mental health being monitored and managed in the workplace? If we think of migrants as a 'reserve army of labor' in traditional Marxist terms, we would not expect their mental states, no matter how bad, to become a matter of concern to authorities: the constant supply of migrant labor ensures that there are always many others to replace those who fall by the wayside, and whose irregular conditions of employment mean that they can easily be dispensed with, cast back into the city and thence to return to the villages from whence they came. However, as we have seen from discussion of events at Foxconn, things are not so simple. The mental health of migrants, at least as it impacts upon the urban factories that employ so many, has indeed become a matter of concern.

Over recent years, psychiatric epidemiologists in China have come to identify the mental health of the rural-urban migrant as something to be researched, even if their lives outside the workplace have not yet become a key focus of organized therapeutic intervention. Researchers have sought to document, if not explain, the mental health consequences of migration from the countryside to the towns. This work "has been particularly focused on the comparison with the population in their hometown or host society, and the effects of different dimensions of social exclusion as stressors" and particular attention has been paid to the *hukou* system (Li and Rose, 2017: 21). The results do not present a clear picture. While one synthesis of the research on the mental health of Chinese migrants suggested that they experienced a greater severity of most psychiatric symptoms than the general population (Zhong, Liu, et al., 2016), a second, more recent synthesis painted "a complex and contradictory picture, both for the mental health status of migrants in relation to non-migrant residents in their locality, and for migrant mental health status in relation to their rural counterparts" (Li and Rose, 2017: 22): some studies showed migrants had better mental health than did those from the areas from where they migrated, but others showed the reverse, depending on the scales used, the nature of the comparison, the regions and cities in question, and much more.

These differences are not surprising, given the variations in the migrant journey and experience that we have already discussed, the dates of the surveys, the particular population of migrants surveyed, the diverse scales and measures used to assess mental health or psychiatric symptomatology, and the circumstances in which the assessment was made—in a migrant's own quarters, a professional's office, or, in some cases, in a room in a factory with managers looking on. Nonetheless, Li and Rose suggest that we can glean something from this research: dimensions of social exclusion, such as limited access to labor rights and social stigma from their host communities, when these were explicitly specified and analyzed, did have negative consequences for migrant mental health, as did aspects of migrants' own self-identity, such as their perception that they were 'outsiders' and distinct from 'locals.'

Following that review by Li and Rose, our colleagues in the School of Public Health at Fudan University carried out a number of studies using conventional mental health measures, and they did indeed find that these showed higher levels of mental ill health among migrants in China.[30] Thus, a survey of 3,286 workers in work units in Shanghai using a number of standardized scales found that migrant workers had a slightly higher prevalence of depression than non-migrant workers, with a notably poor mental health among participants over age forty-five (Li, Dai, et al., 2019).[31] A cross-sectional study of 3,038 migrants conducted in five cities from June 2017 to Spring 2018—Shanghai, Zhengzhou, Xinzheng, Xingyang, and Baoji—found that there was a strong relationship between subjective well-being and high levels of perceived social cohesion, and that the relationship between perceived social exclusion and poor mental health was much higher than that of their counterparts (Zhu, Gao, et al., 2019). A further study of 4,648 migrants to Shanghai recruited from five factories and public places in different districts in Shanghai found that "Chinese migrant workers who were younger, had insufficient self-rated income, had worse self-reported health, used alcohol and were unmarried had a high risk of mental health disorders" (Wang, Chen, et al., 2019: S45).[32] These results undoubtedly suffered from the kinds of methodological problems we remarked on earlier, in their use of a range of scales and measures, and in the sites in which the questionnaires were administered and the assessments were made. Nonetheless, the results from migrants' self-assessments are suggestive: perhaps what is happening here is that the surveys and scales are translating the everyday experience of hardship, and the tensions of the migrant life, into the language and diagnostic categories of psychiatry. Hence the findings point beyond the bare statistics to the need to explore the experiences of the migrants themselves and how they viewed their own situation.

Did these migrant factory workers themselves feel the pressure of their precarious working circumstances, of their fraught relations with the 'locals,' of the dislocation from the settled lives that they could have lived back in their villages? Are their contemporary experiences similar to those described by Pun and Chan, who paint a bleak picture of suffering and exploitation, relieved only, for some, by overt, or somatized, acts of resistance? Or was the experience more like that described by Bao-Liang Zhong and colleagues, who carried out focus groups with a number of urban migrant workers in Shenzhen: stress—work-related stress, family-related stress, financial stress, and the stress of feeling that they did not belong in the city that they now inhabited (Zhong, Liu, et al., 2016). The troubles expressed by members of those focus groups were not framed in the language of mental health, but neither were they framed in the language of subjugation and resistance. People complained of the effects of noise, traffic, crowds, polluted air, and strange tasting water, and ascribed various medical conditions to them. They complained about the harshness of their working environments, strict discipline, and penalization of those who violated regulations on time or output quota. They worried about their parents left behind in their home villages and about their children's academic performance. And they felt the burden of the demands placed on them by the need to provide financial support for their family back home. Many mentioned their feelings of distance from other urban dwellers, not least because they were often forced to move from city to city. As one man put it, having done more than twenty jobs in many different cities: "For many, many years, in many many cities, I work, I get fired, I start a new job again, and I get fired again . . . I look like someone loses his heart, work here, work there, come here, and go there. . . . I never know when there is an end to my wandering" (ibid.: 10). For Bao-Liang Zhong and colleagues, the common theme here was "acculturative stress" caused by the disjuncture between the natural environment of rural existence and that of the city, the disparity between agricultural production and factory work, and the conflict between traditional Confucian values of loyalty to family and modern urban individualism—people no longer felt that they belonged either in their home villages or in the cities to which they had migrated. Their unmet psychological needs, concluded the authors, should be dealt with by specialized mental health services for migrants, focused on "dynamic evaluation of rural-urban acculturative stress and health education on stress management, and, when necessary, individual psychosocial assessment and treatment" (ibid.: 12).

Whether such a 'psychologization' of the ailments of migrant workers is desirable or not, we saw few signs of it in own research in Shanghai. Indeed, the issue of migrant mental health hardly featured at all in the priorities of either healthcare professionals or public health researchers, despite the fact that around one-third of the city's population at any given time was made up of rural-urban migrants. It is true that some migrants who were perceived as disturbing public order were hospitalized.[33] In the 1990s, as Lu and colleagues suggest, you "had to behave quite 'crazily' in order to gain access to medical care, and so most migrant workers in that period remained silent sufferers" (Lu, Lee, et al., 1999: 102). However, even then, 'socially intolerable' behavior did result in hospitalization, usually with a diagnosis of 'schizophreniform psychosis,' and often treated with chlorpromazine.[34] But because migrants lacked health insurance, and employers were unwilling to pay for extended treatment, they were often discharged from hospital against medical advice—while it is not clear what then happened to them, in the absence of any other community treatment it is likely that they were fired from their jobs and returned to their villages (ibid.: 102). More recent studies, however, show that migrant workers do have a higher risk of hospitalization than non-migrants. For instance, a study of patients hospitalized with acute schizophrenia at four psychiatric hospitals in Changsha, in Hunan Province, showed that "Chinese migrant workers, especially women and older male migrant workers, have higher risk of hospitalization for schizophrenia, and greater severity of symptoms once hospitalized, than local residents" (Zhu, Hu, et al., 2018: 97), no doubt because, as in the earlier studies, most migrants lack insurance coverage and delay access to formal mental health services for as long as they can.

Outside hospitalization, it seemed to us that migrants rarely, if ever, made use of the services of the Shanghai Mental Health Centre, which provided 'out-patient' mental health services from assessment to medication monitoring. There were drop-in sessions one afternoon a fortnight in some of the Health Centers in the areas where migrants lived, but it was not clear how widely such sessions were publicized, and they seemed to be sparsely used. And while migrants made such extensive use of their mobile phones that some researchers have identified a high level of 'problematic smartphone use' bordering on addiction, and suggested that usage might be linked to one or other mental health diagnoses (Wang, Lan, et al., 2019), there is little evidence that Shanghai migrants used their phones to access psychological support; rather it seems that smartphones were used to call friends, access social networks and social media, to surf the internet, play games and watch videos.

It is not as if migrants to Shanghai, especially those of younger ages, were unconcerned about the effect of migration on their mental lives. Thus, for the adolescents aged around seventeen and eighteen who participated in the study of perceptions of health and health-seeking behavior conducted by Chunyan Yu and colleagues in a migrant community in Shanghai in 2011, mental states were certainly an issue (Yu, Lou, et al., 2019).[35] "Nearly every adolescent talked about frustration, low self-esteem, mood swings and other issues related to mental health when being asked about their prominent health challenges," they report, and indeed they quote one adolescent as saying that mental health would be their priority for "a program to improve the well-being of floating adolescents in this community" (ibid.: 342). Not that this young woman was very clear about the problem with mental health, although she was apparently wiping tears when she explained that: "Life is really had for migrant parents and it would definitely affect their children . . . Parents are tired and kids would feel unhappy every time when they see their parent's fatigue" (ibid.: 342). Another young woman, enumerating the health problems that migrants have, said "the first one should be smoking, second is violence, and the third is psychological problems" (ibid.: 343). However, the young people interviewed believed that mental health was a personal matter; they were reluctant to seek support from counselors or use community facilities, especially if they involved traveling from their own neighborhood. Those working in factories believed they would get no help from their employers even for physical injuries, let alone for mental health issues, and fear of discrimination meant they were very unwilling to approach any formal health services. Both subjectively and structurally, for good or for ill, they were excluded from the expanding realm of 'therapeutic governance' in China.

Let us return to the Tongli Road, where our collaborators Lisa Richaud and Ash Amin carried out part of the ethnography that was part of our wider study of mental health and migration to the Chinese megacity. As we have already mentioned, the situation of the migrants in Tongli Road in late 2016 was one of great uncertainty, constant change and insecurity, not just because of the normal migrant experiences of demanding but insecure working conditions, low wages, and so forth, but also because the policies that sought to move urban labor 'up the value chain' required sustained efforts to reduce the low-skilled migrant population by outlawing the factories that attracted and employed them.[36] Following the destruction of the factories that had brought so many to the Tongli Road and provided the wages that they would spend there, one shopkeeper commented to Richaud and Amin: "There used to be so many people around here, you couldn't even walk through the street, but now business is no good, everybody has left." As Richaud and Amin report, "over and again, as we walked from one shop to another in June 2017, we heard of the 'pressure' (*yali*) caused by economic collapse and existential uncertainty. Yet revealingly, we also heard of the futility of fretting and feeling low. We witnessed the persistence of routines and lively sociality alongside and within uncertainty, confirming our sense that the destructions, laid over years of tough living as rural-to-urban migrants, fell short of generating sustained and severe mental distress" (Richaud and Amin, 2020: 78).

The remaining inhabitants of Tongli Road were thus not passive in the face of the destruction of their previous way of life. Despite the fact that "for the many rural-to-urban migrants living, working in, or running a business in the neighborhood, everyday life has unfolded since amidst fields of rubble," our colleagues did not find an outbreak of symptoms of stress-related disorders, anxiety, depression, and the like. And despite the undoubted feelings of pressure and strain that they experience, the remaining inhabitants of Tongli Road did not look to the internet psy experts for advice and guidance as to how they should manage their mental health in these situations of 'pressure' and uncertainty. Everyday practices of endurance and fortitude seemed to prevail. Despite references to 'pressure' (*yali*), the management of the everyday was made up by a range of mundane activities—playing cards, joking with others, filling empty time, but not dwelling on one's misfortune: downplaying bad moods with a view that "dwelling on one's suffering was of little help" (Richaud and Amin, 2019: S11). Thus, the inhabitants of Tongli Road adopted a variety of minor tactics to manage themselves in the present in the face of an undecidable future: "'small scale,' and 'barely perceptible' practices of endurance producing moments of being that potentially enable those who find themselves stuck in a destroyed yet still place to feel and act otherwise" (Richaud and Amin, 2020: 79). It is not, of course, that they were unaware of the challenges they might face at any moment: uncertainty is a constant topic of conversation. They certainly say that they feel pressure, but they suppress distress, "swallow it back into their heart" and practice endurance, while finding ways of making life manageable, tolerable, and even sometimes enjoyable notwithstanding the objectively dire situation in which they find themselves.

"Migrant lives," as Lisa Richaud and Ash Amin argue, "are not only lived through difficult experiences and perceptions relating to institutional and material circumstances, social status and belonging, hopes and expectations, or inner deliberations over the 'meaning of migration' . . . The minutiae of the everyday [disturb] easy equations between urban life, stress and mental health, they may well constitute the very site through which migrants learn to negotiate their precarious conditions, rendering them more habitable" (Richaud and Amin, 2019: S12). Reflecting not merely on the situation of these specific migrants but of others, they conclude:

> even for workers in the fast-paced service industry, or for those in the motor factory, where the noise of industrial equipment and the 'squalor' . . . challenge the senses of the newcomer, there is room for adjustment. Habit (*xiguan*) is invoked as a key process through which endurance is forged, as one learns to disattend or dis-sense, as well as to undertake small acts of self-preservation, finding ways to erect boundaries, albeit often porous, between one's body and polluting matters. And, in between moments of fatigue, there are the shared meals with fellow workers, the outings to a nearby shopping area, the evening dance gatherings, the cigarette breaks and all that can offer temporary reprieve. (ibid:. S11)

Perhaps, then, rather than re-interpreting what migrants tell us of their lives in terms of psychological or psychiatric notions of 'mental health,' we would do better to think of the range of techniques for interpreting and managing oneself that are deployed by those living in situations that are uncertain, precarious, and nerve-wracking, making their lives in milieu that are unpleasant, sometimes dangerous, often polluted, and sometimes frankly toxic. The challenge is to understand the ways that subjective states are shaped within these forms of inhabitation through which people, often collectively, make their lives bearable in deeply precarious modes of urban existence replete with biopsychosocial exposures that threaten their bodies and souls.

Migrant experience in China, whether in the factory, the construction site, or in the face of everyday challenges such as those of Tongli Road, thus entails constant states of 'pressure' or, in the words of the resident of Kaula

Bandar (KB) who we quoted in the previous chapter, of 'tension'—a tension that is sometimes so intense that it can injure, and even kill. Would it be legitimate, then, to think of this pressure, this tension, in terms of the English word with so many similar connotations: stress? And if we were to do so, might we not be able to reopen the dialogue among epidemiologists and ethnographers by focusing on the ways in which those in difficult and uncertain situations manage that stress? Surely stress is, if nothing else, a useful way of describing the experience of migrants, and indeed of many if not all those caught up in today's megacities. And surely stress and health are intimately connected. While a little bit of stress might be motivating, who does not find continued stress enervating and exhausting, damaging to both our physical and our mental health? Perhaps, then, stress can provide a helpful route into understanding more about the mental lives of those who move to, are born in, or live in megacities. Indeed, if we wanted to identify the ways that so many laypeople and experts, in India, China, the United States, Europe, and elsewhere, have blurred distinctions between brain, mind, body, and environment, tried to encapsulate the embodied nature of the experience of adversity, as well as the pressures of urban life, we might look no further. Stress, it seems, is both an objective feature of urban life and an experience of almost anyone who lives, works, or tries to travel in megacities. Stress is not just a part of the language with which they describe the feelings of pressure, anxiety, tension, strain, and hassle that pervade urban existence; nor is it only a state of mind, but it is also a state of the body—of blood pressure, hormones, nerves, and neurons. So let us turn to examine the thorny issues that have long surrounded this word that has borne so much explanatory burden: stress.

4

Everyone Knows What Stress Is and No One Knows What Stress Is

"Americans Are Among the Most Stressed People in the World, Poll Finds," read the headline in the *New York Times* on April 25, 2019. Americans, according to this Gallup Poll, "reported experiencing stress, anger and worry at the highest levels in a decade" and were now "among the most stressed people in the world . . . In the United States, about 55 percent of adults said they had experienced stress during "a lot of the day" prior, compared with just 35 percent globally. Statistically, that put the country on par with Greece, which had led the rankings on stress since 2012.[1] A few months before, the report of a survey for the UK's 2018 Mental Health Awareness Week appeared under the headline, "Stressed nation: 74% of UK 'overwhelmed or unable to cope' at some point in the past year." The survey found that "almost three quarters of adults (74%) have at some point over the past year felt so stressed they felt overwhelmed or unable to cope . . . [it] also found that almost a third of people (32%) had experienced suicidal thoughts or feelings because of stress. Meanwhile one sixth of people (16%) said they had self-harmed as a result of feelings of stress."[2]

But what is this 'stress' that is overwhelming so many?[3] Why would people in a country as wealthy as the United States report higher levels of it than people in a much more straitened country, such as Albania?[4] Why should so many people in the United Kingdom feel overwhelmed with stress in 2018, even to the point of contemplating taking their own lives? Of course, most of us think we know what stress is—who has not felt it as we struggle through a crowded daily commute and coped with cancelled trains, as we try to meet the often impossible demands of often precarious work environments, as we juggle the unremitting pings of a hyperconnected world, relentlessly flooded by messages from an ever-growing volume of channels? Everyone knows what stress is. Or do they? In their survey, Gallup assessed stress with one question: *"Did you experience the following feelings during a lot of the day yesterday? How about stress?"* This is, self-evidently, not very specific about what exactly is being assessed. But could we ever assess 'stress' objectively? Could we map its pathways and trace its effects into the body and brain? If we could, would we then find the key to understanding how adverse experiences get under the skin? Could stress research help us get some purchase on the simultaneously neurological, psychological, and sociological experience of living in a city?

There is, as we will see in this chapter, a long history of research on stress, much of which has focused on the stresses of urban life and their implications. This is also a long history of disagreements, false paths, and blighted hopes. No wonder that Hans Selye, probably the best known stress researcher, remarked to reporters that "everyone knows what stress is" and also "no-one knows what it is" (Selye, 1973: 692). Is my stress like your stress? Is stress a result of objective features in the world, or a subjective experience? Is stress a psychological experience or a set of biological processes—or both? Can one speak of stress in the singular, or are there multiple different experiences that can be 'stressors' dependent on one's culture or personality? Is there any experience that cannot be stressful for some people, at some times? Debates about these questions have continued for at least a century. Across these debates, that word, 'stress,' and its cognates have kept their resonance in the everyday language of emotions in almost all countries, even as the biological meaning accorded to stress is constantly reformulated in the course of research. This word thus remains a potent way of pulling together the biological, the psychological, the social, the biographical, and the experiential. Could it create the groundwork for a neurosocial understanding of urban inhabitation where the experience of urban life produces measurable effects, not just corporeal, but psychological and indeed cerebral? Could such an approach not only help us understand the patterns of mental disorder and mental distress among city dwellers, but also ground a new approach to the creation of mentally healthy urban environments?

As we will see in the chapter, we are certainly not the first to ask these questions. We will thus develop our argument through an historical account of the way in which stress has become linked to distress, and especially the ways in which urban stress has been linked to mental distress, in the physiological, psychological and social sciences. We will track the implications drawn from stress research from an early interest in particular forms of behavioral pathology, through the analysis of the mental and psychological consequences of the experience of stress, to its current embodiment in the neurobiology of the 'urban brain.' And we hope, at the end of this journey, that we can begin to identify a way of thinking about neurosociality that can underpin our claims for a new progressive, vitalist, urban biopolitics.

General Adaptation Syndrome

Stress was not the term that was used by Baudelaire, Benjamin, or Simmel, or even the urban explorers of the Chicago School, when they reflected on the impact of the urban experience on the mental lives of migrants to the cities of Northern Europe and the United States. Yet, as Mark Jackson points out in his comprehensive history of stress, the links between stress and disease were being made in the English-speaking world as early as early as the 1870s, with newspapers such as *The Times* suggesting, in 1872, that the apparent increase in deaths from heart disease may have arisen, in part, from the "great mental strain and hurried excitement of these times" (Jackson, 2013: 58). By the early twentieth century, stress figured prominently in the 'energetic' style of thought that underpinned much contemporary physiology, not just in general speculations about the health consequences of modern living, but in specific concerns about the consequences of war on the health of soldiers, and of factory labor on the health of workers. Thus, George Crile (Crile, 1915) argued that stress could give rise to a whole range of pathological manifestations; Clifford Allbutt, William Osler, and William Sadler made links between physical and mental exertion, nervous conditions and heart disease; and D'Arcy Power and Herbert Snow were linking mental troubles to the development of cancer; indeed many came to believe that the link between an individual's life and their physical disorders were, as Jackson puts it, "mediated primarily by the nervous system" (Jackson, 2013: 59ff.).[5]

However, it was Walter Cannon, above all, writing in the early decades of the twentieth century, who laid the foundations for biological thinking about stress for the next fifty years. As John Mason pointed out in 1975, in the first installment of his two-part review of the stress field in the first issue of the *Journal of Human Stress* (Mason, 1975a), Cannon initially used the term 'stress' in a rather casual manner in phrases such as 'great emotional stress,' or 'times of stress' (Cannon, 1914). In subsequent publications, Mason points out, he continued to use similar phrases, such as 'stress of excitement' or 'times of need or stress,' as in "the conventional use of the term 'stress' during that period" (Mason, 1975a: 6). Nonetheless, for Cannon, stress *did* have a more precise biological meaning. He followed Claude Bernard's classic conception of the *milieu interior*: the capacity of the internal environment of the body and its fluids, to compensate for external disturbances, and to maintain an internal equilibrium (Bernard, 1878). Stress, for Cannon, thus indicated a potentially critical disturbance, either emotional or physical, to the mechanisms of checks and balances that managed the body's own regulatory systems: for these physiological processes that maintain the body in its steady state he coined the term *homeostasis*.[6] As Mark Jackson puts it, emotional experiences "comprised a combination of subjective feeling, bodily changes, and instinctive behaviour that was initiated and coordinated centrally by 'the archaic or primitive nervous system' in response to 'great emotional stress', but was executed peripherally by sympathetic stimulation of the adrenal medulla, the thyroid gland, and the liver" (Jackson, 2013: 71).[7] The body itself contained multiple mechanisms for maintaining its dynamic stability in the face of all manner of environmental and emotional stresses, coordinated and regulated by the autonomic nervous system, and largely effected by hormonal cascades. However, when the breaking point was reached, disaster could result.

For Cannon, from his earliest work through his later classic papers such as 'Voodoo Death,' stress was not simply an 'objective' phenomenon. Indeed, it was the culturally shaped subjective perceptions of situations—such as the belief that one has violated a taboo—that initiates and prolongs the disturbance of the sympathetico-adrenal complex that explains the phenomenon. For instance, in explaining the fact that people in some places can indeed be brought to death by being subject to a curse, Cannon writes "'voodoo death' may be real, and . . . may be explained as due to shocking emotional stress—to obvious or repressed terror" (Cannon, 1942: 180). Cannon undoubtedly laid the foundations for stress as a *biological* style of thought. But when most people think about the origins of our contemporary concerns with stress as a biological and hormonal phenomenon, it is another figure that comes to mind—that of the Hungarian-trained doctor who spent most of his working life in Montreal, first at McGill University and then at the University of Montreal: János Hugo Bruno—generally known as 'Hans'—Selye.

Hans Selye did not start his life as a stress researcher—rather, he was trying to discover a new sex hormone (Selye, 1979).[8] But when he administered one potential candidate—an ovarian extract—to rats, he found a 'triad' of pathological changes in his animals—enlargement of the adrenal cortex, atrophy of various lymphatic structures, and bleeding ulcers of the stomach. Selye tried to identify and eliminate the substances that caused these pathological reactions, but to his disappointment he discovered that all sorts of noxious elements—injections of formalin, adrenaline, insulin, extremes of heat and cold, mechanical injury and forced exercise—produced exactly the same changes. According to his own account, this apparent failure suddenly led to a different realization, set out in his letter to the editor of *Nature* in 1936: it appeared that there was what he termed 'a general adaptation syndrome' in his distressed rats—a seemingly identical hormonal response to exposure to a whole variety of noxious agents (Selye, 1936).

This claim—that whatever the external and provoking cause, a similar internal physiological process resulted as the organism's dynamic internal hormonal systems sought to adapt—initiated a burgeoning research program led, most publicly, by Selye himself. Initially based at McGill, Selye moved to the University of Montreal in 1945, where, at one stage, he employed forty assistants and was working with 15,000 laboratory animals on what he now came to term 'the stress response' (Selye, 1956). It seemed that a whole range of pathological conditions could be explained by a process in which "exposure to stress triggered a chain of protective hormonal events that ultimately defeated its own purpose. Intended to preserve functional stability under stress, chronic stimulation of the pituitary-adrenal axis, as it became known, eventually led paradoxically to disease and death" (Jackson, 2013: 115). The physiological non-specificity of the stress response was the key: a similar set of physiological processes was elicited by a whole range of physical or emotional challenges to the organism from the outside world.

At Montreal, Selye was able to expand his group of researchers through the acquisition of many large grants, not just from national research councils and medical institutes, but from medical charities, pharmaceutical companies, and tobacco corporations.[9] He and his colleagues were highly prolific, publishing "over 785 original articles and 12 books" and "pursuing investigations into . . . the properties of cortical steroid hormones; . . . the mechanisms of stress reactions; the development of stress tests; . . . the use of certain compounds such as chlorpromazine, barbiturates and rauwolfia as 'antistress drugs'; and the pathogenesis of endocrine disorders, cancers, hypertension, arthritis and kidney disease" (Jackson, 2013: 147).

Selye's work attracted praise and criticism in more or less equal measure. He had a high public profile, and according to Mark Jackson, he was nominated seventeen times for a Nobel Prize. Yet his critics were fierce, arguing that he was making wild extrapolations about the consequences for human diseases of all manner of pressures, strains, and anxieties, from limited data largely based on animals—rodents—subjected to physical, chemical, or hormonal traumas of various sorts, and that his terminology was constantly shifting, not least in relation to the use of the word stress itself, sometimes as the external and provoking stimulus, sometimes as the internal organic response. Although, by the 1950s, Selye sought to distinguish between 'stressors'—the external agent or event that triggers the response—and the biological stress response itself, the terminology remained slippery. Jackson quotes Ffrangcon Roberts, whose concise assessment predates many similar, but less incisive, critiques: "Therefore stress . . . in addition to being itself and the result of itself, is also the cause of itself" (Roberts, 1950: 105 quoted in Jackson, 2013: 154).

Nonetheless, by the 1950s, the language of stress had become a potent and highly transferable framework for coding the challenges of human conduct in multiple domains: in the military, the factory, in everyday life in the modern world—and in the city. In the United States, Harold Wolff, President of the Association for Research in Nervous and Mental Diseases, who—together with Stewart G. Wolf—became a key figure in US stress research in the 1950s, brought together researchers from many disciplines at a conference in New York in 1949 and co-edited the volume on *Life Stress and Bodily Disease* that resulted (Wolff, Wolf, and Hare, 1950). Its fifty-nine chapters, covering well over a thousand pages, dealt with life stress and disorders of growth and development, diseases of the eye, the airways, the stomach, the colon, the muscles and joints, cardiovascular disease, the skin, and genital and sexual disorders. Wolff summed up the arguments in the closing chapter: "constituted as he is, man is . . . vulnerable because he reacts not only to the actual existence of danger but to threats and symbols of danger experienced in his past, which call forth reactions little different from the assault itself" (ibid.: 1059). Thus, he suggests that an array of different medical conditions arise from the protective reaction evoked by the perception of such threats or symbols when sustained over long periods of time, although noting that they are responded to in different ways depending on culture, character, and constitution. For Wolff and his colleagues, the fact that stress was simultaneously bodily, symbolic, cultural, and social was exactly why it helped conceptualize the relations between the form of life of the individual and the forms of their diseases. But these same advantages of the language of stress are also, all too often, disadvantages. Stress seems to be the key to all the ailments that human flesh is heir to; stress is the cause, and also the consequence; stress is a response to an actual situation but is also infused with meaning from personal biography and cultural symbols—and so on.

Locating Stress

Wolff and his colleagues make copious references to the significance of 'life stress' and 'life situations.' Yet these stresses and situations are seldom discussed in detail and there are no references to the city or urban life. Surprisingly, there is also little discussion of mental health. It is true that this massive collection contains a chapter by Mandel Cohen and Paul White subtitled 'anxiety neuroses, neurasthenia and effort syndrome.' But the main title of this chapter is "Life situations, emotions and neurocirculatory athenia," and the overwhelming problem for the physician is taken to be differentiating the complaints of breathlessness, chest discomfort, dizziness, faintness, and 'anxiety attacks' (scare quotes in original) from other medical diagnoses. Indeed, although the patients themselves characteristically ascribe their symptoms to emotion-provoking situations, military service, and so forth, the authors remark that these correlations have not been verified; after thirty pages of detailed presentation of all manner of physiological tests, they conclude that "The cause and specific treatment of the disorder are as yet unknown" (Cohen and White, 1953: 865).

Others working at about the same time were less circumspect about the reality of the mental conditions brought about by stressful experiences, and more specific about the 'life situations' that were involved. War posed one obvious set of problems that were amenable to stress research. From the 1940s onward, military research in the United States explored why certain men can stand up under the stress and strain of combat, while others suffer from neuropsychiatric disorder as a result of their experiences (Needles, 1945). Stress in military personnel during the Korean War was discussed at a symposium at the Walter Reed Army Medical Centre in 1953 (Davis, Elmadjian, et al., 1953; Davis, 1956) and studied through measures of corticosteroid levels (Howard, Olney, et al., 1955), though Selye's work was not cited. A number of experimental studies followed (reviewed in Pronko and Leith, 1956), for example, seeking to examine the ways that behavior sometimes disintegrated under stress.[10] Stress also found its place in studies of the malaise of work—an area that had long been concerned with questions of the adaptation and maladaptation of the factory worker: in 1952, Lawrence Hinkle and Norman Plumber "published the results of an investigation into life stress and absenteeism amongst 1,297 female employees of the New

York Telephone Company" claiming to show that stress both at home and at work contributed to absenteeism by increasing both physical and psychiatric disease (Hinkle and Plummer, 1952: quoted from Jackson 2013: 157–158).

But if war and work were two key places where stress emerged as a problem in the context of the challenges of managing human conduct, the city was not far behind. In 1944, the epidemiologist Jerry Morris and his long-time friend, the social researcher, Richard Titmuss, collaborated on a paper about the reasons for increasing mortality in peptic ulcer—published in the *Lancet* (Morris and Titmuss, 1944).[11] They would go on to be recognized as major figures in their respective disciplines: Titmuss is generally credited with founding the discipline we now call social policy, while Morris's textbook, *Uses of Epidemiology* (Morris, 1957) ,was for some decades the standard text in preventative medicine. In the 1940s, the two were in an early stage of what would be a lengthy collaboration in a relatively new specialty, 'social medicine'—and peptic ulcer, a kind of open sore affecting the lining of the stomach, turned out to be a very suitable case for setting out what it might achieve (see Oakley, 2007).

Mortality from peptic ulcer had been getting worse since before the Second World War (recall, this is 1944), and had increased even further since (Morris and Titmuss, 1944: 841). However, this increase seemed, on the face of it, not just the unfortunate fact of more pathological cases of ulcer, rather it was more rooted in historical circumstance and social change: relative income, for example, seemed to have an effect on morbidity (the poor got it worse, and earlier); so too did being subject to heavy air attacks, the experience of social change (security of employment seemed to matter), and so on. But perhaps the most striking finding of the paper was geographic: male mortality in urban areas was more than double that in rural—and, further, this effect declined with population density: men of age forty in London showed the same morality as men of age sixty in country districts (ibid.: 843). These effects, Morris and Titmuss argue, "clearly demonstrate the importance of metropolitan life" in peptic ulcer mortality (ibid.: 845). Such a finding, they continue, "is in harmony with the modern picture of peptic ulcer as being often a *psychosomatic* disorder (ibid., our emphasis). Treatment, after all, is hardly likely to be worse in cities. Something else must be at stake. But what? Here we quote these pioneers of social medicine at some length:

If, as social physicians, we keep a weather eye open for new nervous strains and stresses that may be contributing to the obstinate increase of this disorder, the most glaring, it must be admitted, are associated with urban and industrial life. The managerial revolution, speed-up in the factory and on the road, the fungus growth of examinations, the squeezing out of the small shopkeepers all assist in making up what Ryle calls "the mental and physical fret and stress of civilised city life" . . . the restless, energetic and the ambitious types who make up a substantial fraction of the ulcer population will be attracted to the cities and the cities will drive them relentlessly . . . it is hard to resist the conclusion that urban life nowadays is an ideal soil for the flowering of the ulcer temperament. There is room for much clinicosocial investigation of such interplay of constitutional and environmental forces. (ibid.)

In other words: city life, in its 'mental and physical fret,' imposes a particular form of stress on those who are most frenetic and restless; this stress, through some kind of psychogenic mechanism, then gets into the body, and into the stomach, becoming registered, finally, as an open sore on the flesh. What we see in these stomach ulcers is nothing less than the psychic wounds of the urban form of life.

By the time Morris and Titmuss were writing, the theme of the stressful city was almost a cliché; the city seemed obviously to be a 'stressful' environment for those who lived and worked in it. But we still have not established what stress actually is, and through what 'psychogenic mechanisms' it gets into the flesh. To explore the answers that have been given to such questions, we need to turn from epidemiological studies on humans, to research on animals—in particular to research on rats. This will lead us to the question of whether stressed rats are models for stressed humans, and hence whether the pathologies of rats under stressful conditions might help one understand how humans can suffer physical symptoms from environmental stressors. The answer to this question became central, not just to arguments about the biology of stress, but also to problems of planning and managing human urban life.

Rat Cities, City Rats

Studies of environmentally stressed rats began, not in Selye's lab in Montreal, but in Curt Richter's laboratory at Johns Hopkins in New York (Schulkin, 2005). Richter moved from Harvard to Johns Hopkins after the behaviorist psychologist John B. Watson resigned following a 'sex scandal' (Scull and Schulkin, 2009). Richter, whose 1921 Ph.D. thesis was on 'The Behavior of the Rat: A Study of General and Specific Activities,' was recruited to Johns Hopkins by Adolf Meyer, whose own commitment to psychobiology was fundamental to the growth of academic psychiatry in the United States during his lifetime but whose influence faded rapidly after his death. Indeed, as Richter points out in his memoir, charmingly entitled 'Experiences of a Reluctant Rat-Catcher,' it was Adolf Meyer, then a newly arrived Swiss neuropathologist, later Professor of Psychiatry and Head of the Phipps Psychiatric Clinic at the Johns Hopkins Hospital and longtime "Dean of American Psychiatry," who first brought laboratory rats from Europe—specifically, from the Department of Zoology at the University of Geneva—to the United States for studies on the brain (Richter, 1968: 403).

Richter proved a meticulous and inventive laboratory researcher working with his favorite model animal. According to Scull and Schulkin, "his first series of publications, appearing between 1921 and 1925, adumbrates themes that would resonate through all his later work, extending even into the 1980s: the determinants of spontaneous activity; the importance of biological clocks; endocrine control of behavior; the origin of the electrical resistance of the skin; brain control of the motor system; and a device to aid in the measurement of salivation" (Scull and Schulkin, 2009: 21). The question of the responses of rats to stress was a recurrent theme in Richter's work; he concludes his discussion of the effects of domestication (by selective reproduction) on the hormonal system of the Norway rat with the hope that studies of this species may "give us data that will help us to study the effects that the controlling of the environment may have on man" (Richter, 1952: 45). And it was, in part, thanks to the work of Selye and Richter on the response of rats to stress that the rat became, for a while, the model for the urban human.

As Ed Ramsden and his colleagues have shown in a series of detailed studies, this recurrent link between rodents and humans was established in the context of a heated debate in the United States about the best way to design for dense habitation in the city (Adams and Ramsden, 2011; Ramsden, 2011; Cantor and Ramsden, 2014; Ramsden, 2014).[12] The figure of the rat was omnipresent. While many thought that the high-rise blocks then favored in programs of urban renewal would displace the disordered streets where people lived 'holed up like rats,' others argued that these new modernist 'machines for living' would produce their own pathologies; in the words of H. L. Menken, "when they begin to live in houses as coldly structural as step-ladders they will cease to be men, and become mere rats in cages" (Menken, 1931: 165, quoted in Adams and Ramsden, 2011).

But the rat was not merely a metaphor adopted to debate the best and worst forms of urban living in the 1930s and 1940s. As Christine Keiner put it, "[h]istorians of technology, biology public health and the environment have lavished attention on the new chemicals developed to fight mosquitoes and lice, but have neglected the less famous, non-insect pest of World War II: rats!" (Keiner, 2005: 119).[13] On the one hand, thousands of US troops contracted rat-borne diseases in the South Pacific, leading also to the fear that rats might be used in germ warfare "as vectors to spread the plague." On the other hand, according to Keiner, it appeared that rats were a significant economic burden on the US economy: the annual cost of rodent damage in the United States in the 1940s was estimated at US$200 million. It was in this context that Baltimore was chosen as the site for one of the first citywide experimental rat-control efforts, and the person charged with overseeing it was Curt Richter (Richter, 1968).[14]

Richter had spent much time in the 1930s studying how a rodent's selection of foodstuffs was determined by taste, and eventually alighted on a substance called phenyl thiourea which was tasteless but lethal to domesticated rats, although wild rats could taste it and so avoided it. His technicians examined many variants of this compound and eventually found one, ANTU (α-naphthylthiourea), that was both tasteless and toxic to *wild* rats—in fact specifically to the Norwegian rat (*Rattus norvegicus*), which had become the most common rat species in urban areas in the United States as well as in most of the rest of the world. Richter was put in charge of what eventually became a Baltimore citywide program to bait and trap rats—with the quid pro quo that he could keep some of the rats for his own laboratory experiments. But while the results were initially promising, it soon became clear that the rats eventually developed the ability to detect the toxic substance and so avoid the poisoned bait; the population of rats resurged, and indeed grew back to its original level.

That regrowth of population to a stable original level turned out to be important, hinting that there might be some 'ecological' factors that limited population size. When poisoning proved to have its limits, a new project was begun at the Johns Hopkins School of Hygiene and Public Health, which aimed to expand the research started by Richter but now took an 'ecological' approach. The Rodent Ecology Project sought to explore whether the relation between population density, territoriality, and aggression could itself be an effective means of controlling rat populations. In his account of the origins of the idea that aggressive behavior can regulate population size, David E. Davis (Davis, 1987) identifies the work of two individuals working in Baltimore as central: John B. Calhoun and John Christian. Calhoun had joined the Johns Hopkins School of Hygiene in 1946 to study the behavior of colonies of Norway rats in various sizes and types of pens, starting from the question of what limited the size to which the rat populations grew. It was not food, nor was it obvious predation. It might therefore, he reasoned, have something to do with the frequency of contacts between individuals. But rather than studying this in the wild, where there were too many uncontrolled variables, Calhoun "decided to set up a pilot experiment, borrowing some of the techniques of laboratory sciences, in order to study the role of distribution of availability of food and harborage on the growth of a population of rats" (Calhoun, 1950: 113).

Calhoun enclosed a small number of rats in a compound and provided them with all that they needed for their healthy survival: he had anticipated that this would be a 'rat utopia,' but the behavior that emerged produced something very different. As John Adams and Ed Ramsden describe it:

> As the community grew into a "rat city," this became increasingly problematic. Dominant rats were able to secure territories in the corners of the pen, where they lived relatively normal lives with a "harem" of females. Crowding elsewhere prevented the emergence of dominance hierarchies, ensuring that the rats' lives were marked by constant violence, struggle, and disruption. Thus, it was Calhoun's rat city that allowed ecologists to observe directly, and for the first time, the potential of hierarchy, territoriality, and competition for reducing rat numbers. (Adams and Ramsden, 2011: 665)

In a series of additional 'rodent cities' that Calhoun built after moving to the psychology laboratories of the National Institute of Mental Health in 1954, the 'rodent universe'—now also populated with mice—was divided and configured to mimic stereotyped aspects of the human urban environment: relatively spacious cells in high-rise apartments occupied by dominant males with female mates, alongside extremely crowded conditions that Calhoun deliberately created through specific feeding practices. These highly crowded locations seemed to aggravate the kinds of pathological behavior that mirrored the fears of bourgeois urban citizens in the 1950s: aggression, hypersexuality, homosexuality, withdrawal. Calhoun coined the potent term 'behavioral sinks' to characterize the locations that produced these effects on his rats. If rats were models for humans, the dire consequences of high population density in particular parts of American cities seemed plain to see; reciprocally there was now a biological explanation for aggression, sexual license, and all sorts of immoral conduct in the enticing but dangerous zones of the inner city.

At this point, according to Davis, the team at Johns Hopkins drew on research from John Christian on hormonal feedback mechanisms, following which Christian began to work with the Hopkins team.[15] In his 1950 article in the *Journal of Mammology*, 'The Adreno-Pituitary System and Population Cycles in Mammals,' Christian focused on the phenomenon of 'die off' that afflicted many mammal populations once they reached a certain size. Simply put, at a certain level of population, many individual creatures start to die despite the fact that no infections or pathogenic organisms can be found. It is worth quoting his conclusion at length:

> The onset of symptoms, terminating in convulsions, shows a similar pattern in every case, and all would appear to be hypoglycemic in nature. All authors pointed to the increased susceptibility to stress . . . In searching for a common cause for these changes we find that Selye's adaptation syndrome . . . provides us with an answer to the problem. In other words we are probably dealing with the symptoms of adrenal exhaustion on a population-wide basis . . . The adaptation syndrome is the sum of the non-specific physiological and morphological responses to stress other than the specific adaptive reactions (such as sero-logic reactions to specific antigens). Selye has divided these into (1) shock, (2) counter-shock (these two combined are the "alarm reaction"), (3) resistance, and (4) exhaustion phases. Here we are probably dealing with the exhaustion phase, where the animal is no longer able to react to added stress after long, continued stresses, and the whole mechanism breaks down. (Christian, 1950: 250)

As Ramsden points out: while John Christian did not conduct research on humans himself, he was certainly willing to speculate about the human—and specifically urban—implications. For example, in invited lectures that he gave on the CBS television series *The House We Live In*—in which the landscape architect and ecological thinker, Ian McHarg, invited "prominent theologians and scientists of the day to discuss the human place in the world"[16]—he reflected on the ways in which the planned housing development would curtail outlets for the emotions, and speculated that this would limit the growth of human populations "as happened with the experimental animals" (Adams and Ramsden, 2011: 739). Indeed, according to Adams and Ramsden, architects and planners in the United States in the 1960s, faced with the repeated outbreaks of urban unrest and apparent breakdown of civic values in the heart of many of their great cities, turned to the behavioral sciences, and to "the crowding studies of Christian and Calhoun" to argue that such problems arose because cities had not been designed "in accordance to humanity's biological needs as a mammal" (ibid.: 736). For many sociologists and behavioral scientists, the implications of the links between density and pathology that were demonstrated in these rat cities seemed almost self-evident.

However, as it developed in the following decade, the extensive sociological literature on the psychological and behavioral consequences of urban density and crowding reveals much disagreement as to its individual and social consequences. For example, Jonathan Freedman explored crowding and density in relation to a range of urban problems such as aggression and personal space, but doubted the extrapolations from animal studies to humans and concluded that crowding itself was neither good nor bad, but that it intensified the effects of preexisting good or bad social conditions (Freedman, 1975). Galle and Gove took a different view (e.g., Galle, Gove, et al., 1972): drawing heavily on the results of Calhoun's rat studies they argued that the relation between crowding and pathology was not a direct and unequivocal one, but it was mediated by "the subjective experience of overcrowding" (Gove, Hughes, et al., 1979: 62).[17]

Not all urban sociologists accepted lessons from the rat studies. Many argued that, in fact, the evidence ran in quite the opposite direction, that the rodent experiments were no model for humans, and that what had emerged was "a modern folk myth about the evils of crowding" (Porteous 1977: 176, quoted from Adams and Ramsden, 2011: 748). Indeed, urban density had its strong proponents: notably Jane Jacobs and William Whyte. As Jacobs put it, in *The Death and Life of Great American Cities*: "High dwelling densities have a bad name in orthodox planning and housing theory. They are supposed to lead to every kind of difficulty and failure. But in our cities, at least, this supposed correlation between high densities and trouble, or high densities and slums, is simply incorrect, as anyone who troubles to look at real cities can see" (Jacobs, 1972: 202). The word 'stress' does not appear in Jacobs's account of what makes cities great; crowds and strangers do not mean stress, but are rather the eyes on the street that keep a person safe, the source of a certain vitality and unpredictability.

William Whyte, by contrast, based his conclusions concerning the problems of the city on sixteen years of "walking the streets and public spaces of the city and watching how people use them." His first studies "were concerned with density":

They had to be. In the late sixties and early seventies the specter of over-crowding was a popular worry. High density was under attack as a major social ill and so was the city itself. 'Behavioral sink' was the new pejorative. The city was being censured not only for its obvious ills but for the compression that is a condition of it. (Whyte, 1988: 4)

White considered that the utopias that were proposed as alternatives were also underpinned by rodent studies of density, notably "the work of Dr. John Calhoun of the National Institutes of Health" (ibid.). He also derided "university studies on the effects on people of different space configurations, such as how twenty people in a circle in room A performed a task as compared with the same number performing the same task in a square in room B" or those that tried "to monitor people's physiological responses as they were shown pictures of different spaces, ranging from a crowded street to a wilderness glade (ibid.).

For Whyte, the problem with studies of rats and university students was that the research was "vicarious . . . once or twice removed from the ultimate reality being studied. That reality was people in everyday situations." And when one studies people in everyday situations, one discovers that they find all sorts of unplanned ways to make use of the city and its street corners, ledges, pavements. It was not crowding that was the problem, but the emptiness of the streets at the center of great cities, he argued, for the street is "the river of life of the city, the place where we come together, the pathway to the center" (Whyte, 1988: 7) and in fact so many American cities have emptiness, rather than crowds, chaos, and confusion, at their core. Density, in short, was not the problem; indeed, when one actually examined how people made use of city space, the link between crowded streets and neighborhoods and stress was hard to sustain.

The Meaning of Urban Stress

The language of stress seemed to enable conversations across disciplinary boundaries and to link together multiple problems associated with city planning and urban life. Yet many questions remained about its meaning and implications. In 1956, in an attempt to resolve some of these issues, John Calhoun, together with Leonard Duhl, a social psychiatrist, brought together a group of leading biologists, psychologists, sociologists, and urban planners who would meet twice a year for the following twelve years (Duhl, 1963).[18] Duhl adopted what he called an "ecological approach" to mental health—"the study of the multiple factors of the environment that affect the normal development and behavior of the individual and society" (Ramsden, 2014: 293). The specific aim of the work of this 'Committee on Physical and Social Environmental Variables as Determinants of Mental Health'— colloquially known as 'the Space Cadets'—was to provide scientifically based advice to policymakers, architects, and planners on the design of buildings and space to promote mental health.

Stress was, once again, the key. It seemed to link bodies and populations, individuals and environments, physiology and behavior, to reach across the boundaries of social and biomedical sciences and city planning, and to connect with so-called urban renewal policies. The central theoretical framework was that of overload; as Ramsden puts it, "excessive and unwanted social interaction, mediated through a range of social, psychological and physical factors, could result in *crowding stress* and its concomitant psychophysiological pathologies" (Ramsden, 2014: 293), but that these stressors could be mitigated with the support of social networks, peer groups, and subcultures that inhabited specific urban spaces. The language of stress facilitated debate and enabled conversation across disciplinary boundaries, linking the arguments of those who prioritized the physical environment with those who prioritized the social environment, and those who emphasized the role of subjective perceptions as opposed to objective situations. But stress-based ways of thinking could also serve radically opposing agendas; they supported the arguments of those who thought policies should focus on individual psychological issues in mental ill health, as well as those who argued for the need to address the roots of problems of mental ill health in social inequality, poverty, segregation, and discrimination.

The problematics of stress were, of course, not specific to the United States. As Robert Kirk and others have pointed out, in Britain, as elsewhere, by the 1950s, it had become "fashionable to assert" that there was "an increase in the incidence of mental disorders and that the cause of this is the increased stress of modern life," and some medical professionals warned that "mental health propaganda" was "instilling a phobia for the inevitable stresses of life" (Kirk, 2014: 241).[19] Here too, the language of stress appeared to link the concerns of clinicians, biologists, physiologists, endocrinologists, psychiatrists, psychologists, and sociologists—although at the price of significant uncertainty. Kirk draws our attention to one exemplary meeting, in July 1958, when the Mental Health Research Fund organized a conference aiming to "arrive at a synthesis of the concepts used in different branches of the behavioral sciences when discussing stressful effects." Held at Oxford

University, the conference hosted prominent participants, including "the psychiatrists Aubrey Lewis, W. Linford Rees, and Martin Roth; the psychiatrist, psychoanalyst, and ethologist John Bowlby; the ethologists and animal behaviorists Robert A. Hinde and Oliver L. Zangwill; the Pavlovian psychobiologist Howard S. Liddell; the cyberneticians William Ross Ashby and W. Grey Walter; and Hans Selye himself" (ibid.: 241). Kirk's conclusions in relation to the "stressed animal" apply more generally: the language of stress enabled something widely discussed in everyday speech to be "codified within an apparently scientific language . . . subjective states such as pain and suffering could now be quantified, each of which in turn allowed ethical concerns previously limited to the realm of political-cum-philosophical rhetoric to be reconfigured as material practices within, and of importance to, the experimental work of the laboratory" (ibid.: 259).

Many were aware of the diversity of meanings of stress, and of the problems of extrapolating from Calhoun's rat cities to actual human urban environments. However, for researchers trying to understand the consequences of urban environments for those who inhabited them, the term proved hard to avoid, and the literature on urban stress developed rapidly. In the UK, many drew on Selye's arguments that reactions to stress were neurohormonally mediated, but also on the belief that such reactions were dependent on subjective perceptions, feelings, and beliefs: they linked stress reactions to organic disorders from gout to cancer as well as to mental illness (see Jackson, 2013: 172ff.). David Glass and Jerome Singer, for example, edited a 1972 volume that brought together a series of laboratory experiments on urban stress, focusing on stress as a psychological reaction to noise and other stimuli, rather than simply an effect of the aversive stimuli themselves—they measured such physiological indices as galvanic skin response and muscle action potentials in reactions to noise, but found that responses were greatly reduced if the individuals believed that they could turn off or control the noise levels, and in any event most individuals soon adapted to such 'stressors' (Glass and Singer, 1972).

Glass and Singer were not alone in rejecting the simplifications that constantly beset stress thinking. Indeed, as early as 1945, reflecting on the consequences of wartime stress, Grinker and Speigel were clear that whether the stimuli of the battlefield had pathological consequences depended on whether individuals perceived them as a stress, and whether they felt confident that the threat posed could be neutralized (Grinker and Spiegel, 1945: 122). The psychologist best known for his work along these lines was Richard Lazarus, who had himself served in the US Army during World War II

(Lazarus, 1998; Lazarus, 2013). For Lazarus, the meaning that an individual gave to an experience resulted from an assessment, often unconscious, of the situation and the threat that it may pose. What was crucial in all cases was not the stimulus itself, but the cognitive *appraisal* that people made of what they perceived (Lazarus, 1966). It was the appraisal that mediated the reaction, and appraisal was an individual psychological process, which reflected "the unique and changing relationship taking place between a person with certain distinctive characteristics (values, commitments styles of perceiving and thinking) and an environment whose characteristics must be predicted and interpreted" (Lazarus and Folkman, 1984: 24), monitoring both subjective stress and autonomic disturbances. Appraisal—primary, secondary, reappraisal—and their links with adaptation and coping became the abiding concerns of the research of Lazarus and his group, consolidated in their work in the UC Berkeley Stress and Coping Project. It was not just that stress itself was the outcome of cognitive appraisal; the belief that one could cope with a situation itself depended on a cognitive appraisal of the extent to which one had the resources to deal with some challenge or event in the environment. The individual thus suffered from stress when they believed that they did not have the resources—of whatever sort—necessary to deal with the threat that event seemed to pose to their own well-being or that of those who they cared about (Lazarus and Folkman, 1984).

Lazarus and his group were far from alone in reframing stress in terms of culturally shaped, and often unconscious, cognitive processes of meaning attribution and threat prediction. Thus, when John Schopler from the Department of Psychology at the University of North Carolina and Janet Stockdale of the London School of Economics worked on stress in the 1970s, they could confidently assert that research had demonstrated that the effects of crowding density in humans—as opposed to the animals studied by Calhoun—depended on multiple cultural factors, on architecture and design, and on the sex of subjects. These studies, they argued, "completely undermine the intuitive assumption, which has been regularly verified by the animal research, that crowding stress is a monotonically increasing function of density": the effects of crowding depended, not on density itself, but on multiple subjective factors such as a desire for privacy or the extent to which contacts with others were deemed inappropriate (Schopler and Stockdale, 1977: 81).

Despite or because of these ongoing disagreements, some researchers continued to explore the links between social, psychological, and biological stress pathways. Sheldon Cohen was one of the most consistent.[20] Over the next four decades, his lab for the Study of Stress, Immunity and Disease at Carnegie Mellon studied "the role of psychological and social factors in health [and focused] on the possibility that our psychological states and traits may influence our immune systems in a manner that might alter our bodies' abilities to fight off infectious disease."[21] The core of this work, according to their own description, was "the identification of the behavior and biological pathways that can account for relations between psychosocial factors and susceptibility to infectious illness." Cohen also developed a number of widely used scales for measuring 'perceived stress' and used those in research on the effects of environmental stress in multiple areas, for example on 'task performance' (Cohen and Lezak, 1977). His group explored the consequences of interpersonal relations and similar social dynamics on perceived stress. They investigated the biological pathways through which stress was linked to disease, and ways that psychological states and traits influenced the immune system's capacity to resist disease, and the social factors that might mitigate those stress responses. They framed their core question in terms that are now familiar: "how do psychosocial environments get inside our bodies?"

In Canada, Zbigniew Lipowski, who had found his way to Montreal having escaped Nazi-occupied Poland, linked stress research to his own interests in psychosomatic medicine. Working at the Department of Psychiatry at McGill, Lipowski proposed that the stresses caused by an overload of conflicting information were "far-reaching for contemporary youth and contribute to the alienation, unrest, and confusion which is common among them. This conclusion calls into question the capacity of the affluent society to survive the psychosocial complications of its own making" (Lipowski, 1971: 467). These 'psychosocial complications' of an overload of information and sensation were studied in depth in the United States, the health effects of the daily stressful commute being a constant theme (Bellet, Roman, et al., 1969; Singer, Lundberg, et al., 1974; Lundberg, 1976; Schaeffer, Street, et al., 1988), as were comparative studies of rural and urban stress that used the number of prescriptions of psychiatric drugs as their measure (Webb and Collette, 1979). Lipowski himself, who was to become a key figure in psychosomatic medicine, focused on the relations between individual differences and life events (Lipowski, 1985). As he put it in 1977, psychosomatic medicine asked "why a person responds to particular social situations and specific life events with a given pattern of psychological and physiological changes" (Lipowski, 1977: 136).

Lipowski believed that psychosomatic medicine was making a "spectacular comeback" and that a holistic and ecological approach to mental disorders had triumphed: it seemed to mark "the twilight of the golden age of reductionism, of an intolerant and narrow approach to the study and treatment of disease" (Lipowski, 1977: 71). This assessment proved to be premature. As far as stress itself was concerned, perhaps the situation was stated most clearly by Amos Rapoport, another Polish emigre whose work focused on the importance of culture in the built environment and architecture. In a special issue of *Urban Ecology* on 'quality of life' in 1978, Rapoport argued that a subjective perception of particular urban features and cues modulated the stress relationship. Stress, he argued, "impairs psychological functioning or causes a deterioration in goal-oriented tasks . . . it occurs when the organism's homeostatic mechanisms are unable to maintain a state of dynamic equilibrium." Three different elements are at stake: environmental stimuli, organismic factors, and cultural variables. Rapoport pointed out that individuals actively sought out environments that had culturally appropriate levels of environmental stress for particular kinds of activities: thus, noise and density might well be stressors to be avoided in a residential area, but they might equally be actively sought out in a theatre district (Rapoport, 1978: 242–243). One is struck, reading Rapoport's paper, by the dizzying complexity of emic and etic factors, defense mechanisms, the role of norms, the stabilizing consequences of hierarchies, the salience of sense of control, symbolism, rituals, and much more. While Rapoport, like so many others, felt that it was important to design urban environments that were stress reducing, it was not clear why, given the layers of complexity that had now been introduced, the usual suspects of urban design–"courtyard cities ('inside-out' cities), low density, green residential areas and urban villages (homogeneous neighborhoods)"—should be the ones to favor (ibid.: 261). By the 1980s, at least when it came to humans, the radical simplicities of Selye's 'a general adaptation syndrome' and Calhoun's rat cities seemed to belong in the past.

Stress and Beyond: Toward the Urban Brain

We have skated rather lightly across a complex history in this chapter: our goal has not been to offer an exhaustive or novel account of the science of stress; rather, it has been to show the waxing and waning of the concept in the middle decades of the twentieth century as it became attached to multiple, often mutually incompatible, scientific, cultural, and architectural agendas. Many researchers in the latter decades of the twentieth century abandoned stress-based hypotheses for the exploration of the psychosocial shaping of human mental disorders precisely because of these complexities, ambiguities, and uncertainties. This was especially the case in psychology. Reviewing the field in 1975, John Mason concluded that while "the popularity of stress concepts has gradually dwindled in the physiological field during the past 15 years . . . the use of stress terminology and concepts has continued to flourish in the psychological and social sciences . . . with the impact of psychosocial influences upon the organism" (Mason, 1975a: 11). Mason, whose own work focused on the relations between the emotions and the endocrine system, argued that one of the major developments in stress research over the preceding twenty years "has been the increasing awareness of the remarkable sensitivity of the pituitary-adrenal cortical system to psychological and social influences even of a relatively subtle nature. It is now known that emotional stimuli rank very high among the most potent and prevalent natural stimuli capable of increasing pituitary-adrenal cortical activity" (Mason, 1975b: 23). Yet the field, in Mason's view, remained traversed by terminological confusion, and by the growing belief that it was, in fact, the psychological factors—that is to say an individual's *perception* of a particular situation—rather than some 'objective' feature of the situation itself that was decisive in provoking a stress response. Far from resolving the issue, it was precisely this question of individual perception, and the explanatory difficulties that it causes, that led Kristian Pollock to argue, a decade after Mason, that stress was a 'modern mythology'—that "the presence of stress can only be inferred back from an outcome which is prejudged to be the result of exposure to stress, the nature of which remains subjective and uncertain" (Pollock, 1988: 385).

Yet stress seems able to resist these recurrent dismissals. New promises of objectivity, new experimental technologies, and new hypotheses about mechanisms have led to stress theories of mental disorder once again achieving prominence. There are now believed to be measurable biological correlates that indicate that a stressor has 'got under the skin.' Further, it seems there are identifiable pathways through which the effects of stress on the immune system and variations in immune responses can be linked both to physical disorders via chronic hormonal changes and to mental disorders via effects on neurotransmitters, neuronal epigenetics, and neurogenesis. The rat returns, once more, as the prime object of neurobiological experiments that, for ethical reasons, cannot be done on humans; for example, it seems that repeated or prolonged stress in laboratory rats "causes functional changes in neural circuitry in the hypothalamus" (Senst and Bains, 2014: 102). Nowhere was this 'objective' basis for the measurement of stress and for its locus of activity more significant than in the study of the mental effects of urban life. It is to this new object of analysis and intervention—the urban brain—that we now turn.

5

The Urban Brain

It is . . . time for an interdisciplinary neurourbanistic approach that connects public mental health to urban planning to create better environments that will improve the mental wellbeing of individuals and communities in cities, and strengthen the resilience of high-risk individuals and children.

—(ADLI, BERGER, ET AL., 2017: 184)

In 2017, a group of German psychiatrists, architects, and urban planners published a letter in *The Lancet* calling for the formation of a new discipline: 'neurourbanism' (Adli, Berger, et al., 2017).[1] Starting from the now familiar refrain about the proportion of the world's population living in cities and the links between urban living and mental health, they called for an inter-disciplinary collaboration between the planning and health disciplines to develop tools that would meet the challenges posed by mental ill health in urban environments. Whether or not one needs a new discipline is not the important issue from our perspective; what is significant is the emergence of a new style of thought, in which 'the urban brain' functions as the meeting point between the citizen and the city. It is worth paying attention to the ways of seeing and thinking that have provoked this uneasy combination, as well as the new forms of intervention that are now being assembled within it.

In much contemporary research in neurobiology, the brain is taken out of its corporeal, interpersonal, social, cultural context and isolated in the laboratory, studied in model animals, and increasingly *in silica*—which is to say, outside its location in time, space, and language (Rose and Abi-Rached, 2013; Mahfoud, McLean, et al., 2017).[2] But what is interesting about the emerging focus on 'the brain' in contemporary urban neuroscience is that brains are *not* imagined as isolated and enclosed organs. Rather, the complex of neural circuits that constitute the brain is understood to develop over time and in space, within an organism that is in receipt of continuous inputs from the environment, not just through the senses but through its interactions with its material environment and with its conspecifics, its encounters with other humans.[3] In this chapter we look in some depth at the contemporary scientific developments that are constituting this urban brain—new modes of visualization, new understandings of stress, recent work on the epigenetic modification of gene expression resulting from environmental exposures, findings on the social modulation of neuroplasticity, research on the role of the 'atmosphere' of the urban or the urban 'sensorium'; and evidence about the biosociality of exposures. We go into this in some detail to show how the urban brain has come to inhabit an explicitly *neurosocial*—even *neuroecosocial*—space of thought and intervention. While we will also point to the ways in which, all too often, the research on the urban brain falls back into various kinds of reductionist neurocentrism—nonetheless, taken together, and transformed through their relations with the social and human sciences, we argue that these new ways of thinking can enable us to re-cast the experience of living in cities as it becomes visible in the body and brain. This will then form the foundation for our final chapter, where we show how a livelier urban biopolitics, a new way of thinking about inhabiting urban space, might *also* be underwritten by this approach.

The Urbanicity Effect

In 1992, a new collaboration was established between researchers at the Institute of Psychiatry in London and the Karolinska Institute in Sweden. As is well known, many Nordic countries have kept meticulous church, census, and other records on their populations since the eighteenth century; this practice then morphed into the Central Population Registers in the 1960s, in which each resident was given a unique personal identification number, making it possible to link together a range of administrative information on each member of the population, including their health data. In their collaboration, the researchers used linked data drawn from the Swedish National Register of Psychiatric Care to challenge the "'geographical drift' hypothesis," that is to say, the argument discussed in a previous chapter that the higher rates of psychosis in certain areas of the inner city arise because schizophrenics drift into these areas "because of their illness or its prodrome" (Lewis, David, et al., 1992: 137). Arguing that most psychiatrists had given too much weight to endogenous genetic factors in schizophrenia and neglected environmental factors, they found that "The incidence of schizophrenia was 1.65 times higher (95% confidence interval 1.19—2·28) among men brought up in cities than in those who had had a rural upbringing," and that this association persisted even when they adjusted for "factors associated with city life such as cannabis use, parental divorce, and family history of psychiatric disorder. This finding cannot be explained by the widely held notion that people with schizophrenia drift into cities at the beginning of their illness." Hence their unequivocal conclusion: "undetermined environmental factors found in cities increase the risk of schizophrenia" (ibid.). These factors, they went on, may have their effects through 'urban stress' along the lines of the 'stressful life events' previously identified in the work of George Brown and Tirril Harris (Brown and Harris, 1978).

By the turn of the century, this 'urban effect' on health had become widely known as *urbanicity*. In 2001, Carsten Bøcker Pedersen and Preben Bo Mortensen, drawing on data on 1.89 million people from the Danish Civil Registration System, classified everyone on a five-level scale of 'urbanization during upbringing' and linked this to the Danish Psychiatric Register— claiming to find what they termed a 'dose response' relation between urbanicity and schizophrenia. They concluded that "[c]ontinuous, or repeated exposures during upbringing that occur more frequently in urban areas may be responsible for the association between urbanization and schizophrenia risk" (Pedersen and Mortensen, 2001: 1039): their candidates for the unhealthy exposures of urbanicity include infections, diet, and exposure to pollution.

Four years later, Lydia Krabbendam and Jim van Os (Krabbendam and Van Os, 2005) agreed that research did not support the 'urban drift' hypothesis and suggested that a significant proportion of the incidence of schizophrenia may be related to as yet unknown environmental factors in urban environments interacting with genetic risk. While many studies offer clues about the key contenders for these environmental factors (drug use, size of social network, neuropsychological impairment, air pollution, childhood social position), Krabbendam and van Os argued that these tend to homogenize the urban environment and failed to recognize small neighborhood variations, the most important of which might be the level of 'social capital' in these small areas. Other groups of researchers developed this line of argument, hypothesizing that high levels of social capital would be present when people find themselves among a community of others who came from similar backgrounds. Perhaps the migrants who suffered most from adversity were those who found themselves in a small minority in their new neighborhood, poorly scaffolded by previous generations of movers. These positive and negative influences are sometimes described as 'the ethnic density effect' (Schofield, Das-Munshi, et al., 2016: 3051). Peter Schofield and his colleagues, for example, once again made use of the unique identity number given to all Danish residents: they linked data from the Danish Civil Registration System, which includes demographic details and links to parents as well as continuous updates on place of residence and vital status, to data from the Danish Psychiatric Central Register, which covers all psychiatric in-patient admissions (Schofield, Thygesen, et al., 2017). And, indeed, they showed that living in an area where there are a large number of fellow migrants was associated with a lower rate of psychosis, while migrants who lived in areas with a low 'ethnic density' had higher rates. Despite the fact that the findings for psychosis did not hold for the so-called common mental disorders, they once more argued that the reasons that high ethnic density was protective against the urbanicity effect was because it was an indicator of 'social capital.'

But what is 'social capital'? The idea seems simple and plausible: if you live in an area where there are shared values, and where you trust your neighbors, that feels supportive, and perhaps it is a kind of 'resource' that you can draw on in times of stress. If you had such a resource, such 'capital,' and found yourself in a stressful situation, others would be around to offer comfort, a shoulder to lean on, giving you a sense that you are less alone with the trouble, providing moral, emotional, and even practical support and so forth. No wonder, then, that a common theme in research on mental health and urbanicity is that high levels of such 'social capital' protect against mental ill health, while low levels amplify it (Ehsan and De Silva, 2015).[4]

The term 'social capital' has a convoluted history, arising on the one hand from Pierre Bourdieu's attempts to suggest that the 'capital' that affected an individual's life chances was not merely economic, but also arose from networks of social relations of mutual recognition, group membership, and the symbolic accoutrements of being a valued member of society, etc. Here social capital "is the sum of the resources, actual or virtual, that accrue to an individual or a group by virtue of possessing a durable network of more or less institutionalized relationships of mutual acquaintance and recognition" (Bourdieu and Wacquant, 1992: 119). The American sociologist, James Coleman, had a similar idea: social capital, he argued, is a set of obligations and reciprocities in networks of persons in social systems, arguing that individuals benefit in many ways from being part of networks of trust and reciprocity (Coleman, 1988). Arising from these twin sources, many others have sought to develop this idea that humans benefit from their embeddedness in groups, and that they suffer when there is an absence of such embeddedness. Soon the simple idea at the basis of this argument began to fragment, and researchers began to argue that there was not just one form of social capital, but a variety—bonding, bridging, linking, cognitive social capital. Unsurprisingly, these were then transmuted into a variety of instruments and scales claiming to measure them. In this process of 'operationalization,' social capital was transformed from a resource that inheres in social relations, culture, and material conditions, to a factor or variable that is 'possessed' by an individual (for helpful reviews, see Almedom, 2005; Moore and Kawachi, 2017).

But is it definitely the case that togetherness is beneficial? As Kawachi and Berkman (Kawachi and Berkman, 2001) point out, perhaps togetherness is important because of a kind of imitation effect, it may be beneficial when one is 'together' with others who espouse healthy or beneficial behavior—but of course, where others espouse unhealthy or dangerous behavior, togetherness might have just the opposite consequences. Extreme togetherness may help mitigate depression, as Brown and Harris found in the Outer Hebrides, but it also can lead to anxiety about whether one is able to conform to prevailing values (Brown and Harris, 1978). And what is this 'togetherness' anyhow? Is it the *reality* of communal support, or is it more a *feeling* of trust and reciprocity—that is to say a perception, a set of beliefs, or what some refer to as 'cognitive social capital'? If so, how is that to be understood—as a psychological condition or as a social relation that emerges from the rituals embedded in social encounters, as explored by Erving Goffman and Randall Collins (Goffman, 1967; Collins, 2004). And extreme 'togetherness' is often the flip side of extreme exclusion, marginalizing those who are not part of that tightly bonded group; so perhaps what is damaging to mental health is not the absence of social capital but social exclusion in and of itself (Morgan, Burns, et al., 2007; Wright and Stickley, 2013). All these complexities threaten to ruin a good hypothesis. But what becomes clear is that, for this literature, the mental health of those who migrate depends, not so much on the fact of migration itself, but on the conditions—physical, personal, social, economic, cultural—that people experience on their arrival, as they come to inhabit particular geographical and ecological places and spaces.

Understanding Urbanicity—To a New Style of Thought?

In the three decades since the publication of the *The Lancet* paper on "Schizophrenia and Urban Life" that we cited earlier (Lewis, David et al., 1962), thousands of articles have been published on the relationship between urbanicity and mental health or mental disorders. Almost all of the studies are epidemiological in character, using statistical correlations to evaluate associations between urban living, or one or another aspect of urban living, and particular psychiatric diagnoses. Almost all start by repeating the familiar theme that this issue is important because global urbanization trends mean that increasing proportions of the population live in cities. And almost all reviews of this body of research agree that it is difficult to draw firm conclusions because of the dearth of good evidence, the variations in measures and definitions between different studies, and the complexity of the associations that seem to be involved.

Let us take a few examples. In a recent special section of *Current Opinion in Psychiatry* on the theme of Urbanization and Mental Health (Szabo, 2019), a series of scholars reviewed the evidence on the relationships between urban living and psychotic disorders, mood disorders, substance misuse, eating disorders, and anxiety and stress-related disorders. Most of the studies reviewed point to the need for better data and the difficulties of undertaking comparisons between different pieces of research; thus, in the case of dementia—where rates seem lower in urban settings than in rural settings—there are pervasive problems of definitions of urban and rural, and definitions of the disorders in question vary greatly between studies (Robbins, Scott, et al., 2019). There are repeated references to the supposed benefits of 'green space'—in reviewing neighborhood-focused research on the consequences of urbanicity for anxiety and stress-related disorders, authors conclude that "physical (e.g. green space), social (e.g. social cohesion) and biological (e.g. stress response) factors—are directly linked to the presence and severity of anxiety disorders . . . architectural and space design elements . . . can either increase anxiety and lead to trauma triggers or relieve symptoms and reinforce safety" (Ventimiglia and Seedat, 2019: 248). The allure of the microbiome is powerful with "emerging evidence that being raised in urban environments with a wide range of microbial exposure dampens the immune response to psychosocial stressors" (ibid.).

As for mood disorders, it seems that only depression has been seriously explored; the reviewers find that "individuals residing in urban areas experience increased risk of depression. Mechanistic pathways include increased exposure to noise, light and air pollution, poor quality housing, reduced diet quality, physical inactivity, economic strain and diminished social networks" (Hoare, Jacka, et al., 2019: 198). In a later review of the global literature on depression: Laura Sampson and her colleagues find "higher adjusted odds and/or severity of depression in urban areas compared with rural areas in the Netherlands, the United States, India, and Vietnam"; in China, depression was less common in urban than in rural areas, while studies in Ghana, South Africa, and the Netherlands showed no clear relationship (Sampson, Ettman, et al., 2020: 233). It is worth quoting their remarks on these complexities at some length:

> Given the many different aspects of urban living—some of which promote and some of which inhibit mental health—a focus on more manageable, modifiable factors may be fruitful, while simultaneously appreciating the full framework of multilevel influences on health. There are two major challenges to studying the relationship between urbanicity and depression. First, it is difficult to separate the effect of living in an urban area from the effects of higher income or other resources that are often necessary for someone to either migrate to or remain in an urban area. . . . Similarly, for those who migrate, it can be difficult to disentangle effects of urban living from effects of the process of migration itself or the underlying reasons for migration. . . . [The] ubiquity of urbanization presents a challenge for traditional epidemiologic study. Given the many possible mediators and moderators on the complex pathway from urbanization to depression (Galea and Vlahov, 2005) researchers should apply solid theoretical frameworks and causal thinking approaches . . . and move beyond single exposure–outcome association studies. At the same time, more granularity in defining and measuring specific exposures of interest may be warranted; simply comparing large urban areas to large rural areas may mix together many different exposures. (ibid.: 242)

A similar conclusion can be found in the review of urbanicity-psychosis associations in high-, middle-, and low-income countries by Anne-Kathrin Fett, Imke Lemmers-Jansen, and Lydia Krabbendam—showing "complex patterns of urbanicity–psychosis associations with considerable international variation within Europe and between low, middle and high-income countries worldwide" (Fett, Lemmers-Jansen, et al., 2019: 232). They suggest that social and economic stressors such as migration, ethnic density, and economic deprivation, exposure to nature, and access to resources could only explain part of the urbanicity effects: "Urbanicity–psychosis associations are heterogeneous and driven by multiple risk and protective factors that seem to act differently in different ethnic groups and countries" (ibid.). The way forward, in their view, lies in interdisciplinary research "combining approaches, for example from experimental neuroscience and epidemiology . . . to unravel specific urban mechanisms that increase or decrease psychosis risk" (ibid.).

What might such an interdisciplinary approach look like? A later paper by Lydia Krabbendam and her collaborators sketches out one answer (Krabbendam, van Vugt, et al., 2021). The authors are moved by E. O. Wilson's 'biophilia' hypothesis that humans may not be evolutionarily equipped for urban living, given the short history of cities. Indeed, they suggest that humans have an innate love for nature that is disrupted by urban existence, and that urban environments tax our cognitive resources which are restored by contact with nature. One might wonder whether the words 'nature' and 'green'—while they may connote a certain bucolic vision of the forests and fields of northern Europe—adequately capture the evolutionary landscape within which the first hominids emerged. No doubt it is true that many people today find images or experiences of cultivated forests, parks, and gardens restful, yet it seems doubtful that they would feel the same if in an unmapped rain forest or on the featureless bush, however green they were. Indeed, we should hesitate before drawing universal conclusions about an innate love of green nature from research with modern urban humans, many of whom are themselves imbued with a historically and culturally shaped romance of the natural. Arguments about 'cognitive overload' in cities surely need a more subtle approach to the structured and systematic differences in inhabitation and the very different relations to urban space that they entail.

While in 2005, Krabbendam had speculated about the importance of genetic risk, by 2020 she and her colleagues doubted that genetics played a significant part in these urban-rural differences. On the contrary, they return to the theme that while city living may produce 'cognitive overload,' the natural environment has 'salutogenic effects.' These effects might include better immune function, lower blood pressure, and enhanced physical and social activity, as well as alterations in the volumes of grey and white matter in the brain; they might also affect the activity of the neural receptors responsible for social stress processing, and these might have effects beyond the individual exposed to their unborn offspring. Drawing on a number of neuroimaging studies, they suggest "stress sensitization through environmental stressors, neurotoxicity and neuro re- and degeneration as possible neurobiological pathways that mediate urbanicity effects on cognitive functioning and mental health. Future studies need to systematically investigate multiple mechanisms that could underlie the urban effect on the brain (e.g. exposure to toxic or noise pollution, social stressors) . . . To improve our insight into which specific urban features are involved, experimental and experience-based studies that investigate immediate responses to specific physical and social characteristics of urban environments will be indispensable" (Krabbendam, van Vugt, et al., 2021: 1014).

Krabbendam and her colleagues thus recognize the importance of engaging with disciplines such as sociology, anthropology, urban planning, and geography; they conclude their review by suggesting that researchers need to start from the position that "the lived experience and sense-making of subjects are crucial for analysing the effects of urban or natural milieus on mental health." They thus suggest the use of ecological momentary assessments, which sample individual experiences of their urban environment in real time, and map these using GIS and other data, combined with the use of mobile EEG devices that can directly monitor the psychological effects of urban stress on the brain, and allow their correlations with psychological indices of stress—thus to unravel the "multiple interacting pathways and reciprocal relations of the urbanicity–mental health conundrum" (Krabbendam, van Vugt, et al., 2021: 1016). What would we find, then, if we really did venture beyond the correlational styles of thought in epidemiology and focused on what was really going on in individual urban brains in 'real time'— as their human bearers lived, moved, inhabited, experienced urban space?

Seeing the Urban Brain

Of course, there is a long history of brain visualization, of attempts to see human characteristics, and human pathologies in the cerebral tissues themselves. In the nineteenth and early twentieth centuries, the dead brains of criminals, the mad, and the brilliant were extracted, preserved, classified, mapped, and anatomized in attempts to correlate the intellect with the size or weight of the brain or the topography of the cortex (Hagner, 1997; Hagner, 2001; Hagner and Borck, 2001; Hecht, 2003). Those dead brains sadly failed to give up their secrets. Only in the twentieth century were technologies developed that could overcome the seemingly impenetrable barrier of the skull, to visualize the living brain in situ (Kevles, 1997). We moved rapidly from techniques that involved the painful injection of air or dyes into the vessels that entered the skull to technologies such as Positron

Emission Tomography (PET) and functional MRI (fMRI) that seem to show the activity of the living brain as it thinks, feels, desires, decides, and experiences the world around it (these are reviewed in Rose and Abi-Rached, 2013: ch. 2). Most of those technologies are 'heavy' and tied to the laboratory. PET scans require a person to be injected with radioactive tracers that bind to certain biological molecules, and then to lie in a large machine that takes images that show the take-up of the 'tagged' molecules in different areas of the body or—in our case—the brain (Dumit, 2003). fMRI requires the subject to remain motionless in a large and noisy scanner while a powerful magnet takes advantage of the fact that de-oxygenated hemoglobin is more magnetic than oxygenated hemoglobin, visualizing variations in oxygenation thus serves as a proxy to show increased brain activity in certain regions (Beaulieu, 2000). However, newer, 'lighter' technologies have been developed, such as mobile EEG devices that enable patterns of brain waves to be monitored and recorded during activity,[5] or Near Infrared Spectroscopy (NIRS), which can monitor and record levels of blood oxygenation in the layers of the cortex just beneath the skull, thus providing a proxy measure of brain activity, especially in the frontal cortex (Denault, Shaaban-Ali, et al., 2018). For researchers, despite the limited penetration of these devices into the depths of the brain, the advantage is that both increase the capacity for mobility, enabling the research subject to move around an environment (Bunce, Izzetoglu, et al., 2006).[6] It seems that, at last, one can see the urban brain in action.

In 2005, in Chiba prefecture in Japan, a team of researchers took seventeen female participants out for a walk.[7] First they went to a forested area. Then they walked around an urban station in Chiba City. At different points during the day, the researchers used NIRS to measure hemoglobin in cortical tissue in particular brain regions in real time—thus comparing the effects of walking in the two different areas, in terms of the participants' brain physiology (Tsunetsugu and Miyazaki, 2005). Much to the pleasure of the researchers—who were, not coincidentally, from Japan's Forestry and Forest Products Research Institute—significantly lower levels of oxygenated blood were detected for the forest as opposed to the city areas after walking—showing, the authors argued, "that in a forest environment, the activity in the prefrontal region was calmer than in a city environment" (ibid.: 469). Indeed, these researchers were not concerned with the neural effects of urban experience, but with that of the *forest*. This was just the start of a series of studies on 'the physiological effects of *Shinrin-yoku*'—that is to say, the effects of immersion in the forest atmosphere or forest bathing. Most of these did not access the brain directly but used other physiological measures such as salivary cortisol, blood pressure, pulse rate, and heart rate variability (Park, Tsunetsugu, et al., 2009; Hansen, Jones, et al., 2017) to assert the importance of "increased awareness of the positive health-related effects (e.g., stress reduction and increased holistic well-being) associated with humans spending time in nature, viewing nature scenes via video, being exposed to foliage and flowers indoors and the development of urban green spaces in large metropolitan areas worldwide" (Hansen, Jones, et al., 2017: 895).[8]

Some continued to try compare the 'urban effect' and 'the rural effect' using brain imaging laboratory studies. Thus, a group of researchers at Chonnam University in Gwangju, South Korea, used fMRI to measure the brain activation of a series of participants, while they looked at images of variously rural ('forests, gardens, parks and hills') and urban ('high buildings, offices, electrical cables, garbage collections') scenes (Kim, Jeong, Baek, Kim, et al., 2010). In this case, while viewing rural scenery, the participants showed greater activity in areas of the basal ganglia, "important for positive emotions"; by contrast, when looking at urban scenes, participants showed activity in brain areas associated with aversive imagery and with evaluating cues that might predict danger (ibid.). Thus, the authors argued, participants showed "an inherent preference towards nature-friendly living" (ibid.: 2607). Their findings, they concluded in another paper published the same year,

> support the idea that the differential functional neuroanatomies for each scenic view are presumably related with subjects' emotional responses to the natural and urban environment, and thus the differential functional neuroanatomy can be utilized as a neural index for the evaluation of friendliness in ecological housing. (Kim, Jeong, Kim, Baek, et al., 2010: 507)

The belief that while the city jangles the nerves, swards of green have the opposite effect seems to have been the intuition behind an experiment conducted in Edinburgh a couple of years later, reported in an article entitled "The Urban Brain" (Aspinall, Mavros, et al., 2013). These researchers equipped their participants with a portable Emotiv EPOC™ 'wireless EEG' headset—which recorded electrical activity at fourteen different locations on the skull, using a proprietary algorithm that translated EEG data into four "emotional parameters," viz. frustration, engagement, excitement, and meditation. They then walked twelve people (individually) through three distinct areas of Edinburgh: an urban shopping street with light traffic, a green space with lawns and trees, and a busy commercial district. Following the walk, the researchers correlated the output from the devices with the participants' presence in the different zones: how did different experiences of the environment correlate with the algorithms representing people's emotional states? The most significant finding showed a marked difference in activity as people moved from busy streets to quiet green areas: "the transition from Zone 1 to Zone 2 (urban shopping street to green space) . . . [shows] reductions in arousal, frustration and engagement (i.e. directed attention) and an increase in meditation" (ibid.: 5). The authors proposed that, in the future, studies like theirs might be "particularly beneficial in exploring the health improving potential of environments while people are on the move" (ibid.: 5).

Many similar studies followed, some seeking to directly measure urban effects in the brain, others using different physiological measures to support the view that, while urban living rattled the nerves, experiencing, seeing, walking in nature was good for the brain (Kondo, Jacoby, et al., 2018). There are enormous technical issues in these studies—in particular, issues around the sensitivity of mobile measures. Nevertheless they seek to go beyond a general belief that experiences of rural or urban environments must somehow be inscribed in the brain, to render such beliefs technical so that these inscriptions can be measured in real time by brain reading devices.[9] Urban experience has become neural.

These studies—and we have offered here only a small selection—provide a novel way of imagining and mapping the experience of cities. They encourage us to see those cities in terms of levels of stimulation, to map the spaces of the city in neural terms. We are urged to see the city *in the brain*, as urban citizens wind their way from place to place—here, noisily frustrated; there, calmly restored—often simplified into the differences between 'grey' and 'green' spaces. Stress is, once again, at the heart of these arguments. On the basis of their systematic review of studies of stress in relation to various outdoor environments, Michele Kondo and colleagues conclude that there is "convincing evidence that spending time in outdoor environments, particularly those with green space, may reduce the experience of stress, and ultimately improve health" (Kondo, Jacoby, et al., 2018: 136). They suggest that exposure to stress is "one of the ways that environmental and neighbourhood conditions 'get under the skin' and lead to poor health and associated health disparities . . . Conditions such as blight, segregation, poor social cohesion, and violence combine with personal experiences like job insecurity and discrimination to produce a range of persistent stressors"(ibid.: 148).

A novel field of intervention on urban mental health is thus opening up within the nexus of urban subjectivity, neural circuits, and urban design—and their associated regimes of governance. This argument was catapulted into popular debate by some research from Andreas Meyer-Lindenberg and his group based at the Central Institute for Mental Health in Mannheim, Germany. The study that they published in 2011 (which has since been cited more than 1,000 times) was reported not just in journals such as *Science* ('The Mental Hazards of City Living')[10] and *Nature* ('City Living Marks the Brain')[11] but also in *Wired* ('City Life Could Change Your Brain for the Worse')[12] and many similar semi-popular outlets. The claim made by these researchers was that they had begun to identify the *mechanisms* that accounted for the fact that, while urban dwellers were, by and large, better off than their rural cousins, they experienced poorer mental health (Lederbogen, Kirsch, et al., 2011). And we will not be surprised to learn that these hypothesized mechanisms revolved around 'stress.'

Recruiting volunteers from cities, towns, and rural areas in Germany, the Mannheim group put their subjects into fMRI scanners, and set them a task of solving an arithmetical problem. They subjected them to various levels of 'stress' by putting increasing pressure on them to complete the task rapidly and to do well. As this pressure increased, so did heart rate, blood pressure, and cortisol levels—taken to be measures of stress. But also, as 'stress' increased, it seemed that different patterns of brain activation occurred depending on the extent and timing of exposure to an urban environment; in short, they processed stress differently:

> Our results identify distinct neural mechanisms for an established environmental risk factor, link the urban environment for the first time to social stress processing, suggest that brain regions differ in vulnerability to this risk factor across the lifespan, and indicate that experimental interrogation of epidemiological associations is a promising strategy in social neuroscience. (Lederbogen, Kirsch, et al., 2011: 498)

According to a report in *Nature* by Alison Abbott, one of their leading science journalists, Meyer-Lindenberg had first thought of the cerebral effects of city living while studying in New York, where he was "struck by the number of homeless mentally ill people on the streets," and began to wonder "if city living was somehow making the brain more susceptible to mental-health conditions" (Abbott, 2012: 164). Meyer-Lindenberg's surprise suggests that some neurobiologists are less than fully immersed in the heated debates on mental health policies and their consequences. Nonetheless, the research itself painted a picture of mental life in the city that many commentators found compelling. Accompanying Abbott's report was a highly stylized and abstracted model of an 'urban habitat,' showing a small, triangular, green space, boxed in by grey buildings. A series of blacked-out human figures are dotted around, with captions describing their affective states: one, marked as 'Relaxed,' is depicted on a green square beside a tree; a huddle of figures in the middle distance are identified as 'Anxious,' while two more forlorn figures, far off to the right of the image, are marked as 'Isolated' and 'Lonely,' respectively. A caption above the last of these informs us that "feeling different to neighbours—owing to socioeconomic status or ethnicity—may be a factor. Immigrant populations have an increased risk of psychiatric disease" (ibid.). The urban, here, is not a space of cosmopolitan mingling, of civilized living, commercial vitality, cultural effervescence, and so on. On the contrary, reduced to a cartoon that bears no relation to the lived experience of any city dweller, it is represented as an array of potentially pathogenic neurobiological spaces.

If we return to the research itself, we can see that the way that stress was actually simulated in the laboratory experiments was as abstracted from lived experience as are these cartoons of urban life. The Meyer-Lindenberg group, like others, simulated stress in laboratory conditions because this was necessary if they were to visualize stress while their subjects were in fMRI scanners, which of course allow much more detailed mapping of brain activation than the EEG devices used in the naturalistic research described earlier in this chapter. The experiment used the Montreal Imaging Stress Task (MIST), "a social stress paradigm where participants solve arithmetic tasks under time pressure," giving them negative feedback on their performance by showing them a 'performance scale' and providing further negative feedback through headphones. This setup produced the fMRI images that were interpreted to show different patterns of brain activation for those who had been *brought up* in cities and those who *currently lived* in cities. They suggested that chronic activation of stress pathways at different stages in brain development had led to different ways of processing stress in the two groups. For those brought up in cities, they claimed to have found a "regionally specific effect on the pACC [the pregenual anterior cingulate cortex], a major part of the limbic stress regulation system that exhibits high neuronal glucocorticoid receptor expression, modulates hypothalamic–pituitary–adrenal axis activation during stress, and is implicated in processing chronic social stressors such as social defeat." On the other hand, the high levels of amygdala activity they found in those who currently lived in cities when subjected to stress "signals negative affect and environmental threat" and might be related to "anxiety disorders, depression, and other behaviors that are increased in cities, such as violence" (Lederbogen, Kirsch, et al., 2011: 499).[13] This research thus seemed to show that there were indeed 'urban brains' that took different forms depending on the timing of exposure to urban stressors during one's life course.

We will, again, leave to one side the many technical objections one might make to this laboratory research and its extrapolation to everyday urban existence. What is more interesting is that, despite these issues, an array of psychiatrists, planners, architects, and urban policymakers began to argue—in scientific journals, the mass media, and an array of conferences and reports—that the research provided the basis for new practices for intervention and management. Launching a program by the International Council for Science in late 2014, for example, Anthony Capon explained to journalists how cities were associated with growing problems in non-communicable disease and mental health: "The essence of this programme," Capon said, is about "scientists working with urban decision makers. It is about identifying problems together, and how we might better understand those problems and developing better ways of responding to rapid urban population growth" (quoted in Kinver, 2014). Richard Coyne, a professor of architectural computing at Edinburgh College of Art, and a co-author of the paper that tracked mobile EEG measures in Edinburgh, was clear about the implications of the kind of work that he and his colleagues were doing. 'Our study,' wrote Coyne on his blog in 2013:[14]

> has implications for promoting urban green space to enhance mood, important in encouraging people to walk more or engage in other forms of physical or reflective activity. More green plazas, parkland, trees, access to the countryside, and urban design and architecture that incorporates more of the atmosphere of outdoor open space are all good for our health and wellbeing.

This first wave of research, which compared neural responses to stress in those born in or living in cities, and which urged planners to provide access to green spaces to mitigate the stresses associated with noisy, crowded, and overstimulating urban environments, was hardly adequate to what we know of the multiplicities of urban habitats and the diversity of those who inhabit them. It did not give us much specificity about the kinds of urban experience that are hinted at in ideas like 'social exclusion,' 'social capital,' and 'social defeat' and their role in mental ill health. Nor did it help us understand who, among those who inhabit cities, might fare best and who might fare worst, let alone why. The urban inhabitant was depicted as an interchangeable data point—as if the distribution of the environments of inhabitation across the contemporary city was not—and had not historically been—distributed unequally through hierarchies of wealth, race, and class.

Subsequent research has tried to offer something that we might consider more 'ecologically valid.' In a special issue of the journal *Current Opinion in Psychology* on socio-ecological psychology, Markus Reichert, writing with co-authors including Meyer-Lindenberg, argues for "ambulatory assessments," which use smartphone-based ecological momentary assessments, smartphone diaries, various monitors of physiological function such as accelerometers, ECG monitors, and fitness trackers combined with highly accurate GPS-based location tracking. Belatedly recognizing the limits of laboratory-based studies and retrospective reports of emotions, this group now argues for the ecological validity of real life measures that "capture how emotions, thoughts and behaviours fluctuate across time . . . modulated by biological, cognitive and contextual factors" (Reichert, et al., 2020: 159). But if the strength of the real-time ecological assessments is precisely that they map stress—and associate emotions and thoughts—in real time, this is also their limitation. 'Real time' is, of course, not a continuous flow of presence— humans live in the confluence of the currents of manifold pasts, ambiguous presents, and the shadow of multiple potential futures. For a sociologist or a philosopher, the presence of the past is a matter of memories, associations, sedimented meanings in streets and artefacts, stories, and myths. For neuroscientists, by contrast, the past is present because of its sedimented consequences in the human brain. And, for most, that sedimentation is a result of one major factor—stress.

The Biopolitics of Stress

If stress theories of mental disorder have achieved prominence once more, it is in part because of a hypothesis that has become widely accepted about the biological mechanisms by which a subjective perception of stressors can act on the brain. In the familiar 'fight or flight' response, something that is experienced by an individual as 'stressful' results in the increased production of cortisol, a glucocorticoid that is produced in the adrenal gland. Cortisol has a wide range of effects on the body, the most significant of which is the increased production of glucose, together with an inhibition of the production of insulin, thus preventing that glucose from being stored. This increase in blood glucose prepares the organism for 'fight or flight' by providing the muscles with an easily available energy source and simultaneously narrowing the arteries, and generating increased production of epinephrine, which raises heart rate and blood flow. However, if high levels of glucocorticoids continue over time, this leads to the production of cytokines—small molecules that act as signals between cells and are especially important in immune and inflammatory responses. While the consequences are complex, continued production of cytokines upregulates the immune response, producing inflammation.[15] Sustained activation of these cytokines has a wider impact. In particular, it leads to changes in the size of the amygdala, the medial-frontal cortex, and other brain regions by modulating the HPA axis—the connections between the three adrenal glands of the hypothalamus, the pituitary gland, and the adrenal glands. Contemporary stress researchers argue that it is these effects on the brain that lead to changes in mood, emotion, and behavior, and that studies—once more mostly carried out in rodents—show that prolonged high levels of cytokine activation are associated with symptoms similar to those of certain psychiatric conditions (Dantzer, O'Connor, et al., 2008; Pariante and Lightman, 2008; van der Kooij, Fantin, et al., 2014; Sandi and Haller, 2015).

Bruce McEwen was one of the most tenacious researchers seeking to draw conclusions for physical and mental health from thinking about the neurobiological effects of stress. He argued that the evolved response to stress—'allostasis' or stability through change (Sterling and Eyer, 1988)—is protective; however, prolonged or repeated elevation of stress hormones has long-term consequences, increasing what he termed 'allostatic load,' that raises future risks of developing disease (McEwen, 1998; McEwen and Lasley, 2002; Lupien, McEwen, et al., 2009; McEwen, Bowles, et al., 2015). Further, seemingly appreciating the psychological and sociocultural evidence that what is crucial is not objective circumstances but the cultural shape of one's perception of a situation, McEwen insisted that "[s]tress is a state of the mind, involving both brain and body as well as their interactions," and it is the brain that is "the central organ of stress and adaptation" (McEwen, 2012: 17180). The social and physical environments get 'under the skin' through the neuroendocrine, autonomic, and immune systems, both in the course of early development and during later experience. Over time, stress has enduring effects through a hormonal cascade which acts on the structural plasticity of the hippocampus and other brain regions, notably the amygdala, the prefrontal cortex, and the nucleus acumbens. Its consequences for neuronal changes are not merely shown in animal studies but are supported by neuroimaging studies in humans: both acute and chronic stress inhibit neurogenesis, and affect synaptic turnover, spine density, branching and length of neuronal axons (Davidson and McEwen, 2012). While a perception that one is in a dangerous, precarious, or threatening situation for oneself or those one cares about normally produces adaptive change, when such a perception is chronic, stress becomes 'toxic' and toxic stress has "implications for understanding health disparities and the impact of early life adversity and for intervention and prevention strategies" (McEwen, 2013: 673).

Thus, a mechanism by which a variety of subjective experiences, perceived as stressful as a result of individual socio-biographically and socio-culturally shaped meanings, can be translated into neurobiological configurations with deleterious consequences for brain and body. Of course, the argument that stress is a subjective response to external 'stressors' does not by any means imply that the distribution of such stress is independent of the actual distribution of potential stressors such as lack of money, insecurity of employment, bad living conditions, isolation, noise, pollutants, problems with traveling to work or walking to the shops, threats of violence, and so forth. While those external stressors inescapably increase the likelihood that individuals will perceive themselves as subject to stress, they do not inevitably determine those perceptions. On the one hand, as we saw in our discussion of the migrant experience in Shanghai, people may become inured to them or stoical in the face of them. On the other, experiences that many would find entirely acceptable, such as walking into a crowded space, taking public transport, or encountering strangers on the street, may appear exceptionally threatening to some.

This focus on 'toxic stress' and specifically 'toxic stress' in childhood, is shared by many who adopt a broadly 'neurodevelopmental' approach to mental disorders. Consider, for example, the way that the issue of stress, and of toxic stress, is framed by the World Health Organization Report on *The Social Determinants of Mental Health* (World Health Organization, 2014). This report first reviews the evidence that has unequivocally established that common mental disorders such as depression and anxiety "are distributed according to a gradient of economic disadvantage across society" (Campion, Bhugra, et al., 2013), and that there are consistently strong associations between poverty—in particular food insecurity, poor housing, financial stress, and similar indicators of a precarious and demanding form of life—and 'common mental disorders' (Lund, Breen, et al., 2010). Having painted social factors in such broad terms, and pondering which of these broad demographic indicators might be most important, we will not be surprised to find that the authors of the WHO report settle for a common explanation for the effects of these different forms of adversity: stress.

Of course, stressful experiences do not always lead to mental disorders, and such disorders can occur in the absence of such experiences, so the report invokes the notion that social supports 'buffer' against stress: "the level, frequency and duration of stressful experiences and the extent to which they are buffered by social supports in the community" is what counts. And, in its view, those "lower on the social hierarchy" are more likely to be subject to such experiences and have access to fewer buffers and supports (World Health Organization, 2014: 17–18). Their choice of the term 'buffer'—rather than the psychological language of appraisal, adaptation, and coping— invokes familiar arguments about 'social capital,' now wrenched from its roots in the work of Bourdieu and Coleman in order to allude to the extent of strong social ties of reciprocity in particular communities. Indeed, echoing Richard Lazarus but without referring to his work, what turns out to be crucial is 'cognitive social capital'—the *belief* by individuals that such ties exist and that there are others to call on in times of difficulty.

The WHO report echoes the "ecobiodevelopmental" framework of Jack Shonkoff suggesting that "toxic stress" can occur "when a child experiences strong, frequent, and/or prolonged adversity—such as physical or emotional abuse, chronic neglect, caregiver substance abuse or mental illness, exposure to violence, and/or the accumulated burdens of family economic hardship— without adequate adult support" (Shonkoff, Garner, et al., 2012: e232).[16] The Report thus paints both 'the environment' and 'buffers' in terms of very broad factors, while recapitulating some rather old arguments about the importance of 'adequate' support in early life for future mental health.[17] However, we can see some of the problems of such an analysis in stress-based arguments that try to explain the fact that children from poor families tend to end up as poor adults, or, to put it more generally, why the social class of parents is predictive of the social class of their children. For example, Bruce McEwen,[18] in a paper co-written with his sociologist brother Craig McEwen (McEwen and McEwen, 2017), draws upon the work of a number of neuroscientists to argue that development of the prefrontal cortex in infants is "involved" in "observed SES disparities" (Hackman and Farah, 2009: 68).[19] They argue that toxic stress "alters its structure and functioning through the release of hormones and neurotransmitters by nerve cells" (McEwen and Morrison, 2013), and refer to the work of Shonkoff cited above in concluding that the consequences include compromised capacities for behavioral and emotional self-regulation, including working memory and executive function.

The emphasis on the enduring neural consequences of events in the early years of a child's life are part of a wider style of thought that is having significant policy impact in a number of countries, including those in the Global South (see Pentecost, 2018). Shonkoff's own work (Shonkoff, Garner, et al., 2012) underpins the school of thought and intervention that focuses on Adverse Childhood Experiences, or ACEs.[20] A related school of thought, framed in terms of the Developmental Origins of Health and Disease (DOHaD), has its origins in David Barker's work on the correlations between birthweight and later ischemic heart disease (Barker, 2007), or 'the foetal origins of adult disease' (Cooper, 2013), proposes that exposures in utero or 'the first 1000 days' has a 'programming effect' on the brain that establishes the foundations of optimum health, growth, and neuro-development across the lifespan.[21] These movements seem full of virtuous intentions, for example wishing to draw attention to the need to remedy the social disadvantages experienced in early childhood that inhibit neural development. However, as Daniel Hoffman and his colleagues point out, "while a large number of studies provide evidence that supports the concept of DOHaD," most of these have focused on poor early nutrition, drawing on data from children exposed to famine or from longitudinal studies and arguing that these are 'risk factors' for later chronic diseases; researchers have had to extrapolate from animal studies to support their postulations of the potential epigenetic, metabolic, and endocrine mechanisms involved (Hoffman, Reynolds, et al., 2017). Whether or not extrapolation from laboratory research with rodents—mice, rats, and sometimes guinea pigs—is valid in the case of Type 2 diabetes, hypertension, or coronary heart disease, such extrapolations are certainly perilous in the case of mental disorder. The almost ubiquitous dependence on animal models for neurobiological conclusions is sometimes acknowledged in this literature (Shonkoff, Boyce, et al., 2009: 96), but the implications are almost never addressed.[22] For example, the widely cited 2013 paper by McEwen and Morrison, to which we have just referred, relies entirely on evidence from animal models for its claims about the vulnerability of the development of the prefrontal cortex to stress (McEwen and Morrison, 2013).[23,24]

More promisingly, perhaps, Susan Prescott and Alan Logan have called for attention to 'ecological justice' in what they term the 'dysbiosphere' (Prescott and Logan, 2016).[25] Their proposal takes a much broader view of the developmental origins of health and disease, addressing "the forces—financial inequity, voids in public policy, marketing and otherwise—that interfere with the fundamental rights of children to thrive in a healthy urban ecosystem" while also focusing on the "grey spaces" of socioeconomic disadvantage that "insidiously reinforce unhealthy behaviour, compromise positive psychological outlook and, ultimately, trans-generational health" (ibid.: 1075). Not only do Prescott and Logan suggest that "greater focus on positive (beneficial) chemical and non-chemical, biotic and abiotic, family, neighbourhood and societal 'exposures' might uncover mechanisms of resiliency that go far beyond disease prevention and extend into health" (ibid.: 1076)—but also that we need to attend to how already disadvantaged populations bear a dual burden because they tend to inhabit urban "grey space", areas that "may include disproportionately higher industrial operations, commercial activity and major transportation routes, with resultant noise stress and excess light at night," as well as "residential proximity to higher levels of grey space and less equitable access to biodiversity," as well as large numbers of "bars, liquor stores, convenience stores, fast-food outlets, and tobacco vendors" coupled with "profit-driven marketing, billboards, sidewalk signage, in-store magnification of unhealthy products and targeted screen media delivery that make grey space an entirely different 'mental' environment" (Prescott and Logan, 2016).

The seemingly inescapable recurrence of the opposition of grey space to green space is at least given some substance here—grey space is not bad for one simply because it is not green, but because, because of the highly inequitable distribution of populations across urban space, the 'grey spaces' in which most disadvantaged people live are characterized by a high likelihood of toxic exposures. Here we can see how such an approach to what Prescott and Logan term "mental environments" might help us make our way through the pathways between specific modes of urban life and particular forms of physical, mental, and societal health. It is crucial not simply to pathologize neighborhoods because they do not conform to a certain bourgeois idea of good urban life. Yet we need to attend to the shaping and constraining of forms of life by discriminatory politics, policies, and planning over many generations; policies that have emplaced social exclusion and racism deep into the fabric of our cities, affecting not merely 'the first thousand days' but the whole course of the lives of those who have no option but to inhabit them. From this perspective, stress does not need to be an individualizing notion or one that roots all subsequent problems in early experiences of adversity. Precarity—in housing, employment, finance, and basic security—together with high levels of toxic ambient exposures, is endemic in the lived experience of those most excluded, including many communities of migrants and refugees.

If we want to figure out the pathways for the embodiment of adversity, then we need to start from these ecosocial questions—rather than from the premise that the line of causation begins with toxic stress in inadequate families that damages the developing brains of individual children and dooms them to a suboptimal future in physical and mental health and intellectual development. An ecosocial account of the shaping of the urban brain would map out the shaping of stressors through collective experiences of poverty, exclusion, isolation, racism, violence, and environmental degradation. It would deepen such an understanding by exploring how these experiences get understood, and the ways that these are assigned meaning in specific groups and communities. It would seek to identify what there might be within urban life that mitigates against stress, whether that be the physical environment of individual apartments or houses, the layout of streets and the organization of public space, mundane experiences in cafes and shops and informal friendships, as well as more substantial forms of collective organization and mutual aid. And all of this leads us to a different question: what kind of biopolitics might such a neuroecosocial understanding of urban existence enable? Let us turn to some further research that can help us to think through these questions.

Epigenetics: Beyond the Genetic Program

As we know, there is a long history of the belief that madness—and all its synonyms from lunacy to mental disorder—is hereditary, or at least that individuals inherit a constitutional susceptibility to mental disorder that can be triggered by adverse circumstances of various sorts. From the inception of modern psychiatry in the mid-nineteenth century, most psychiatrists held to something like this view at least when it came to serious mental disorders. From the 1930s onward, there was much research that sought to demonstrate it—for example showing that if one of a pair of identical twins developed a mental disorder, the other was highly likely to develop a similar disorder, and that this concordance was much more likely than in the case of non-identical twins. Research tried to locate the gene or genes that were responsible, often announcing the discovery of 'the gene' for this or that condition, only to discover later that their findings were not replicated.[26] Many psychiatric geneticists, like other life scientists, thus moved away from simple genetic determinism to argue for the importance of gene-environment interaction, in which individuals inherited, not a 'gene for' a condition, but a genetic sequence that increased the likelihood of developing such a condition where an individual was exposed to familial or environmental adversity at particular periods in their life course (Tabery and Griffiths, 2010). As sequencing of the human genome advanced, much effort was expended to try to identify the variations at the level of DNA sequences that were linked to suscepti- bility to mental disorders, again with little success.[27] While some thought that better results would be obtained with larger samples, better diagnoses, and more sophisticated algorithms, others sought to find different ways, for instance those based on large, long-term cohort studies that combined gene- tic data with information on key life events to disentangle themselves from simplistic genetic arguments about causation, some suggesting a reversal of terms, such that environmental factors like childhood maltreatment were construed as causes that led to mental disorders only in the presence of certain genetic variants (Caspi, McClay, et al., 2002; Caspi, Sugden, et al., 2003; Caspi and Moffitt, 2006).

But another way to think of the relations between genetics and environ- ment has come to the fore in recent years, with significant implications for thinking about urbanicity and mental health. The basic argument is far from new: from the 1960s onward, evolutionary and developmental biologists were highly critical of the 'genetic program' approach which assumed that inherited DNA simply expressed itself in the process of development of body and brain (Jablonka and Lamb, 2014). They argued that it painted an entirely misleading picture of the ways in which genes and environment interacted with one another from the moment of conception onward—environment here embracing everything from the cellular to the social milieu. And, as we moved into what some have called 'the postgenomic era,' it turned out they had the evidence on their side. Today, even the most committed proponents of psychiatric genetics recognize that, with the exception of a few very rare conditions, there are no 'genes for' mental disorder, and at the very least many genetic variations of small effect are combined in the development of mental disorders, even for those diagnosed as psychoses, let alone for the more common forms of distress such as depression and anxiety (Plomin and McGuffin, 2003). In addition, it has become clear that what is crucial is not merely the inherited DNA itself—the genome—but the ways in which particular genetic sequences are expressed or suppressed over the course of development, and the ways that this process is shaped by the constant transactions between the developing organism and its environment. It is this that has come to be termed epigenetics.

As usual, epigenetics is a contested concept (Carey, 2012; Landecker and Panofsky, 2013; Lappé and Landecker, 2015; Lock, Burke, et al., 2015). For present purposes, we will take epigenetics to mean the processes by which gene sequences are activated or deactivated across the life course, largely through mechanisms of methylation and demethylation, in certain cells in particular regions of the body, under environmental influences.[28] Some of the most widely referenced epigenetic research relating to brain development came from a Canadian group led by Michael Meaney: their experiments with rodents showed that the earliest relation that a mother has to her pup can shape the expression of genes in its brain and therefore shape the way in which that pup's brain develops into adulthood; this shapes the way in which that pup treats its own pups, which in turn shapes the development of the next generation of pup's brains and so on and so on, down the generations (Meaney and Stewart, 1979; Meaney, Aitken, et al., 1985; Champagne, Chretien, et al., 2004; Pruessner, Champagne, et al., 2004; Weaver, Cervoni, et al., 2004; Cameron, Champagne, et al., 2005; Champagne and Meaney, 2006; Szyf, Weaver, et al., 2007; Szyf, McGowan, et al., 2008). Meaney and his colleagues were not slow in arguing that these findings could be extended to humans, for example arguing that specific epigenetic patterns could be found in suicide victims with a history of child abuse (McGowan, Sasaki, et al., 2009; Meaney and Ferguson-Smith, 2010). This research led to much publicity. An article in *Nature* playing on a reversal of the normal cliché of nature versus nurture was entitled 'in their nurture' (Buchen, 2010). Other research, also carried out in rodents, seemed to show that factors such as diet and exercise led to epigenetic changes that might increase brain health, for instance generating epigenetic changes that increase the production of a protein called BDNF (brain-derived neurotrophic factor) which enhances the growth of nerve cells (Sleiman, Henry, et al., 2016). These and many other similar experimental findings, usually on animals such as mice, rats, and guinea pigs, led to a widespread belief that genes—in the sense of the inherited sequences of DNA bases—are *not* determinant—that the way in which they play out in any cell of the body is also a matter of milieu.

For many social scientists, epigenetics signals a radical revolution in genetic thought (Lock, 2013; Meloni, 2014; Lock, Burke, et al., 2015; Niewöhner and Lock, 2018). However, a number of cautions are in order. First, we need to remind ourselves that, as developmental biologists have long known, the contributions of extra-corporeal environmentally triggered epigenetic changes over the life course, while undoubtedly significant in the development of pathologies, are dwarfed by the role of inherited gene sequences, with largely standard and predictable patterns of gene activation and de-activation, thus shaping the basic features of an organism in regular and predictable ways (Jacob and Monod, 1961).[29] This regularly ends up in the emergence of a stable and fully formed organism, despite the fact that, for example, no two lungs are identical, even for monozygotic twins. This is also true for brain development: a large proportion of coding sequences in the human genome are expressed in the brain, and there is certainly much similarity between individuals in the overall architecture of brains, but no two brains are identical, either in general structure or in patterns of connectivity and neuronal circuitry, even for 'identical' twins (Van Essen, 1997; Devlin and Poldrack, 2007). Epigenetic processes are responsible as much for broad uniformity across individuals as for variations between them.[30]

Second, and perhaps more important for our question, we must point out once again that most of the research that underpins these arguments has been carried out in laboratory experiments on small animals, bred specially for research over dozens of generations, and kept from birth (and before) in laboratory cages (Rader, 1998; Rader, 2004). Extrapolation from the brains of such animals to 'wild type' animals, let alone to wild type human brains, needs to be undertaken with great caution, if at all. As we have already pointed out, there are huge differences between rodent and human brains, and these differences are not just in scale, but in the fundamental organization and capacities of 'the brain.'[31] Even if one was to stay with the etiolated conceptions of the social environment common to much psychiatric research, most would find it difficult to draw a parallel between the feelings that a guinea pig pup might have to its con-specifics and evidence that an individual's trust in the social support offered by others in their community might mitigate the effects of stressors on mental health. The slide from evidence about the effects of environmental adversity in rodents to those in humans is highly problematic, but nonetheless routine (to take just one of numerous examples, see Yam, Naninck, et al., 2015).

Some researchers avoided the many problems of such extrapolations by looking directly at epigenetic changes in adult humans who have experienced various forms of urban stress. Thus, Sandro Galea and his colleagues carried out a number of studies on urban mental disorder, which sought to examine such epigenetic changes in adult humans who have experienced urban stressors. Galea's group examined the epigenetic profiles of residents of a Detroit neighborhood and found distinctive gene methylation profiles in residents who had been assaulted: they suggested that "cumulative traumatic burden may leave a molecular footprint in those with [PTSD]" (Galea,

Uddin, et al., 2011: 402), and more generally that "different aspects of the urban environment are distinctly and variably linked to brain structure, function, and hence phenotype" (Goldmann, Aiello, et al., 2011: 859). Further research from Galea's group linked long-term epigenetic changes to risk and resilience in trauma (Sipahi, Aiello, et al., 2013), argued that childhood maltreatment was associated with epigenetic differences in hypothalamic-pituitary-adrenal (HPA) axis genes (Bustamante, Aiello, et al., 2013), suggested that epigenetics may explain the prevalence of respiratory symptoms in those responding to disasters such as that at the World Trade Center (Gonzalez, Guffanti, et al., 2014), and proposed that psychosocial stress accelerates immunological aging, perhaps through epigenetic mechanisms (Aiello, Dowd, et al., 2016). Indeed, a decade ago, on the basis of a review of studies of schizophrenia, major depressive disorder, posttraumatic stress disorder, anorexia nervosa, and substance dependence, this group argued that "dysfunction of epigenetic mechanisms offers a plausible mechanism by which an adverse social environment gets 'into the mind' and results in poor mental health" (Toyokawa, Uddin, et al., 2012: 67).

There are, therefore, plausible mechanisms linking environmental exposures to neurobiological changes that can be taken seriously by thoughtful social scientists. Yet not all agree that social scientists committed to countering the effects of social inequity on mental health should concern themselves with a search for pathways and mechanisms. Thus, for more than a quarter of a century, Bruce Link and Jo Phelan have argued that we should not spend our time and energy trying to identify specific risk factors or untangling the minutiae of causal pathways, but we should continually stress the macro-social character of social inequality, notably socio-economic status. We should focus on 'the causes of causes,' they argue, and recognize that socioeconomic status is a 'fundamental social cause' of mental ill health (Link and Phelan, 1995; Phelan and Link, 2010; Phelan and Link, 2013). Dismissing the view that such measures are 'mere proxies' for the true causes in the causal chain leading to disease, they argue that it is crucial to attend to the processes that lead people to be exposed to these more proximate risk factors, that put those of lower SES "at risk of risk" (Link and Phelan, 1995: 81).

Few would disagree with the general argument that poverty and lack of material and social resources negatively influence health—indeed, this is the basic premise of arguments about the social determinants of health, and of mental health (Allen, Balfour, et al., 2014; World Health Organization, 2014; Marmot, Allen, et al., 2020). But the links with socioeconomic status are actually an artefact of the ways—actually the variety of ways—in which epidemiologists have created and used versions of this measure as a variable in their correlational approach to mapping diseases across populations. It is true that this way of highlighting the impact of social conditions on health sounds compelling in contrast to the individualistic focus on health behavior that has become so common in advanced liberal societies such as the United States. But it has many weaknesses—not least failing to recognize that, as Jonathan Wolff and Avner de-Shalit put it, the many determinants of well-being are "not all reducible to a common currency" (Wolff and de-Shalit, 2013). Moreover, while Link and Phelan's position may well be radical in the United States, the social determinants of health, and of mental health, are well accepted by researchers and policymakers in most other regions of the world. There is no doubt that increasing social equity would have significant beneficial consequences on the incidence of ill health. But, given the likely persistence of a heterogeneous array of inequities in the distribution of resources, powers and capabilities for the foreseeable future, the question of pathways and mechanisms remains highly important, conceptually, politically, and for specific policies such as those involved in planning and managing urban spaces.

In 2013, Bruce Link collaborated with Sandro Galea, in an article setting out six paths for the future of social epidemiology (Galea and Link, 2013). The two authors agreed on the weakness of approaches that limited themselves to factors and correlations and on the need to move beyond this correlational style of thought. Four of their six potential paths focus on the need for more research on the social determinants of population health. However, two of these paths move further in the direction that interests us here: first, the need for the development of theory to open the 'black box' of correlational thinking, and second, a focus on 'mechanisms.' Galea and Link argue that the emphasis on macro-social factors has now been widely accepted, but it has led to the dominance of "social epidemiologic work that constrains itself outside the skin, with an interest in social processes without much concern with why these processes may matter . . . attending to mechanisms can help epidemiologists sort out which of their plausible social determinants are the most compelling ones" (Galea and Link, 2013: 846). As we have seen, Galea's work, with its focus on epigenetic changes consequent on trauma, had already made contributions in this respect. In a later paper, Galea and Katherine Keyes argued that what was needed was attention to what they termed "causal architecture" which enables us to move away from the epidemiological focus on risk factors. Rather than focusing on associations between factors, "a causal architecture approach . . . would ask: What is the structure of causes that underlie disease? Do these causes work together or separately? And most importantly, which causes are the most prevalent in the population" (Keyes and Galea, 2017: 4).

There are many methodological and conceptual difficulties to overcome in thinking through how one might establish such a causal architecture in any particular case. Nonetheless, the work of Galea's group on the epigenetic pathways that embody—or 'embrain'—the impact of urban exposures to trauma provides a compelling example of how we might begin to understand some of the biological pathways and mechanisms entailed in the experience of adversity. This might enable us to work out ways in which the everyday experience of social adversity and social suffering that is so well described in ethnographic research can engage with the new 'social' styles of thought just beginning to take shape in the contemporary neurobiology of mental disorder, in which the human brain in particular is 'plastic'—modulated by its dynamic transactions with its milieu, at timescales ranging from the millisecond to the decade, from conception onward.

Neuroplasticity: The Modulated Brain

We have known for many years that while the human brain develops significantly in utero, it develops further, and rapidly, in the first two years of life, reaching around 80 percent of its adult weight by the age of two. While there is little change in the volume of the brain after five years of age, at the gross level of neuroanatomy there are changes in the relative proportion of grey matter (which reduces after 12 years) and white matter (which increases over development up to puberty and indeed well into adulthood). There are also changes in the size of various brain regions, for example in the hippocampus and the amygdala, which appear to be sex related and may be hormonally controlled (Casey, Giedd, et al., 2000). But crucially, synapse formation— that is the formation of the webs of connections between neurons—is central in neurodevelopment and occurs well before birth and throughout early life. There is an overproduction of synapses during this period, many of which are 'pruned' in the first years of life, presumably in response to experience and in the process of learning. To put it simply, synaptic connections that are regularly used will strengthen—as argued long ago by Donald Hebb (Hebb, 1949) and summarized in the well-known aphorism 'what fires together, wires together.' On the other hand, those connections that are not used will be pruned. There is extensive synaptic plasticity—that is to say, the formation and pruning of synaptic connections—in the period leading up to puberty, linked to experience, habit formation, and learning, and, around the time of puberty, there is another intense phase of synaptic re-organization (Blakemore and Choudhury, 2006).

It is thus well recognized that the formation and stabilization of synapses is experience dependent, and that in this sense there is synaptic 'plasticity' throughout the life course. However, for a long time it was thought that *structural* plasticity—the development of new neurons and their integration into functional circuits—was limited to early childhood and a few 'critical periods' in development, notably in 'adolescence.'[32] Only relatively recently has it been accepted that there is considerable structural plasticity in the human brain through adulthood. This first became evident in neurological studies of patients who had suffered stroke or other forms of brain damage, which showed that, on occasion, patients could recover some of the functions that had been lost, presumably because other areas of the brain somehow acquired the ability to undertake them. Hence, researchers began to suggest that, in certain circumstances, perhaps with specialized training and exercise, the brain was capable of 'rewiring' itself.[33]

There is, however, a significant distinction between such 'rewiring' and the development and incorporation of new neurons, that is to say neurogenesis. Until the 1980s, most leading authorities argued that neurogenesis occurred rarely if ever in the adult mammalian brain, even though it had been found in the brains of birds and a few other species (for a good review, see Fuchs and Flügge, 2014). There were good reasons for believing this, because it seemed very likely that the generation of new neurons would disrupt existing neural circuits, for example those that had developed as a result of learning (Rakic, 1985). However, Elizabeth Gould and her group, overcoming much scientific skepticism and considerable technical challenges, demonstrated clearly that such neurogenesis did occur in adults, working initially with rodents (Gould, Tanapat, et al., 1999) and then with primates (Gould and McEwen, 1993; Cameron and Gould, 1994; Cameron, McEwen, et al., 1995; Gould, Reeves, et al., 1999). Rodent experiments also showed that neurogenesis was enhanced by training and exercise and adversely affected by early adversity and by adult social isolation and stress (Mirescu, Peters, et al., 2004; Stranahan, Khalil, et al., 2006; Opendak, Briones, et al., 2016).

Gould and her colleagues were initially cautious in any extrapolation to humans. However, some human studies, for example of examination of postmortem brains, did suggest that neurogenesis occurred in some regions of the adult human brains, and some suggested that measures of stress, as shown by levels of the glucocorticoid cortisol in human blood and saliva, provided indirect evidence to support the extrapolation of the rodent research on environmental stimulation of neurogenesis to humans (for a good review, see Chen, Nakagawa, et al., 2017). Many, however, remained skeptical of such extrapolation, given the differences in brain size and complexity in rodents that we have already discussed. In 2018, a study by a large international group of researchers concluded that "recruitment of young neurons to the primate hippocampus decreases rapidly during the first years of life, and that neurogenesis in the dentate gyrus does not continue, or is extremely rare, in adult humans" (Sorrells, Paredes, et al., 2018: 377). This critical conclusion provoked Gould, together with a number of researchers, to review the field and argue that, to the contrary, "there is currently no reason to abandon the idea that adult-generated neurons make important functional contributions to neural plasticity and cognition across the human lifespan" (Kempermann, Gage, et al., 2018: 25).[34]

Despite these unresolved controversies, a new popular image of 'the plastic brain' is taking shape, with authors enthusiastically claiming scientific support for their claims that 'the brain' is open to molding by its milieu from conception up until late adulthood, and that we can influence this by our own actions (Doidge, 2007; Begley, 2009; Arden, 2010). The suggestion that aspects of 'lifestyle' might increase neurogenesis has been enthusiastically taken up in the fantasy world of health on the internet. However, we need to exercise extreme caution. Aside from the problems of extrapolation, there is a strong temptation for individualization when the researchers seek to draw social and policy implications from this research. As with the use of rodent evidence in arguments about the developmental origins of health and disease, some researchers have found it a short leap from ambiguous experimental evidence produced in laboratory studies of the effects of various environmental manipulations on rodents to speculation that poor parenthood might inhibit neurogenesis, and hence lead to lifelong disadvantage (Leuner, Glasper, et al., 2010) leading to interventions that focus on those parents—usually the mothers—themselves, and sometimes even on young women prior to conception (Sharp, Lawlor, et al., 2018; Pentecost and Meloni, 2020). Perhaps the most we can say at this stage is that, while it is clear that neural circuits in the human brain transform in timescales from milliseconds to decades across the life course, and are thoroughly enmeshed in a milieu that is not bounded by skull or skin, we need collaborative research to explore the mechanisms and consequences for humans in the real world of their lived experience, whether in cities or elsewhere. And, of course, if plasticity does occur in particular situations and is inhibited in other situations, we still need to identify the forces that place people, and hold people, in those plasticity-inducing or -inhibiting situations in the first place.

The Exposome: An Urban Sensorium

We may now smile knowingly at the miasmatic theories of disease that were prevalent for so long, with their explanations of ill health in terms of the potent mixture of noxious odors from corrupting matter and the foul exhalations of one's fellow citizens (Nash, 2006), exacerbated by defective morals and lax habits in the perilous but seductive lanes and alleys of the 'cities of dreadful delight' (Walkowitz, 2013). But perhaps we should pause before consigning everything involved in those past beliefs to ignorance and prejudice. Districts really do have their own atmospheres after all: on the one hand, a mixture of affects and emotions, of feelings of calmness or excitement, of melancholy or joy, holiness or eroticism (Anderson, 2009).[35] We are becoming increasingly aware of another component of atmospheric exposures—of noxious pollutants in the air, the water, the ground, the buildings and more. For our current purposes, we can think of an 'atmosphere' as the sensory and affective, bodily, cerebral, largely non-conscious milieu that suffuses those who inhabit a particular spatial position or trajectory. To understand such urban atmospheres, we need something like an ecology of the senses.

We can start from the classic arguments of Jakob von Uexküll (von Uexküll, [1934] 2010) that require us to recognize that humans, like other organisms, inhabit and create a specific *Umwelt*, a 'biosemiotic' world made up of the aspects and attributes that are meaningful for us humans with our specific senses of touch, taste, smell, hearing, and vision, attuned by evolution, development, and our own cultures to those dimensions that are salient for our own existence (Kull, 1999; Kull, 2003). When we recognize the characteristics of the *Umwelt* within each human organism exists, the distinction between the neurobiological and the cultural ceases to make sense, for together these create our own perceptual and sensory universe. The human *Umwelt*, the ways we attend to and make meaning of that which threatens us and that which we desire, the perceptual cues that enable us to locate ourselves, our own bodies, and to navigate ourselves through our own milieu, is not that of a tick, a fly, a mouse, or a dog. What, then, of the *Umwelts* of the cities that we humans have created for ourselves? What role do the different human senses—sight, touch, smell, hearing—play in our urban *Umwelt*, in the spatializations of life in cities (Urry, 2003)?[36] The senses that orient people in space and in time, flowing through the 'portals' to the body and mind—the eyes, the ears, the nose, the skin—bring present and past inextricably together. Each hour, in each room, house, street, office building, shop, or factory, is not only visually specific but carries sounds, smells, the touch of other bodies or their absence—individually or together, these can evoke a whole scenario made real though myth and memory.

Vision and visibility has long been considered the primary sense, and this has certainly been the case for those concerned with urban governance. City planners have often sought to govern by vision, opening up dangerous agglomerations of persons, habitats, and habits to the purifying and civilizing influences of visibility. City spaces also brand themselves by their visual appearance, from the neon lights of city centers, to the little theaters of shop windows, or the enticing lights of cafés and bars. And the visual negotiation of the city is not just a matter of managing one's way across the physical topography of roads, pavements, parks, subways, but of negotiating the gaze of others, creating intimacy or rejecting it by meeting or avoiding eye contact, intensifying encounters with challenging gazes or de-escalating potential conflicts with downcast eyes. Vision, as John Urry remarks in his provocative essay (Urry, 2003), also marks class, not just through the familiar framing of wealth, work, gender, and age by dress, but by the form of the gaze itself. The wealthy watch the heaving masses on the streets from their cars; the genteel enclose themselves in newspapers, books, and reading devices on buses and the metro, the tourists gawk from their coaches and buses. Visitors from afar and travelers from nearby no longer struggle with paper maps furling and unfurling in the breeze, but walk with their gazes fixed on their devices, obeying the instructions as to when to turn or cross a road, inhabiting a space simultaneously physical and virtual.

Moreover, as has been remarked by authors from the earliest times, cities are noisy—the clatter of hooves, the shrieks of street vendors, the whoosh of cars or buses, the blare of radios from cars or of piped music from stores—so much so that the absence of noise, the preternaturally dark and silent street, summons anxiety in the stranger, but familiarity in the local. And in the cities of today, one is never far from the sounds of diggers, pile drivers, road drills, and all the other noises associated with the incessant repair and upgrading of urban material infrastructures. No wonder, then, that so many create their own soundscape, as we have moved from the speaker systems of the 1980s, through the Sony Walkmen of the 1990s, to today's ubiquitous mobile devices. Sound can locate an individual in space or seem to render them placeless, to transport them from their particular patch of asphalt into a despatialized world that they carry in their pockets.

Touch, and the avoidance of touch, also requires mastery of movement in the crowded city, on the pavements, in the shops, in the transport systems. We have some important contributions to the cultural history of touch (Classen, 2005; Classen, 2012) and some discussion of the management of touch in specific professions such as nursing and teaching, but there is little research on the *management* of touch in the city, and in modern life more generally. Such management requires more than a mastery of movement, it requires a reorganization of intimacy—how, for instance, to negotiate the presence of other bodies on public transport, not all of them innocent,[37] or crammed shoulder to shoulder in a small, enclosed elevator with a dozen strangers (Goffman 1963; Finnegan 2005).

And what of smell? Despite it being long considered as the least important sense for humans, the nose plays a very significant role in the differentiations of urban niches (Classen, Howes, et al., 1994; Kiechle, 2017; Barwich, 2020).[38] Smell can evoke places, from a city as a whole to the scents of particular individuals—as the 'hero' of Patrick Süskind's *Perfume*, who has memorized all the smells of Paris, knew well (Süskind, 1986). And there are the characteristic smells of shops and stores—from the Fierce tang emanating from the stores of Abercrombie & Fitch to the sugary aroma characteristic of Lush—now increasingly managed as 'scent marketing' in the service of consumption (Gulas and Bloch, 1995; Krishna, 2011; Spence, 2015).[39] The city has long been associated with inescapable encounters with the smells of others with whom one is almost inevitably forced into contact—an olfactory reality that has long been the friend of racists and xenophobes (Rhys-Taylor, 2013). If modernity is characterized by a war on smell, the smell of human waste confined to the water closet, the smell of perspiration effaced by baths, showers, soap and unguents, the smell of rotting rubbish transported outside the city to spaces of invisibility inhabited only by scavengers, this is a war that, for many, including dwellers in inadequate and overcrowded apartment blocks, let alone in polluted and insanitary slums and favelas, is far from won.

Such atmospheres of lived experience are central to our own neurosocial approach to the vital city, and to its potential transformation in the name of mental health. And the biotic and sensory exposures that characterize each locale are now being captured in the emerging interest in the microbiome and the exposome. As researchers on the human microbiome project remind us, "the microbes that live inside and on us (the microbiota) outnumber our somatic and germ cells by an estimated 10-fold. The collective genomes of our microbial symbionts (the microbiome) provide us with traits we have not had to evolve on our own . . . understanding the range of human genetic and physiologic diversity means that we must characterize our microbiome and the factors that influence the distribution and evolution of our microbial partners" (Turnbaugh, Ley, et al., 2007: 804). Researchers have argued that activities of these microbes shape development, modulate the capacities of the organism, and affect both health and disease, not least through the gut-brain axis (Human Microbiome Project Consortium, 2012; Mayer, Tillisch, et al., 2015), and some have suggested that the "emerging links between our gut microbiome and the central nervous system (CNS) [could be] regarded as a paradigm shift in neuroscience with possible implications for not only understanding the pathophysiology of stress-related psychiatric disorders, but also their treatment" (Kelly, Kennedy, et al., 2015: n.p.)—arguing indeed that stress can affect the permeability of the intestinal gut barrier, permitting "a microbiota driven proinflammatory state with implications for the brain," in particular in relation to depression and other 'stress related psychiatric disorders' (ibid.). However, once more, caution is needed: there has been much premature speculation about the significance of the human microbiome in maintaining physical and mental health (Valencia, Richard, et al., 2017), and there is "a relatively limited understanding of the broader environmental factors, particularly social conditions, that shape variation in human microbial communities" (Herd, Palloni, et al., 2018: 808). Significant methodological shortcomings in this research will need to be overcome if it is to fulfill its promise to be "a new frontier in understanding the biology of human health" (Renson, Herd, et al., 2020: 63). As Herd and her colleagues remark, "fulfilling the promise of microbiome research—particularly the microbiome's potential for modification—will require collaboration between biologists and social and population scientists" (Herd, Palloni, et al., 2018: 808) and such collaborations are currently in their infancy.

Despite these challenges, researchers on the microbiome agree that it is acutely sensitive to changes in the internal and external milieu, in other words to the exposome—a concept formulated "to draw attention to the critical need for more complete environmental exposure assessment in epidemiological studies [and to provide] a comprehensive description of lifelong exposure history" (Wild, 2012: 24). The exposome is "composed of every exposure to which an individual is subjected from conception to death" (ibid.), and research suggests that immersion in an environment, suffused with chemicals, gases, pollutants, pharmaceuticals, radiation, and much more, shapes an organism in ways as fundamental as those attributed to the genome. We thus need to consider the ways that humans' capacities, and health and disease, are shaped and reshaped not just by "processes internal to the body such as metabolism, endogenous circulating hormones, body morphology, physical activity, gut microflora, inflammation, lipid peroxidation, oxidative stress and ageing," and not only "the extensive range of specific external exposures which include radiation, infectious agents, chemical contaminants and environmental pollutants, diet, lifestyle factors (e.g. tobacco, alcohol), occupation and medical interventions," but also by "wider social, economic and psychological influences on the individual, for example: social capital, education, financial status, psychological and mental stress, urban–rural environment and climate" (ibid.). Indeed exposures such as tobacco or environmental pollutants "have specific 'omics' profiles," in other words, they show distinct patterns of transcriptomics, epigenomics, and metabolomics (Wild, Scalbert, et al., 2013: 480). It is exceptionally difficult to measure the exposome, despite the potential combinations of instruments such as sensors linked to geographic information systems (DeBord, Carreón, et al., 2016), and major challenges remain in identifying and distinguishing the multiple vectors involved (Guloksuz, Rutten, et al., 2018). Nonetheless, perhaps miasmatic theory should not be wholly banished to a misguided past: these conceptions of the microbiome and the exposome reframe miasma for the twenty-first century.

Toward a Conception of the Neurosocial City

Many have criticized George Engel's 'biopsychosocial model' (Engel, 1977) on the grounds that, while virtuous in its aims, it is vague, all-encompassing, and can cover a multitude of different and incompatible approaches—so much so that at one and the same time some can claim that both clinical and experimental medicine has long been biopsychosocial, while others can claim that this has never been the case. Borrell-Carrió, Suchman, and Epstein, writing twenty-five years after Engel's initial proposal, try to clarify what this approach entails: "Philosophically, it is a way of understanding how suffering, disease, and illness are affected by multiple levels of organization, from the societal to the molecular. At the practical level, it is a way of understanding the patient's subjective experience as an essential contributor to accurate diagnosis, health outcomes, and humane care" (Borrell-Carrió, Suchman, et al., 2004: 576). But it is hard to see what might be specific to what they term "biopsychosocially oriented clinical practice" except an attention to the patient and their history. From another direction, we are fully in agreement with Nancy Krieger's arguments for an 'ecosocial approach' stressing that health and ill health arise out of the 'embodiment' of a fractal web of transactions between biological and socio-environmental vectors (Krieger, 1994; Krieger, 2001). It is indeed important to understand "how we literally biologically embody exposures arising from our societal and ecological context, thereby producing population rates and distributions of health . . . socially patterned exposure-induced pathogenic pathways, mediated by physiology, behavior, and gene expression, that affect the development, growth, regulation, and death of our body's biological systems, organs, and cells, culminating in disease, disability, and death" (Krieger quoted in Palm, Schmitz, et al., 2013). These are, as Krieger rightly points out, 'theoretical' issues (Krieger, 2014). Yet it would not be too harsh a judgment to suggest that the theories and concepts that are required remain embryonic, and that the studies carried out within this framework are, in the main, descriptive rather than analytical. Hence, as we have suggested, conceptualization of mechanisms and pathways is crucial if we are to identify tractable points within this 'web of causality' where effective transformations should be directed.

We have used the term 'urban *brain*' in this book to stress that our approach is neurosocial, not 'psychosocial.' This is not because we wish to reduce or ignore the role of 'mind' or mental events in these pathways, but because we want to suggest that many, perhaps most, of the processes that are at stake here, even though they are shaped by experience and in turn shape that experience, operate below the level of consciousness that is often implied in references to the mind. In this chapter, we have tried to specify some of the pathways now emerging within contemporary neuroscience: new modes of visualization, new understandings of stress, recent work on the epigenetic modification of gene expression resulting from environmental exposures, findings on the social modulation of neuroplasticity, the role of the 'atmosphere' of the urban or the urban 'sensorium,' and evidence about the biosociality of exposures. We have done so at some length as an attempt to unfold some new ways of thinking that might underpin a new 'neurosocial' conceptualization of the 'urban brain' and, indeed, underpin a new urban biopolitics that addresses the ways that these are lived together in the experience of a form of life actively lived across space and time. Can we give this argument an empirical specificity that would enable analysis and action? It is to this task that we now turn.

6

Another Urban Biopolitics
Is Possible

At present an analytical science of the city which is necessary is only
at the outline stage. . . . The right to the city cannot be conceived of
as a . . . a return to traditional cities. It can only be formulated as a
transformed and renewed right to urban life . . . is it here necessary
to exhibit the derisory and untragic misery of the inhabitant, of the
suburban dweller and of the people who stay in residential ghettos,
in the mouldering centre of old cities and in the proliferations lost
beyond them? One only has to open one's eyes to understand the
daily life of the one who runs from his dwelling to the station, near
or far away, to the packed underground train, the office or the factory,
to return the same way in the evening and come home to recuperate
enough to start again the next day. The picture of this generalized
misery would not go without a picture of 'satisfactions' which hides
it and becomes the means to elude it and break free from it.

—(LEFEBVRE, "THE RIGHT TO THE CITY," 1996 [1968])

Urban thought has long been biopolitical. Politicians, intellectuals, journalists, philanthropists, social reformers, urban planners, sanitary inspectors,
medical officers, and a growing band of social scientists have long worried
about the relations between vitality and urban space—from graveyards,
docks, sewage systems, parks, centers and peripheries, from suburbs, to
apartment blocks, industrial zones, and council estates.[1] These concerns

about governing the vital life of cities have been bound up with particular ways of knowing cities and those who dwell in them, creating a practical expertise of government that draws on philosophy, ethics, sociology, statistics, and politics and links these to low-key, everyday strategies for governing conduct (Osborne and Rose, 1999). In almost all such strategies, even those that deploy authoritarian tactics of law and punishment, individual city dwellers have been a key target for management, urged to work on themselves, their conducts and habits, and to take responsibility for themselves in the name of individual or collective health and life.

In this chapter, we will not revisit the critical evaluations of the many and varied regimes of biopolitics that have taken urban mental life or urban mental disorder as their problem. Rather, we will argue that it is possible to imagine another way of governing the vital and neural lives of urban citizens, based on different knowledges, different strategies, and different forms of subjectification. There are possibilities, perhaps no more than that, in the emerging neurosocial knowledge that we have outlined in this book, for a perception of human vitality that no longer sees individuals as distinct, bounded biological domains but rather as inextricably immersed in, constituted with, even sometimes devastated by, the intra-individual, biological, physical, semantic, and affective worlds they inhabit. Such a perception also sees humans, individually and collectively, as actively making their lives, not just as constrained or enabled by material resources, but also formed by aspirations and judgments, shaped by esoteric meanings and memories. In the urban biopolitics that we imagine, the authorities that would govern mental life and mental distress would no longer be primarily psychiatrists, care workers, or others authorized because of their professional mental health training, but all those involved in shaping and planning the spaces, habits, and exposures that make up the everyday network of niches and trajectories that interlace across every city.

This would be a biopolitics in which individuals did not just have legal, political, and welfare rights to the city (whatever these might mean in practice) but rights, rather, to vitality, and to the affordances that would enable that vitality to unfurl itself. Claims to rights and justice are often asserted, of course, to contest the patterns of capital accumulation and privatization, race- and class-based segregation, and the direct and indirect violence of containment and securitization that have been characteristic of urban development globally since the Second World War. It is important to support those claims, and we certainly do, but not to take the language of rights and justice as exhaustive of a meaningful politics of urban life. We need a biopolitics that brings the living bodies and souls of humans to the center of questions of urban governance, and that addresses injustice, at least in part, in terms of the unequal distribution of bodily encounters and exposures.[2]

Urban Justice: The Right to the City

Urban justice today is, as we have already implied, often framed in terms of claims to 'rights to the city,' with Rights to the City groups emerging around the world, in marginalized communities, not just in the Global North but also, for example, in Brazil and Ecuador (Minton, 2017). But what are these rights? For Peter Marcuse, the right to the city is "a claim and a banner under which to mobilize one side in the conflict over who should have the benefit of the city and what kind of city it should be. It is a moral claim, founded on fundamental principles of justice, of ethics, of morality, of virtue, of the good" (Marcuse, 2009: 192). Marcuse argues that it can unify "those directly in want, directly oppressed, those for whom even their most immediate needs are not fulfilled: the homeless, the hungry, the imprisoned, the persecuted on gender, religious, racial grounds" (ibid.: 19), with "those superficially integrated into the system and sharing in its material benefits, but constrained in their opportunities for creative activity, oppressed in their social relationships, guilty perhaps for an undeserved prosperity, unfulfilled in their lives' hopes" (ibid.). Well, perhaps. But what seems to be at stake here is a nostalgia for a different city—a wholesome integration of humanized space and humanized life in the face of the disenchantment of the actual city: technologized, capitalized, privatized, fragmented, exploited for private profit and social control by technocrats, bankers, constructors, estate agents, and so on. Who, confronted with such a vision, does *not* dream of the city of good citizens, engaged in their polity, caring for their neighborhood, becoming themselves in their relation with their material and interpersonal urban world?

Perhaps Henri Lefebvre was anticipating such arguments when, a quarter of a century ago, he wrote: "The career of the old classical humanism ended long ago and badly. It is dead. Its mummified and embalmed corpse weighs heavily and does not smell good . . . Trivialities and platitudes are wrapped up in this 'human scale.' It is not even an ideology, barely a theme for official speeches" (Lefebvre, 1996 [1968]: 149). Indeed, we could do worse than return to Lefebvre's impassioned text that seems to be the root of later writings that frame the demand for urban justice in terms of a right to the city. For Lefebvre, the right to the city should be posed neither as a demand to restore some traditional city; nor in terms of an opposition between the horrors of urban life and the comforts of nature, in which the countryside appears as a kind of restorative break from the city. These ways of thinking relinquish a claim on the city itself, a claim to inhabit the city well, a claim to "renewed centrality, to places of encounter and exchange, to life rhythms, and time uses, enabling the full and complete *usage* of these moments and places" (ibid.: 179, emphasis in original). We need instead, says Lefebvre, to open our eyes to the real miseries of urban existence as they are lived, the generalized misery that is "the daily life of the one who runs from his dwelling to the station, near or far away, to the packed underground train, the office or the factory, to return the same way in the evening and come home to recuperate enough to start again the next day" (ibid.: 159).

Half a century ago, David Harvey considered these issues in *Social Justice and the City* (Harvey, 2009 [1973]). In arguing for the need to bring together a sociological and geographical imagination of the city, Harvey suggested that this would both "enabl[e] us to grasp history and biography and the relations between the two in society," and help "the individual to recognize the role of space and place in his [sic.] own biography, to relate to the spaces he sees around him, and to recognize how transactions between individuals and between organizations are affected by the space that separates them" (ibid.: 23–24). For Harvey, in 1973, bridging the gap between urban history and urban biography means not only understanding spatial form as a socially symbolic function, but also recognizing that the symbolic dimension was as much a psychological function as anything else (ibid.: 330). He thus believed that we could learn from laboratory experiments on the reaction to various forms of spatially organized stimuli—from "reactions to complexity, depth perception, associations in meaning, pattern preferences, and so on" (ibid.: 33).[3] But he considered that it would be extremely difficult to relate these findings to complex activity patterns as they unfold in the city. Perhaps this is why he posed the question of justice, not in terms of the lived experiences of individuals as they give meaning to the social and symbolic dimensions of their urban habitat, but rather in terms of "territorial distributive justice" which could be assessed by measuring how equitably resources were distributed across some territory. And while, in later writings, Harvey extends this question to ecological justice, thinking in terms of "inequalities in protection against environmental hazards," and their effects on the "marginalized disempowered, and racially marked positions of many of those affected" (Harvey, 1996: 385–386), the question of lived experience in the city remains subsumed with a demand for "a just and ecologically sensitive urbanization process under contemporary conditions" (ibid.: 438).

The challenge, for us, is to place that issue of lived experience at the center of a concern for urban justice, that is, to focus on the ways that urban injustice is deeply enmeshed in the inequitable ways in which we *inhabit* urban space, and in the possibilities and constraints of the human biology that is in a constant state of active co-constitution with such sites and practices of inhabitation. This is what a specifically political attention contributes: a method for grasping the socio-spatially- and socio-politically-shaped distribution of urban exposure, ranging from stress, isolation, and trauma to environmental pollution, air quality, noise, and heat.

Of 'Other' Urban Spaces

Urban geographers seeking to imagine 'other urban spaces' often revisit Michel Foucault's strange essay on heterotopia (Foucault, 1967).[4] In his text, Foucault variously describes heterotopias as 'emplacements' "that have the curious property of being in relation with all the other sites, but in such a way as to [suspend], neutralize, or invert the set of relations that they happen to designate, mirror, or reflect" (Foucault, 1986 [1967]: 24).[5] In a later reflection on the essay, Peter Johnson argues that Foucault uses the idea of heterotopia to contest "utopian forms of resistance and transgression based on a space of liberation"(Johnson, 2006: 82).[6] Heterotopias are "fundamentally disturbing places . . . there is no inevitable relationship with spaces of hope. It is about conceiving space outside, or against, any utopian framework or impulse" (ibid.: 84). But it would be misleading to think of these 'other spaces' as merely the products of Foucault's political imagination.

Consider, for example, the cemetery, which figures prominently in Foucault's analysis. As Johnson points out, referring to Foucault, while on the one hand, a cemetery is an emplacement of "profound spatio-temporal disruption, a place that encloses an 'absolute break with traditional time,'" on the other, the location of cemeteries was the focus of repeated concerns about hygiene in the growing European cities, which led to their removal from the sacred environs of the church to the outskirts of cities (Johnson, 2012: n.p.).[7] Indeed, questions of health in cities—of births and deaths, of illnesses and hygiene—have long been a privileged focus of 'the will to govern.' Foucault's lectures on 'the politics of health in the eighteenth century' could be viewed as the first in his series of thoughts on 'governmentality' and 'biopolitics'; they focus extensively on the ways that urban health became a central concern for authorities—"medical management determined by the authorities, supported by an administrative apparatus, framed by strict legislative structures, and addressing itself to the entire collectivity" (Foucault, 1999: 90).[8]

This new role for medicine as part of the rationalities of 'police'[9] gave a special place to the medicalization of the ordinary family. While the aristocratic family remained, primarily as a mechanism for inheritance, the families of the respectable class and of the laboring poor were now conceived as machines for health, with new rules for parents on the care, dress, and exercise of the child to ensure "the good development of the organism" and on the necessity to maintain a healthy and purified space in the domestic dwelling. But alongside this was a recognition that the city—with its districts suffused by dampness and exposure, its poor ventilation, its potentially dangerous water and sewage systems, the location of cemeteries and slaughterhouses— was both perhaps the most dangerous milieu for the health of the population and a potential locus for their control. Regular panics over urban rates of mortality led—both in France and in England—to the demand for medical surveillance of urban space and its most dangerous locales. It also led to a great concern over prisons, ships, ports, and hospitals, all seen as places that were vulnerable, because they were openings for disease to enter the city. Further, the hospital, while a crucial site for reform and medical improvement, and indeed for medical education, was radically insufficient for addressing the spatial distribution of disease—a perception that gave rise to a series of programs and experiments for disseminating medical persona across the space of the population, in managing towns both large and small, treating indigents, children, and families, and in fact serving to constitute the social body itself.

The medico-administrative complex that began to form, a complex of knowledge, expertise, and intervention organized around towns and cities, served not just as one of the first dimensions of governmentality, but also as the foundation of what would later become sociology: "medical reason was itself a specialising and urbanising science . . . by the 1830s a discourse on the 'medical climatology' of towns had evolved into an empirical medical topography concerned with the mapping of disease in localised spaces" (Osborne and Rose, 1999: 743). This coming-together was not principally a negative program concerned with eradicating disease, but rather a positive program for the promotion of good health: "the task of good government of urban space" in the mid-nineteenth century was not just to minimize disease but "to promote health" (ibid.). The city thus became an 'ethicohygienic' space—a territory in which the moral life of the citizenry was mapped into the spatiality of disease: 'milieu' and 'character' were made into functions of one another until, very gradually, "the spatial relation of citizen to habitat was turned into one that can and should be governed" (ibid.). In this sense, "the healthy city is not a city of minimal disease and social contentment, it is an active organic striving for its own maximisation against all that which would threaten it" (ibid.: 753).

Such a 'will to health' conceives of the city "as a network of living practices of well-being" and aims "to shape the ecology of the city in order to maximise the processes that would ensure the well-being of its inhabitants individually and in their 'communities'" (Osborne and Rose, 1999: 750).[10] All aspects of urban life are to be "mobilized in the name of a norm of well-being," from zoning habitations, managing pollution from vehicles, design of urban spaces were "suffused with this 'ecological' concern for health"—a program that involved alliances between health professionals, non-governmental organizations, community groups, and many others to manage "aspects of urban existence—jobs, housing, environment, public safety, diet, transport—not just to ward off sickness but to promote well-being" (ibid.: 752).

When we speak of our wish for a new urban biopolitics, informed by the new sciences of the living, are we not, then, merely translating this governmental will to health into a new language? In wishing to empower local communities, are we not, once more, allocating them responsibilities for their own healthiness, to strive for well-being in all aspects of their lives, to adopt healthy lifestyles, eat properly, manage stress, activate their self-responsibility? Are we not, yet again, seeking to create and instrumentalize an ethic in which the governing ambition for urban economy—in all senses of that term—is to be achieved by inculcating and activating each individual's aspiration for their own health?

To govern the city in the name of health: this hardly constitutes a radically new politics of life, even if it draws on new ways of framing this issue within the life sciences to explore the relations between bodies and cities. It remains true that, as Austin Zeiderman has remarked, in relation to his research on urban biopolitics in Bogotá, Colombia, "we understand little about how the politics of life functions in urban contexts and how it affects the way cities are planned, built, governed, and lived" (Zeiderman, 2013: 72). And yet, as Zeiderman shows, biopolitics, and in particular the politics of biological citizenship can bite both ways: he gives the example of people living in designed 'high risk zones' in Bogotá who negotiate their claims on the state via their relationship to the specific geological and biological vulnerabilities through which these zones are governed. Such an analysis reframes the idea of 'rights to the city' in an empirically grounded manner, for, as Zeiderman shows, "the right to housing is thus a privilege bestowed on members of a collectivity whose entitlements are grounded not only in shared membership within a political community but also in their common condition of vulnerability" (ibid.: 73).

The shift to a biopolitical point of view, then, shows us how questions of justice and rights can move beyond concerns with distribution of resources or democratic participation, to be connected with concerns about specific forms of bodily vulnerability. If we are going to think biopolitically, we need to expand our horizons beyond the regulatory effects of urban public health, and of the fragility of bodies submitting passively to the normative demands for the management of their corporeal existence. As Elizabeth Grosz puts it, "cities have always represented and projected images and fantasies of bodies . . . the city . . . enframes, protects, and houses while at the same time taking its own forms and functions from the (imaginary) bodies it constitutes . . . cities of the future, like cities of the present, will not be imposed on an unwilling populace, that is, from the outside" (Grosz, 2001: 48–53). With the fantasy of regulatory and normative imposition thus put to one side, we need to think more expansively about how bodies and brains are shaped in and through the space and places we are born and grow in, dwell in, move through, that shape us as we shape them.

Transcorporeal Exposures: Beyond the Binary

We have become accustomed to think of the relations between bodies and environments as a relationship between two domains. Public health officers think of the habits and practices of those who live in particular urban environments, and focus on how the relationships between urban surroundings, on the one hand, and individual behaviors, on the other, can be made more salutary. Geneticists who consider such matters talk of "GxE," and ponder the interaction of genes with the environment. Specialists in human relations think of workplaces as unsafe or demanding environments, and their effects on our minds and brains. We ourselves fall into ways of writing about pollution in our external environment and its effects on our bodies, our diet, our physical health. And so on. It seems hard to escape this dualism of the inside and the outside, the transactions across the seeming natural border of the skin, the organic unity that it encloses and the portals to the external world that it guards. But for a new urban biopolitics, we need to think beyond this binary.

Conceptually, perhaps this is what Gilles Deleuze tried to convey in his account of the fold: "what always matters is folding, unfolding, refolding" (Deleuze, 1993: 137). It is not a matter of "the interaction between a human animal biologically equipped with senses, instincts, needs, and an external, physical, interpersonal, social environment. . . . the inside is itself no more than a moment, or a series of moments, though which a 'depth' has been constituted within human being . . . a space or series of cavities, pleats and fields, which only exist in relation to those very forces, lines, techniques and inventions that have created them" (Rose, 1996: 188). As Stacey Alaimo argues, material interchanges between human bodies and the environment require "corporeal theories, environmental theories, and science studies [to] meet and mingle in productive ways . . . [T]he environment" is not located somewhere out there, but is always the very substance of ourselves" (Alaimo, 2010: 4). A new practice of ethics is required once one recognizes that the human is embedded in, suffused by, constituted through the very stuff of the material world: a "fraught sense of political agency" can emerge "from the perceived loss of boundaries and sovereignty . . . a trans-corporeal subjectivity in which bodies extend into places and places deeply affect bodies" (ibid.: 5). We see the same approach in other authors who have conjoined the histories of environment and health to grasp how the chemical, industrial, and economic transformations that have "so thoroughly shaped modern environments" have also produced a slew of "toxic, over infectious, agents of illness" which, as they come to settle in the bodies of more and more people, may even mark a new kind of "epidemiological transition" in which the body is enmeshed in "a wide range of material flows, from commodities to the inadvertent byproducts of industry and agriculture to more obscure and natural processes that have not always fallen within the analytic domain of human culture" (Mitman, Murphy, et al., 2004: 3; 10).

Michelle Murphy has traced the highly specific ways that such chemical exposures get materialized—what she calls "the historical ontology of exposure" (Murphy, 2006: 7). But how are we to think about the politics of exposure when the flows—both inside the body and around it—are not so obviously 'material'? How should we think about exposure when the psyche is engaged? How should we think about exposure when these transactions—of exposure, and intoxication—seem to involve vectors (stress, fear, anticipation) that are much less easy to grasp? This is not to endorse a distinction between the psyche and the body, but precisely the reverse: to ask how we can think about exposures when the materiality of being exposed is inextricably entangled with both conscious and non-conscious mental processes.

Opening Our Eyes

What would it mean, then, to act on Lefebvre's injunction that we quoted at the start of this chapter—to "open one's eyes to understand the daily life of the one who runs from his dwelling to the station, near or far away, to the packed underground train, the office or the factory, to return the same way in the evening and come home to recuperate enough to start again the next day"? What would it mean to do this with a focus, not only on the strictly corporeal, but also on the psychological, the mental, and the neuro-biological dimensions of transcorporeality? What would it mean to refuse the binary of organism and environment, using the resources offered to us by the emerging 'ecosocial' or 'neuroecosocial' approaches that we outlined in our last chapter? And how might we reconfigure our approach to social justice in the city in this light?

We can start with the argument we have made at various points in the previous chapters: that humans, like other animals, inhabit, develop in, dwell in, move through certain niches, trajectories across space and time that are composed of relations and transactions between humans, and between humans and their non-human companions, and the material environment that both inhabit. Thus, following our argument in the previous chapter, one might 'decompose the city' analytically into a multiplicity of such niches, or 'biosocial localities,' each with its own characteristic forms of life and its characteristic biologies. This would enable us to have a more finely tuned attention to the well-known gross demographic indicators showing how morbidity and mortality take different patterns in different districts or areas within cities.

But these exposures are not merely material. A niche is not simply the 'objective' material space that one occupies, or moves through over minutes, hours, days of the week, months, and years. For humans, at least, one's niche is not a set of extra-corporeal geolocations 'out there.' We suggested in the last chapter that a niche is more like an *Umwelt* as characterized by Jakob von Uexküll (von Uexküll, [1934] 2010). Although the German word '*Umwelt*' simply translates as 'environment,' von Uexküll uses it to emphasize the ways in which a living creature does not just 'interact' with a given environment, but actively transmutes that environment into a milieu for living its own par-ticular form of life. Thus the *Umwelt* for each animal is that which it perceives, senses, renders perceptible in and through its own sense organs—sight, hear-ing, smell, taste, and so on. It is a world of saliences, of the elements that are of salience to a particular creature in its form of life—its sustenance, its threats, its prey, its conspecifics, its points of reference. These *Umwelten* are not quite objective and not quite subjective, indeed not conceptualizable in terms of such an inner/outer binary in the first place. The tick, the bat, the dog, the human . . . each lives in an 'irreal world'—to use the term coined by Nelson Goodman (Goodman, 1978). And for the human, the *Umwelt* is made up of the particular array of saliences, persons, buildings, visibilities, and affects experienced by those who navigate a biosocial niche, not just shaped by the evolution of our species and the characteristics of our sense organs, but also saturated by memories and meanings, spatialized in terms of pleasures and fears, hopes and dreams, real or imagined experiences, and by the resonances of names and stories of places and spaces.

Mental Maps of the Imagined City

How should we proceed to grasp the diversity of these urban *Umwelten*? One might start by examining the method used by Kevin Lynch in his classic book *The Image of the City* (Lynch, 1960). For Lynch, an image was more than a mental representation. What he terms the "environmental image" is an integral part of each culture, and while it may be "less vivid" today than in pre-industrial societies, it "is still a fundamental part of our equipment for living," permitting "purposeful mobility" for those who inhabit it (ibid.: 124).[11] The environmental image acts as an organizer of activity, its patterns provide a basis for the ordering of knowledge—and vice versa—and its symbolic qualities can establish an emotional relationship between an environment and those who dwell within it, whether of fear or of comfort. What one sees, says Lynch, is "based on exterior form," but how an individual "interprets and organizes this" and how they direct their attention "in turn affects what he sees" (ibid.: 131). But more than these reflections on imageability, and indeed more relevant than his much-quoted argument that urban inhabitants make their city by organizing its parts into a coherent pattern, constructed in terms of *Paths, Edges, Districts, Nodes,* and *Landmarks,* is Lynch's method. His research team interviewed "a small sample of citizens with regard to their image of the environment," asking them first to talk about what comes to mind when they think about their city, how they would describe it to another, and then asking them to draw a "quick map" of the central area of the city "as if they were making a rapid description of the city to a stranger" (ibid.: 140–141). They were then asked to "give complete and explicit directions for the trip they normally take going from home to where they work," picturing themselves making the trip and reporting on the things they would see, hear, or smell, the emotional feelings that they would have at each stage of the journey. These interviews—of which we give only a partial account—were followed by what we would now describe as a walking interview or "go along" (Evans and Jones, 2011), actually taking the route they mapped in their imaginary journey, accompanied by the interviewer who used a tape recorder to capture their answers to questions about their feelings as they walked the route.[12]

Lynch was concerned with the "imageability" of different urban forms: the quality that gives them "a high probability of invoking a strong image in any given observer" (Lynch, 1960: 9). He thus drew normative conclusions from the maps that his interviewees and his researchers drew, arguing that cities need to be made legible or imageable to those who negotiate them. His book thus opened—or re-opened—a line of thought about the perception of the city and its relevance to urban design that continues today. However, we would like to take up Lynch's challenge in another way. The 'subjective' maps of those journeys from home to work that are imagined and then walked by his interviewees are maps of the niches they have constructed for themselves, niches filled with memories and emotions that suffuse the material constraints of managing their daily lives in urban space. This approach to mapping the city was taken further by Stanley Milgram. Milgram is best known for his disturbing studies of obedience to authority (Milgram and Gudehus, 1978), but he is less renowned for the psychological maps of New York and Paris that he and his colleagues created in the 1970s (reprinted in Milgram, 1992). These were collected through empirical studies drawing on Lynch's techniques, that aimed to map the 'psychological representations' that each city inhabitant carries around with them, the cognitive picture they build up of how the streets connect with one another, that enable them to move from place to place. Milgram and colleagues were concerned with the cognitive work involved in knowing a city. But they recognized that mapping is not exclusively a 'cognitive' matter. As Milgram puts it, maps are suffused by "attitudes and feelings" toward different parts of the environment based on their childhood neighborhoods, sites of romantic attachment, and so forth (ibid.: 64). Thus, while Milgram is most concerned with the ways that these maps "encode, distort or selectively represent" urban space, and the comparison with "reality," he also recognizes that such maps contain "emotional and intuitive components" and are collectively shaped, symbolic configurations of belief and knowledge (ibid.: 98–99).

For us, it is this dimension that is primary. Mental maps render visible the often non- conscious ways of inhabitation of one's niche, affectively charged memories, neural traces, which include sites of fascination and pleasure, sites of anxiety and dangers, some experienced, some from half-recalled conversations, stories, or myths. Unfortunately, Milgram did not develop this line of thought. Indeed, in his much-cited paper, "The Experience of Living in Cities," he gives priority to the idea of 'overload' in understanding the quality of urban life (Milgram, 1974: 1462). He argues that this idea was implicit in Simmel's account of the urban citizen, who conserved psychic energy by limiting close acquaintances and maintaining superficial relations with others, and devotes much attention to how individuals and organizations protect themselves from overload, at the cost of limiting spontaneous integration with the life of the city, and estranging themselves from their interpersonal and social environments. His examples are now well known: bystanders do not intervene in crises in cities as they would do in small towns and rural areas, they are less willing to trust and assist strangers, they are less likely to apologize if they bump into people in the street, and cities foster a kind of anonymity between inhabitants, an 'impersonality' that leads to tolerance of private lives and eccentricity. Nonetheless, and despite this focus on the cognitive, in his closing remarks, he refers to "the differing atmospheres of great cities such as Paris, London and New York" and the fact that each "has a distinctive flavor, offering a differentiable quality of experience" (ibid.: 1468)—intriguing remarks that, to the best of our knowledge, he did not develop in subsequent work.

Ecological Psychology

From our point of view, mental maps—if 'map' is the right word here—don't just represent, they enable; they make some ways of thinking, feeling, relating to others, managing one's life, possible, and others difficult or impossible. How then can we go forward to a more granular and transcorporeal conception of a niche, that goes beyond a species-wide conception of the *Umwelt*, that is not bound up in Cartesian binaries, that builds on the work of Lynch and Milgram, but that refuses to deploy ancient trichotomies of cognition, emotion, and volition to characterize inhabitation. One place to begin, and indeed one that has become central to the field of 'ecological psychology,' is with James Gibson's conception of affordances (the paragraphs that follow are heavily indebted to Rose, Birk, et al., 2021).[13] James Gibson invented the term 'affordances,' in his endeavor to think perception in a way that was not premised on the idea of an 'interaction' of 'environment' and 'individual.' As he put it:

> The affordances of the environment are what it offers the animal, what it provides or furnishes, either for good or ill. The verb to afford is found in the dictionary, the noun affordance is not. I have made it up. I mean by it something that refers to both the environment and the animal in a way that no existing term does. It implies the complementarity of the animal and the environment. (Gibson, 1979: 127)

For Gibson, certain material features of a niche—those that are salient in particular ways, imbued with particular meanings and affects—engage with humans co-present with them, making certain ways of acting possible (or impossible). The milieu is embodied in such a way to make it possible to walk, run, sit, look, step, stop and talk, gather in a smaller or bigger group, move through or remain—indeed to occupy that space in the kind of ways described, in such detail, in the ecological studies of William H. Whyte (Whyte, 1980; Whyte, 1988). Gibson in fact uses the term 'ecological niche' to characterize the ways that each organism is attuned to, and stimulated by, its affordances to see, think, and act in particular ways: "a niche," he suggested, "refers more to how an animal lives than to where it lives. I suggest that a niche is a set of affordances" (Gibson, 1979: 128).

Barry Smith has given us a useful interpretation of how Gibson's work enables us to grasp the ways that "the sentient organism is housed or situated within a surrounding environment of which it serves as interior boundary":

> In perception, as in action . . . we are caught up with the very things themselves in the surrounding world, and not with 'sense data' or 'representations.' . . . [but a] direct linkage between the perceiving organism and its environment which grows out of the fact that, in its active looking, touching, tasting, feeling, the organism as purposeful creature is bound up with those very objects . . . which are relevant to its life and to its tasks of the moment. (Smith, 2009: 5)

Gibson was primarily concerned with 'perception' which, for him, was not a matter of mental representations but a direct attunement between the organism and its environment in the ways that enabled its specific ways of life. Gibson makes much of the fact that for humans, as indeed for other organisms, we are not only caught up with 'things' but also with other organisms, including but not limited to our conspecifics who are themselves relevant to our lives and to our tasks of the moment. As Rietveld and Kiverstein point out, "The human ecological niche is shaped and sculpted by the rich variety of social practices humans engage in" (Rietveld and Kiverstein, 2014: 325). The many and varied forms of life that humans have made for themselves each involve shared ways of being with others: "Affordances are possibilities for action the environment offers to a form of life, and an ecological niche is a network of interrelated affordances available in a particular form of life on the basis of the abilities manifested in its practices—its stable ways of doing things. An individual affordance is an aspect of such a niche" (ibid.: 330). Humans have to master the skilled practices, corporeal and cerebral, necessary to conduct themselves in specific situations within a form of life. Rietveld and Kiverstein are right to stress that there is a strong normative presupposition involved here, for the implication is that, in each form of life, there are 'socio-culturally' correct ways for any individual to engage with the multiple possibilities available within what they term 'the rich landscape' of human and non-human affordances.[14]

But we need to inject a certain unease into this picture, for affordances are not such for all. While Rietveld and Kiverstein celebrate the multiple possibilities opened by the publicly available character of the affordances of human niches, they do not address the ways that these are shaped by strategies of government, how they embody particular forms of authoritative knowledge, and are suffused with differentials of power. One might think here, on the one hand, of Michel Foucault's microphysics of power—as in his compelling accounts of the normalizing intent built into the design of spaces and buildings, constraining the interrelations of subjects in prisons, factories, schools, and other disciplinary institutions (Foucault, 1977 [1975]). And, on the other, one might think of Erving Goffman's careful descriptions of the ways in which individuals manage their lives in such institutions (Goffman, 1961; Hacking, 2004). But more, we would need to consider the mobile, swarming, ultra-rapid forms of free-floating control of conduct across space and time incessantly modulating conduct that are gestured at by Gilles Deleuze (Deleuze, 1992) and which were, in earlier times, also analyzed so compellingly by Goffman (Goffman, 1963; Goffman, 1967; Goffman, 1983). Normativity is, as always, intrinsically bound with judgments—by self or others—of non-normativity, of the judgment of those who, by design or for other reasons, are either not capable or not willing to manage themselves according to these norms. And it is here, in the strategies for creating and enforcing norms at any one time and place, and in the multiple forms of distress exacerbated by the perceived discrepancy between the norms and the actuality, that we need to focus in any analysis of urban biopolitics.

Thus, while Rietveld and Kiverstein are thinking of Wittgenstein when they adopt the term "form of life," we might do better to conceptualize what is at stake here in terms of what Stephen Collier and Andrew Lakoff term a "regime of living," problematic situations where the question of how to live is at stake, both for those who would govern, and for those who are governed (Collier and Lakoff, 2007). Collier and Lakoff here draw our attention to the work necessary to create and sustain a form of life in conditions of difficulty or uncertainty, and the ways that norms are negotiated by those subjected to them. However rich the landscapes of material and socio-cultural affordances may be, then, they do not always enable lives to be led in ease or in comfort, especially for those whose 'being in the world' is non-standard. As Arseli Dokumaci reminds us, the attunement that Gibson proposes between the organism and the affordances of an ecological niche vary according to the corporeal, and indeed neural, properties, tendencies, and dispositions of the organism—in this case the human subject—at any particular time, and it is these that make it possible or impossible to see, think, and act in particular ways in that situation (Dokumaci, 2020: 397). The constant negotiation required to make a life within a normative regime is highlighted by Dokumaci's examples from the mundane lives of people with various 'impairments': a spoon that does not afford soup-eating for a person with rheumatoid arthritis, a pedestrian road crossing indicated by lights that does not afford safe crossing for those who do not see well, or a room closure—a door—that does not afford opening for someone physically unable to grasp a doorknob (ibid.: 399). Disability, she argues, "involves the making of new affordances that ensure the continuance of mundane living even under conditions in which that living is most devoid of resources. Further, these affordances are not 'normal' living gone awry; they are not yet another body technique; quoting Ayo Wahlberg, she argues that they are "kinds of living" in and of themselves with their own "vital norms" and their own "quality of life" (Wahlberg, 2016: 185). But what, for Dokumaci, is the particular "*precariousness* of the affordances made by a person with disabilities" (ibid.: 407) is also the precariousness of the affordances that have to be made and negotiated by all those living lives in conditions of adversity, and in particular those experiencing mental distress or living under the description of a mental disorder. Hence, we need to move from thinking of 'niches' to thinking of trajectories of niche construction, or what Milena

Bister, Martina Klausner, and Jörg Niewöhner refer to as 'niching' (Bister, Klausner, et al., 2016; Bieler and Klausner, 2019).[15]

Niching

Niches are constructed in action, in the actions that people take to make their lives manageable within their everyday material, symbolic, semantic, institutional, social, and political constraints.[16] While they draw some inspiration from 'niche construction theory' in evolutionary biology, Bister, Klausner, and Niewöhner propose the term 'niching' to refer, not to species or populations, but to the way that people living with a psychiatric diagnosis "constantly negotiate the multiple tensions between both being part of urban assemblages, exploring them, building social networks, conquering unknown urban spaces and engaging in modes of dwelling that close them off from urban assembling, that fold in on themselves and that individualize experiences" (Bister, Klausner, et al., 2016: 191). They argue that while psychiatry frames this in terms of individual coping strategies and the availability of social support, they "introduce the term niching to explore these tensions in relational or ecological terms . . . These ongoing processes of creating viable surroundings are by no means restricted to people with a psychiatric diagnosis. They are necessarily part of everyone's quotidian life" (ibid.: 192).

Niching, then, is the constant work of creating and recreating one's niche, not as a matter of individual agency but as "an embodied and emplaced practice, a continuous work of navigating the infrastructure of care, and the corporeal consequences of medication, that transcends the opposition of individual actor and material environment." We can see this in examples from our own research in Shanghai. As we described in chapter 3, between the time when we chose Tongli Road for our fieldwork and the actual start of the study, the small factories behind the street were declared illegal and bulldozed to the ground, with no notice, as part of Shanghai's strategy to 'move up the value chain.' Time and again, as our colleagues Lisa Richaud and Ash Amin walked from one shop to another in June 2017, they "heard of the pressure (*yali*) caused by economic collapse and existential uncertainty," yet these "forms of distress and illbeing such as low moods, worried, doubts or anxiety" were "managed in such ways that they become absorbed with everyday rituals of living"—what Richaud and Amin refer to as "situated endurance" (Richaud and Amin, 2020: 78). It was not as if the lives of these migrants were previously secure; the situation of rural-to-urban migrants in

Chinese cities, without the formal residency rights granted by urban *hukou*, is always filled with uncertainty, a constant alertness for the recurrent news of events emanating from national or city government, or from the factory owners themselves, that will require movement to another factory, another part of the city, or even a return to their villages. But, in the words of one migrant worker, the stress experienced by the continual requirement to manage one's self in conditions of precarity was "swallowed back inside one's heart" (ibid.: 97).

At least, in 2017, the inhabitants of Tongli Road did not make use of the languages of psy emanating from China's psychoboom (Yang, 2017; Zhang, 2017; Zhang, 2018); they did not translate *yali* into symptoms or seek expert assistance either in person or in the growing availability of therapeutic interventions on the internet, but rather they 'attuned' themselves via the small-scale sociality of everyday life, shared talk, jokes, complaints, and all the mundane activities of daily 'niching.' But their regimes of living were no less embodied and emplaced, and the question of how they should live was, on the one hand, a problem for those who would govern them, and on the other, an ongoing challenge for their self-management. Self-reports from rural-to-urban migrant workers seem to show less acute illness, chronic disease, and disability than either permanent rural or permanent urban residents, perhaps illustrating the so-called healthy migrant effect (Hesketh, Jun, et al., 2008). Yet long-term prospects may not be so benign (Yang, Wu, et al., 2020) if we are to take seriously the links that psychiatric and social epidemiology has identified between social suffering (Kleinman, Das, et al., 1997), structural violence (Farmer, Nizeye, et al., 2006), and the experience of dis-ease (Marmot and Bell, 2012; Allen, Balfour, et al., 2014; Marmot, 2015; Marmot, Allen, et al., 2020).

Greg Downey has given us a very different example of niching in his study of the daily lives of children living on the streets in São Salvador da Bahia, the capital of the Brazilian state of Bahia in the Northeast Region of Brazil (Downey, 2016). Downey refers to the lives of these children as "a limit case showing the challenges of living in the city as an ecological niche" (ibid.: S52).[17] As Rose, Birk, and Manning put it, the niche for these children:

> is both pre-shaped for them, and requires a constant labour of active recreation, encompassing their daily journeys from the favelas, derelict buildings or vacant spaces where they sleep, to the places where they work, to the traffic ridden streets, road junctions, pavements or elsewhere, where they make a bit of money by begging, watching parked

cars, selling sweets on the buses, or by theft . . . They have devised forms of conduct which make their lives possible, in which they forage for food, visit charity kitchens and meal programmes or find other ways of securing their means of subsistence—for example by procuring meals from restaurant left-overs—in this niche they have collectively constructed for themselves. (Rose, Birk, et al., 2021)

But this example illustrates more than the physical demands and dangers of this daily labor, for the material, social, and neurobiosocial milieu of such 'niching' exposes the children not only to constant stress from the possibility of accidents of violence from hostile strangers, but also to a poor diet and lack of sanitation with unknown effects on their health and their gut microbiome, as well as to a range of exposures to traffic fumes, dangerous chemicals, pathogens, and parasites.

Precarious Niching

What, then, are the mental and physical costs of precarious niching? Statistical reports demonstrating the pattern of physical and mental health consequences of the Covid-19 pandemic have shone a bright and painful light on the highly inequitable distribution of precarity, even in wealthy countries with developed welfare and social security systems, and in cities that had previously imagined themselves as well-governed. In the UK, for example, despite the vacuous repetition of the mantra 'we are all in it together,' it is clear that the greatest toll in physical sickness and death has fallen on the many who are forced to make their lives in the most precarious niches, those living in poverty, inadequate housing, financial insecurity, those at risk of domestic abuse, and—in particular—members of black and minority ethnic communities, who are inter alia over-represented in the health service (Laurencin and McClinton, 2020; Office for National Statistics (UK), 2020; Rose, Manning, et al., 2020; Tai, Shah, et al., 2020). Inequities among those infected with Covid-19 and those who get very sick or die from their infection are almost certainly accounted for by the social conditions in which they live—too few rooms at home, frontline jobs that do not allow working from home, exclusion from forms of public support, and underlying medical conditions themselves arising from conditions of precarity. When it comes to mental distress, it is predictable of course that many people are sad, worried, miserable, angry, scared, exhausted, lonely, troubled, distressed, perturbed, apprehensive, dejected because of the pandemic. But it is most likely that these feelings will tip into enduring and serious mental distress among people seeking to sustain their lives in conditions of significant existing structural adversity, experiencing enforced isolation and the evaporation of whatever meager social support was already on offer.

We have already discussed the dilemmas of 'stress' in great detail, but we can now begin to see how we might go beyond the distinction between objective and subjective that it relies upon, in other words between stress, stressors, and stress responses. In an attempt at clarification of the literature on stress "for the twenty first century," Blair Wheaton and colleagues define stressors as "conditions of threat, challenge, demands, or structural constraints that, by the very fact of their occurrence or existence, call into question the operating integrity of the organism" (Wheaton, Young, et al., 2013: 300). Starting from this definition, they argue that there is "a sequence of causation including stressors which may precipitate stress depending on the social circumstances attending the occurrence of the stressor and, therefore, its meaning, which in turn may precipitate distress, depending on the state of coping with resources when the stressor occurs. The multiple contingencies in this process suggest that many things we think of as potentially stressful turn out not to be and, even when stressful, may not translate into increased distress" (ibid.). Reprising Richard Lazarus, these authors argue that an individual organism endows something with meaning through a process of 'appraisal'—"people's evaluative judgment of the situation or event that is influenced by individual-level and environmental factors" (Epel, Crosswell, et al., 2018). It is this reaction that provokes the generalized stress response, with its hormonal cascade via the HPA axis and its neurobiological consequences of gene activation or de-activation. Unfortunately, this endeavor to clarify and simplify the confused literature into a single model is *still* grounded in the idea of some primordial boundary between the external and internal world of the individuated organism, crossed only by an internal evaluative mechanism. For the new urban biopolitics we seek, we would need a conception of stress that refused these distinctions. It would go beyond the suggestion that what was needed was to measure stress in context and the psychophysiological individuation that is their premise (ibid.: 162). It would thus underpin a different urban biopolitics of stress that did not, as Epel and her colleagues suggest, focus on individually targeted interventions that will enhance stress resilience and promote "healthy behaviors" but that would seek to reshape much more fundamentally the conditions of inhabitation of biopsychosocial niches.

To begin this task, we would need sociological and ethnographic investigations to map out the shaping of stressors by collective experiences in specific niches characterized by poverty, exclusion, isolation, racism, and violence. That is hardly new. What we add nonetheless is, first, a recognition that our forms of life have created a material exposome that is toxic not only to our corporeality in general, but to our urban brains in particular. Stress pathways are undoubtedly important here, but so, perhaps, are the disturbances in the microbiome which have been linked with anxiety, depression, and bipolar disorder. A number of researchers are now focusing on exposome-driven brain inflammation and their role mood disorders, neurodegeneration, Alzheimer's disease, and many other forms of mental disorder and distress (Ryu and McLarnon, 2009; Haney, Zhao, et al., 2013; Rosenblat, Cha, et al., 2014; Pariante, 2017). This area of work is marked by overclaiming that goes beyond the findings of research and often neglects the key question of causal direction. There is certainly no one-way path between inflammation and its cerebral and mental correlates: research shows a complex and bidirectional relationship between inflammatory brain markers and negative or positive social experiences, relations with loved ones, or the experience of loneliness (Eisenberger and Moieni, 2020). While researchers struggle with directions of causality, from our own transcorporeal perspective, this actually offers evidence of the pathways that inextricably entangle the cerebral within its ecological niche. It begins to turn theoretical accounts of atmospheres into an empirically tractable understanding of how "humans capacities, and health and disease," are shaped and reshaped by "the extensive range of specific external exposures which include radiation, infectious agents, chemical contaminants and environmental pollutants, diet, lifestyle factors (e.g. tobacco, alcohol), occupation and medical interventions" (Wild, 2012) through mechanisms including "metabolic changes, protein modifications, DNA mutations and adducts, epigenetic alterations, and perturbations of the microbiome" (Niedzwiecki, Walker, et al., 2019: 107).

We have suggested that a new vitalist urban biopolitics might begin with mapping the urban exposome. Perhaps the clearest present-day example is how researchers are currently mapping air pollution (Hoek, Brunekreef, et al., 2002; Guxens, Lubczyńska, et al., 2018), including its relationship to the probability of being diagnosed with a mental disorder (Bakolis, Hammoud, et al., 2020). A renewed urban biopolitics would be open to a range of sensory mapping strategies, coupled with neurobiological assessments of brain development across human lives, to show how precarious and dangerous inhabitations, that entail exposures to soil and water pollution, and to industrial intoxicants, have consequences for brains as well as bodies (Katukiza, Ronteltap, et al., 2015; Porzionato, Mantiñan, et al., 2015; Ahmed, 2020).

But beyond mapping this 'material' exposome, one would also need to map the irreal worlds constituted in the niching trajectories of people living in different forms of adversity. We would thus need to combine 'ecosocial' methods, such as the mental maps of Lynch and Milgram, and the 'walk-along' interviews that have been so suggestive in the 'niching' research of Niewöhner, Bieler, Bister, and Klausner, with the ecosocial momentary assessment capacities of smartphone apps such as 'the Urban Mind' (Bakolis, Hammoud, et al., 2018), which are already being explored by a number of research groups (Erhan, Ndubuaku, et al., 2019; McEwan, Richardson, et al., 2020; Reichert, Braun, et al., 2020: 159). It is now possible to combine smartphone apps that regularly poll their users for 'Ecological Momentary Assessments' of moods and emotions, with monitoring of physiological function such as heart rate and measures of physical behavior, such as accelerometers to track the speeds of walking, non-invasive measures of brain activity such as mobile ECT or NIRS caps, and of course GPS trackers that can accurately identify a location and correlate this with features of the urban environment.

For many researchers with an experimental background, the advantage of these methods is that they enable research to move out of the lab and into real life, while avoiding the reliance on 'subjective assessments' derived from individuals' self-report on their mental state. However, for our point of view, that self-report, that is, the subjective experience of the urban environment, remains crucial. It is to this end that Winz and Söderström, developing the arguments in earlier papers by the present authors,[18] propose biosensory ethnographies that combine continuous measures of electrodermal activity (EDA) with ethnographic observations and interviews to analyze ecological processes in psychosis (Winz and Söderström, 2021). Their aim is "to provide an ecological (temporal and spatial) analysis of the actual encounter of the participants with the urban" with the aim of capturing "the situated experience of persons living with mental health problems" and illuminating "the precise ecology of mental illness" (ibid.: 161).

We take a critical distance from the framing of this work in terms of the problematic concept of psychosis and the suggestion that those living under such a diagnosis have a distinct sensory relationship with urban environments. We are also concerned with the way that this approach seems to regard those who participate in their study as experimental subjects, data points rather than co-researchers. We also remain unconvinced that the apparently objective physiological measure of skin conductance is the most appropriate for assessing 'arousal and stress' as the corporal dimension of urban sensory experience. Nonetheless, our approach has much in common with the strategy of biosensory ethnography that these authors aim to develop. Drawing on many of the sources we have discussed in this book, we share their aspiration to "bring biosocial investigations out of the laboratory and into daily life situations [and] get a better understanding of the intertwining roles of inter-sensory perception, the built environment and spatial transitions in urban mental health" (Winz and Söderström, 2021: 169).

A New Urban Biopolitics?

When David Harvey, in *Social Justice and the City*, sought to bring together sociological and geographical imaginations of the city, his view was that, however important, the 'psychological' dimension of the urban experience, "reactions to complexity, depth perception, associations in meaning, pattern preferences, and so on" would be difficult if not impossible to relate to the actual patterns of activity as they unfolded in urban life (Harvey, 2009 [1973]: 33). If we have now reached a point when those difficulties can be overcome, technically and methodologically, what are the implications for how we might seek social justice in the vital city?

For some, the answer seems simple: if humans benefit, in terms of physical and mental well-being, from green spaces, because of their evolved love of nature, what is needed is to increase access to green spaces. But this would be an urban planner's solution to a problem that lies, not in space itself but in structural and systemic inequities in the experience of the city: the 'structural violence' (Galtung and Höivik, 1971) that is the consequence of economic, political, and legal structures, and gender discrimination and racism, impairing the lives of so many, yet so embedded in our forms of life, in the niches we inhabit and create, that they are normalized and invisible. In this sense, the demand for access to green space can lead us to a dead end. The transcorporeal exposures of bad housing, degraded neighborhoods, overcrowding, financial insecurity, precarious employment, obesogenic and polluted environments, social exclusion, racism, stigmatization, and violence cannot be combated by planting trees, encouraging urban gardening, or designing in parks, however much these might sometimes provide some temporary solace. We should not dismiss the aspirations of those urban 'Thrive' movements that are spreading to many cities across the globe, at least to the extent that they seek to valorize and rebuild the non-professional informal networks of mutual support that are so crucial in the immediate experience of urban inhabitation. But these are not sufficient to redress the systemic inequalities, structural violence, and social suffering ingrained in the socio-spatial nature of most cities.

The need to address these systemic and structural issues does not mean that one should dismiss changes in the 'microphysics of power' materialized in urban design. In the same way as city streets have been redesigned with dropped curbs to enhance the opportunities for mobility of those who use wheelchairs or push buggies, a new vitalist biopolitics would involve multiple redesign of the micro-architecture of signage, pavements, street furniture, pedestrian spaces, transport arrangements, car-free zones, and much more. But it might also involve the kinds of large-scale urban imaginations that, in Europe, lay behind the creation of Garden Cities and New Towns, and which, in countries such as China, are underpinning major innovations in design at the whole-city level today. If it is possible to imagine, and enact, the making and remaking of neighborhoods, city centers, and whole cities for 'ecological' reasons, it is no less possible to imagine and enact the remaking of cities to maximize the vital lives, the mental and neural well-being, of all those who inhabit them.

This is, we think, one way in which, today, we can "open our eyes" to understand and transform the daily lives of those who run from their dwellings to the stations to the packed metro trains, the over-airconditioned office, the increasingly roboticized factory, the intensely surveilled call center, the brutal distribution warehouse, the relentless food delivery scooter and the like, or who are forced by social isolation and environmental danger to shelter in their apartments from morning to evening, day after day, week after week, year after year. Perhaps in this way we can, without nostalgic humanism or utopianism, answer Lefebvre's call to extend the right to the city—the vital, neuroecosocial right to the city—to all its citizens.

Conclusion: Toward a Sociology of Inhabitation

In this book, we have argued for a re-vitalization of social theory and socio-logical research, contending that our understanding of the vicissitudes of human experience, of the actual mental and physical lives of human beings as they make their ways in the spaces and places that they inhabit, will remain incomplete until it accepts the methodological and theoretical implications of the fact that humans are, inescapably, living beings. This requires us to engage, critically but seriously, with the knowledge that is emerging from the life sciences about the entangled pathways enmeshing living organ-isms in their material, social, and symbolic milieus across their lives. We have suggested that the implications of such a biosocial approach to human inhabitation are particularly pertinent for understanding urban lives, that is to say, the abilities and the ailments of the human beings who are born in cities, migrate to cities, and live in cities. We have drawn on insights from ecology to assist us in grasping the ways in which humans transform their urban environment into a setting for living, through the constant process of creation and recreation of niches. And we have concluded that it is through the study of trajectories of neurosocial life within such niches that we can best understand the transcorporeal shaping of urban inhabitation.

Humans share their urban niches with many other forms of life that make cities their home. From rats, to microbes and viruses, the history of human urban inhabitation—vitality, morbidity, mortality—has always been entangled with these other life forms. There has also been the constant challenge of managing the inputs and outputs of vital lives in cities, from securing supplies of food and water to organizing the disposal of excrement. To pursue these issues in detail would require another book. Here, we have followed the threads that can help us understand the mental consequences of inhabiting the multitude of sprawling, noisy, traffic-ridden, crowded, polluted niches that we call cities. To try to make sense of the multiple forces that bear upon urban mental life, we have focused on the migrants who have moved, and are still moving, in their millions from rural villages and small towns into ever-expanding cities. There is, of course, no one story of 'the rural migrant.' However, rural-to-urban migrants—today as in earlier centuries—often occupy marginal, racialized, and stigmatized localities, and so are disproportionately exposed to the vectors that research has shown to be associated with mental distress.

In the field of migration and mental health, most attention has been focused on international migration, for example migration from Europe to the United States in the late nineteenth and early twentieth centuries. However, as we have argued, migration from the countryside drove the growth of European cities in the nineteenth century and was key to the concerns of Walter Benjamin, George Simmel, and other theorists of modernity. It has driven the recent growth of cities like Shanghai, São Paulo, Mumbai, Lagos. This is why we have suggested that the rural migrant—despite the multitude of historical, geographical, cultural, and communal local differences and specificities—is the defining figure of the accelerating urbanization processes with which policymakers have grappled since the mid-nineteenth century, and still grapple with as we write. With colleagues in the United Kingdom and China, we looked in detail at Shanghai, where the metropolis is being transformed by the arrival of millions of migrants from rural provinces; with colleagues in the UK and São Paulo we continue to explore the experiences of those favela dwellers who now consider themselves Paulistas, but whose families migrated, mainly from North East Brazil, one or two generations ago. Together with our colleagues, we have been trying to imagine a critical interdisciplinary sociology of the experience of those who have moved to the metropolis in search of a better life, yet who too often experience adversity, uncertainty, and precarity. We believe that such a sociology can not only tell us a lot about the consequences of such precarity for people's subjective states, or their 'mental health,' but also provide a new vitalist way of thinking about the central questions of our discipline concerning the consequences of adversity—social injustice, social suffering, and systemic violence—for life itself.

We have argued that, in seeking to grasp the subjective consequences of migration to, and living in, cities, we must go beyond the correlational style of thought that has characterized analyses of the social determinants of mental health for several decades. We must also move beyond arguments in both the social sciences and the life sciences that are framed in terms of 'interactions' between individuals and their environment. We consider these to be inadequate for a number of reasons. There is a lack of granularity in the broad-brush correlations between urban living and mental health that such approaches produce. There are also basic problems with the way that interactionist modes of thinking conceive of relations between a coherent individual bounded by their skin and an external social and material environment. There are, of course, many accounts of 'embodiment' in philosophy, anthropology, and feminist theory. There are phenomenological accounts of the experience of one's body, bodily comportment, sociological accounts of the social shaping of the micro and macro management of bodily comportment, feminist accounts of the performativity of gendered bodies, and many more. But in relation to health and illness, references to the need to understand the embodied nature of experiences and adversity have often been more aspirational than mechanistic—that is to say, they have not been grounded in an attention to specific pathways and mechanisms.

However, the kinds of research that we have discussed in this book demonstrate that we are now able to trace out some of these pathways and mechanisms through which modes of urban inhabitation breach the deceptive boundary of the skin, and hence to understand the organism as constitutively enmeshed in its material, transpersonal, cognitive, affective, semantic, remembered, and imagined irreal world. We have used the example of stress as a focus for much of our thinking about the pathways that are involved in this transcorporeality. Stress has been a constant refrain in reflections on urban life since at least the nineteenth century, but the meanings of stress and the mechanisms through which it is transmuted to human bodies and brains have often been unclear and have long been contested. Stress points us to only one of many pathways, of course. But we have argued that contemporary research on stress can help us to make *partial* sense of at least *one* of the ways in which, for many, the everyday experience of the exigencies of urban inhabitation, of affliction, and suffering, is not merely mental and psychological but written in bone, blood, and brain: in lungs, livers, and hearts, in gut microbiomes, in endocrine systems, in the activation of genetic sequences, in synapses, neurons, neurogenesis, and neural circuits.

We use the phrase 'a sociology of inhabitation' to describe our approach—a sociology of what is at stake in the precarious daily work of making a space in the world into a milieu habitable for living. At the heart of such a sociology of inhabitation is our proposal that if we are to understand what it means to inhabit the city today, and especially how multiple forms of urban injustice mark the bodies and souls of urban citizens, the basis for such an understanding might be found in attention to the vital realities of *life itself*. This does not mean that we are dismissive of the legal or philosophical language of rights and justice, or of the claims that people make in the name of equal rights on municipal authorities, on powerful neighbors, or simply on one another. But it comes from a concern, to put it no more strongly, that some of the theoretical and academic literatures that focus on the 'right to the city,' or that pursue 'spatial justice' within it, miss some of the central problems of urban inhabitation today.

We have suggested that, to fully grasp the ways that mental life is marked and often scarred by life in cities, we would do well to turn beyond psychology to emerging theories and concepts in the neurosciences. No doubt much research in neuroscience is vulnerable to the familiar critiques of reductionism and individualism. But we believe it is necessary to engage with developments in neuroscience that do not extrapolate to human societies from laboratory-based research with inbred mice and rats, and which do not study the human being as an isolated individual or a data point in a randomized controlled trial. Researchers in different fields and traditions in neuroscience are grappling with the recognition that, for scientific and not ideological reasons, it is necessary to place human brains in human bodies— bodies with organs, with nerves, with certain sensory capacities, inhabited by billions of microbes—and to place those bodies, in turn, in the niches and milieus within which they have co-evolved. There is certainly a work of 'critical friendship' to do in such collaborations, as we have suggested in previous chapters. But there is also space for a more affirmative engagement.

In proposing such a neuroecosocial approach to urban experience, we are building on the idea of biological localities that we have developed elsewhere (Fitzgerald, Rose, et al., 2016b; Fitzgerald, Rose, et al., 2016a). This concept, in turn, arose from Margaret Lock's anthropological recognition of the fact that there were 'local biologies': that to say a phenomenon such as the menopause is biological does not imply that it is universal (Lock, 1993; Lock and Kaufert, 2001). Our concept of 'biological localities' similarly reminds us that historically and culturally shaped places have both social and biological consequences for the human and non-human organisms who inhabit them, and indeed who co-create them. And if lived space is, at least from this perspective, biological, then a politics of such lived space must also be a biopolitics; the politics of *urban* space must also be an *urban biopolitics*. That means thinking of a good city, a just city, in terms of the capacities of its multiple overlapping populations to live lives, and to go on living lives, that are as unfettered as possible by embodied and embrained forms of sickness, pain, and distress. This is the 'other biopolitics' that we argue for, when we ask what it would mean to produce and sustain 'good' urban life today.

For us, such a biopolitics is not an abstract theoretical proposition—indeed, biopolitics and biopower were not abstract concepts for Michel Foucault, from whom we have borrowed this term (Rabinow and Rose, 2006). Nor does it require some revolutionary rupture or radical break from the past. From the garden city movement of the early twentieth century, to the policies of social housing of the 1950s and 1960s, to campaigns against gentrification and displacement, and to small-scale movements to create urban gardens and the like that are happening today, we have well-established ideas, policies, and practices that take the material environment of the city as *an environment* for *an organism*, and take this as the starting point for a very particular kind of urban politics. These may not think of themselves as biopolitical, but they are. And although an urban biopolitics may well entail the production of a particular kind of governable subject as outlined by Foucault in his analysis of nineteenth-century town planning (Foucault, 1984; Elden, 2016), it is also not reducible to strategies for the creation of docile subjects fit for economic and sociopolitical exploitation.

How, then, can one build on the kinds of insights we have traced in this book to create a new urban biopolitics that places mental life at its heart? We can benefit from examples from developments in architecture and design that aim to provide security and affordance for aging, cognitively impaired, or neurodegenerative communities; for example, using visual and auditory clues to let a person with a neurodegenerative condition know where they are, or interior design without patterns that can lead to disorientation for someone with a brain disorder, and so on.[1] Perhaps this sounds banal. But it seems to us a useful starting point for developing ways to create environments that are co-productive with the actual brains and brain functions of the people who are going to make their lives within those environments. We might also think of the various Maggie's Centres dotted around the UK—a series of carefully designed and landscaped modern buildings, located near major hospitals, and which are intended to provide psychological and social restoration to cancer sufferers and their families, through specific architectural features and careful landscape design.[2] Here again, the specific capacity and frailties of a body-in-need-of-recuperation become the basis from which a built environment takes its rationale. There may be no explicit claim to justice in these strategies for those in the throes of a terrible ailment, except the basic claim that access to treatment should be based on need and not on wealth. Yet these are nonetheless strategies that prioritize what one might call 'the right to the requirements for living' for those making their lives within the new vital norms that such illnesses create.

It is here, we suggest, that consciously addressing the intersection of biology and building may hold some political promise. We might consider the UK National Health Service's 'Healthy New Towns' initiative, which aims to build 26,000 'healthy' new homes on NHS property, as an exemplar to the wider built environment industry: "Places where people live have a significant impact on their mental and physical health but that impact is too often negative," says the leaflet setting out the scheme: "it is essential to help prevent ill health by planning, designing and developing higher quality places."[3] The ambitions are as ordinary and as theoretically unexciting as thinking about safe walking and cycling routes, but they also mean foregrounding buildings that afford socialization, spaces that make leisure possible, integrated primary care health centers, and so on. Why might this not be, just as the program describes, the basis of a wider strategy to create 'healthy, safe and sustainable cities' through architecture and urban design, through housing, through the management of mobilities, through the careful construction and maintenance of biophysical environments from microbes to air quality?

We are not suggesting setting aside questions of urban justice or the 'right to the city'—such rhetorical claims, and the legal and political instruments borne out of them, remain central to debates around access to housing, about the construction and maintenance of high-quality infrastructure, about access to the resources produced *by* the city, and increasingly about the quality of the urban environment and the rights, not only to basic utilities such as clean water and adequate sewage disposal systems, but also to be free from air polluted by traffic fumes and other vectors of what we would term the urban exposome. Our aim, rather, has been to move those questions onto a biopolitical territory; to wonder if a politics framed in terms of demands for urban inhabitants to be able to live as free as possible from debilitating stress—in all its material and social forms—would not serve the ends of justice in a way that is currently under-appreciated. This would also be a politics that placed at its center the actual production of urban habitats that maximized the possibilities for our lives as vital organisms, whether through the formal routes of architecture, urban design, and urban planning, or just the informal arrangements and constructions that individuals use to make their places habitable. What would our focus on pathways add to the examples that we have cited above? Perhaps only this: to start, not from the dreams of architects and planners, but from the experience of those living in adversity as they construct and enact the trajectories of their particular urban niches day by day; to learn the mental maps of their *Umwelts*, and to be led by them in starting any biopolitical reconstruction of the urban experience in the light of their expertise on what, short of fundamental socio-economic transformations, might mitigate mundane everyday urban stress.

It is fair to ask how such an urban biopolitics attentive to the neuroeco-social pathways that underpin distress might address the dire experiences of those making their lives in the slums, ghettos, and favelas of the Global South. One does not need a biomolecular gaze to be aware of the toxic combinations of poverty, overcrowding, dilapidated dwellings, polluted water, sewage, chemical contamination, and the subjective experiences of precarious existence to recognize the multiple potential pathways to disease, disability, and mental distress. But even here, short of complete urban reconstruction, transformation of labor markets, implementing citywide strategies to combat racism, social exclusion, and much more, an urban biopolitics with a neuroecosocial gaze can underpin collaborative work with those who make their lives in those conditions to understand, and to support and develop, all those material and social affordances that can mitigate it. It would, for example, reject, or at least situate, the focus on interventions in 'the first 1000 days' to mitigate the 'toxic stress' that some believe accounts for the reproduction of poverty across generations (Hackman and Farah, 2009; Segretin, Hermida, et al., 2016; Lipina and Evers, 2017; Farah, 2018).[4] While the impact of poverty, malnutrition, poor sanitation, and other forms of adversity on women during pregnancy and in the early years is certainly crucial, it is too easy to blame these for the perpetuation of poverty in families through the years, and to think that interventions focused on the caregiver (usually envisioned as the mother) will overcome the systematic disadvantage and structural violence that continues to adversely affect bodies and brains into adulthood (Sharp, Lawlor, et al., 2018; Pentecost and Meloni, 2020). A neuroecosocial biopolitics such as the one that we are advocating would refuse to make individuals or families take responsibility for their own biosocial fate (Hedlund, 2012; Kelly-Irving and Delpierre, 2019). It would recognize that it is scientifically mistaken to extrapolate from laboratory experiments with rodents to "the entirely different notion that higher quality psychosocial experience in the first 2 or 3 years of life will have a much greater effect than similar experiences later on, because the early experiences bring about a lasting change in brain structure" (Rutter, 2002: 13). Indeed, it remains the case, as Michael Rutter pointed out two decades ago, that while we still have limited understanding of the mechanisms or pathways of structural or functional neurobiological modifications across the human life course, we know that human brain development, including neurogenesis, continues through adolescence and into later years, and we know that even for those whose neurological development has been marred by extreme deprivation in the early years, there is experience-dependent brain plasticity across the life course and rapid and enduring improvements in cognitive functioning if their home environment improves (Rutter et al., 2007). Brain development is not set at infancy but affected by adversity, including environmental toxicity, throughout life. Thus, our neuroecosocial biopolitics would take as its object the mapping and transformation of the structural conditions that not only deny so many decent housing, education, and employment, but condemn them to making their lives within toxic, obesogenic, polluted environments, where they are reliant on cheap but overprocessed food promoted by transnational corporations, undoubtedly negatively affecting their microbiomes and much else—together denying them what some have termed 'ecological justice' (Prescott and Logan, 2016).

In the cities of the Global North, perhaps the clearest example of concerted strategies to address urban mental health are those developed under the title of Thrive: the loosely associated movements that have spread from New York (ThriveNYC)[5] to London (Thrive LDN),[6] Toronto (ThriveToronto),[7] and elsewhere. Each of these initiatives is different, but we will focus here on ThriveNYC, the first of these Thrives, which was initiated in 2015 and became the subject of much criticism.[8] The strategy arose from the perception that on the one hand, as many as one in five New Yorkers were experiencing mental health problems that were not just deeply troubling for individuals and their families, but were exacting a social and economic cost on the city itself. Yet, on the other hand, the resources of the city could and should be mobilized to tackle that problem at a population-wide level, not just to address mental illness but also to support and promote mental health.[9] Thus, in the words of ThriveNYC's *Roadmap for Mental Health for All*, "our ability to thrive—as human beings and as a city—is closely tied to our mental health" (Thrive NYC, 2019: 10). The *Roadmap* sets out the six "Guiding Principles" that underpinned its approach. *Changing the culture* to enable New Yorkers to have an open conversation about mental health and training people in ways of responding to those in mental distress; *Acting early*, prioritizing preventive intervention especially in families and for children in schools; *Closing treatment gaps* by providing mental health care provisions locally in every community and thus improving access and impact, especially in relation to homelessness and opioid addiction; *Partnering with communities* by 'embracing the wisdom and strength of local communities,' creating what were termed 'culturally competent solutions' seemingly focused on pathways to specialist care to improve use of services by those from black and minority ethnic groups with mental health needs; *Using better data* by collecting reliable citywide data on the health and emotional wellness of children and the factors affecting it, and establishing a mental health innovation lab to analyze and interpret the data; and, last, *Strengthening the government's ability to lead* by creating a mental health council to engage the community and implement the plans.

Gary Belkin, then Chief, Strategy and Policy officer of ThriveNYC, together with Chirlane McCray, First Lady of New York City and one of the key initiators and supporters of the strategy, suggest that these are key elements in what they term a public health approach to mental health, one that is focused on solutions that are "large scale and generally operate outside the context of individual medical treatment, although they also identify better design and equitable access to effective treatment and services [and] therefore engage a range of policy, health system, and social levers for mitigating illness and poor outcomes, and remove obstacles to living in preventive and health-promoting environments" (Belkin and McCray, 2019: S156). Yet, despite these aspirations, the initiatives that they highlight focus on identifying those in need of specialist services and facilitating access to treatment. They barely touch on the 'neuroecosocial' imperatives for a new urban biopolitics that we have aimed to highlight in this book.[10] They devote one sentence to acknowledging that the built environment and the social environment of cities may be linked to mental health,[11] but despite referencing many papers on these issues, their multimillion-dollar strategy does not include measures to address the role of the urban milieu itself in exacerbating or mitigating mental distress.

Our focus on material affordances suggests that a truly 'public health' approach to urban mental health would have very different priorities. It would need to look much more closely at the actual trajectories that are lived by those in adversity, as they inhabit, create and recreate their urban niches, to identify which affordances exacerbate or mitigate stress, perhaps employing some of the methods for the ecological assessment of experience that we have discussed in this book. It would need to work, not just with mental health and social work professionals, or even just with public health officials, but with architects, planners, builders, managers of offices and workplaces, and indeed all those who should be involved in the redesign of urban niches and regimes of urban inhabitation. This requires addressing issues very distant from those prioritized in standard psychiatric interventions. These might include attention to the minutiae of the design of street furniture so that one can walk on pavements without obstructions. They would certainly focus on traffic flows, to ensure that as many urban citizens as possible, and particularly those living in adversity, could make their lives free of traffic noise, and free of pollution from traffic fumes. They would need to address the dumping of chemical effluent and other toxic waste from factories and other industrial activities. They would need to take seriously the architectural and spatial underpinnings of anxiety, designing spaces without blind corners and dark alleys, and free from the health-destroying presence of betting shops, pawn shops, or shopfronts defaced with violent or offensive graffiti. Perhaps as with dementia-friendly cities, they would recognize the need to incorporate clear signage, designed to make sure that however distressed one is, on can know one's location without having to resort to a smartphone. Perhaps they would need to take account of the fact that respite from urban stress sometimes lies simply in the availability of small corner shops, local cafes (not chain) where one receives a simple nod of recognition from a familiar face and can pause a while over a cup of tea or coffee without feeling obliged to buy food or to be transfixed by a laptop. Perhaps they would need to design well-lit, clean, and managed squares with comfortable benches and other affordances of relaxation for those who wish, not to consume, but to merely rest awhile.

Lives at work would also need to come under biopolitical attention, for example investigation and rectification of the pathogenic character of workspaces, whether these be Amazon warehouses, polluted factories, air-conditioned offices, or food processing plants. Questions would need to be asked about the lives of those driving Uber taxis and riding Deliveroo cycles that increasingly form the workspaces of so many of those who work in our cities. Lives within the home would also need to be prioritized in such a neuroecosocial biopolitics. For example, it would need to give a high priority to addressing the challenges to loneliness, thinking not simply about the right to have a secure roof over one's head but also the right not to be constantly alone under that roof—to be a visible and valued member of a social community, a right to be part of all the mundane interactions and encounters through which communities are produced (Cacioppo and Patrick, 2008; Jo Cox Commission on Loneliness, 2017; Mann, Bone, et al., 2017). In many dimensions of such a biopolitics, urban design and urban architecture play an important role. For example, lonely-proofing communities is not only an architectural question, but it is *partly* an architectural question. One can thus see how an architecture engaged with the kind of renewed biopolitics we promote here would be concerned with producing shared spaces that afford informal everyday encounters, housing developments that are amenable to people at very different points in their lives, creating inclusive city centers that do not give priority to the consumption habits of shoppers, tourists, and young people, and so on.

Of course, none of this is in opposition to or a substitute for the need to address those macro-level stressors that are experienced disproportionally by those living with mental distress. Some of these are obvious, in the large-scale issues of design and availability of decent housing to ensure security, and the use of concierges to manage them. One can add to all the other arguments for something like a universal basic income, an evidence-based claim that the stresses that are a consequence of financial insecurity and precarity are major factors in generating and sustaining mental distress. One can also underpin arguments for tackling structural racism and systemic violence with evidence demonstrating clear and intelligible neurobiosocial pathways that link these to mental distress and often to frank mental disorder. One can point to the effects that food poverty, especially in obesogenic environments, has on mental as well as physical well-being through its consequences for the microbiome. One can map the distribution of toxic atmospheres across urban space and reveal how many of those who experience all those other disadvantages also have to make and enact their niches in habitats suffused with both visible and invisible pollutants known to have malign neurobiological consequences. This does not simply reduce the politics of the city to the experience of stress. But it does ask us to think more critically, and more expansively, about what it is exactly that we are claiming a right to. It asks us to take seriously the proposal that the right to the city is also an ecological claim—indeed, one might say, at least in Lefebvre's formulation, it is an ecological claim *first*. Hence, if one were to think of the right to the city in vitalist terms, it becomes amenable to an ecological politics that takes the indivisible imbrications of organisms and environments as its primary—if not its only—point of intervention.

This book is only an attempt to establish the historical, scientific, and theoretical credentials of such a project. It is not the place for an extensive account of what that looks like in practice. But we recognize that it might lead us onto some uncomfortable political terrain. It might mean, for example, transforming the political desire for the state to engage in the construction of large-scale affordable housing developments, by considering whether alternative approaches might be better able to innovate the internal design and the external environmental configurations of housing to mitigate stressful effects for some people. Perhaps strategies involving multiple small-scale architects and builders might produce housing that better recognizes how a sense of insecurity in and around a person's primary dwelling can be implicated in sustained low mood, and how designing in certain forms of conviviality might ameliorate that stress. Some, such as John Boughton (2018), have suggested that these concerns amount to a stealth critique of public housing. But housing is not a social good simply by virtue of being public or being affordable. Perhaps we need to abandon our laments about the privatization or quasi-privatization of particular urban spaces, to explore whether formally private but nonetheless 'publicly accessible' parks might do the job better. And, more generally, perhaps we might abandon a sentimental attachment to a leading role for public authorities in favor of an enhanced imagination of what affordances the inhabitants of a space—even transient inhabitants—require.

We could go on. But we leave the fleshing out of such ideas for future, less speculative, and more richly empirical projects to come. In any event, what makes such proposals meaningful for us—whether they ultimately prove achievable or not—is that they speak to our commitment to thinking about justice in the city not simply as an assertion of legal rights and entitlement, but rather as the capacity to live well, as a biological person, in a habitat that brings comfort and pleasure. What holds them together is a recognition that urban dwellers are living organisms before they are citizens; that where they live is a habitat before it is a house or apartment; that the space in which they walk to work or go shopping or bed down for the night is an ecological niche as much as it is a neighborhood. There are dangers—and dangerous simplifications—in turning urban thought in this direction. We have discussed many of those dangers already. But the hope underpinning the approach we have advocated in this book is that the benefits of such thinking might outweigh the costs, not just for those already enjoying the benefits of the wealthy cities of Europe and North America, but rather for those systematically and structurally excluded in so many ways from those benefits: those living precarious lives in run-down social housing projects, and the banlieue of the urban penumbra, and especially for those migrating to the great megacities of 'the Global South,' anticipating that the opportunities of the urban milieu will enable them to improve their own material and vital lives and those of their children and families. If we start from these concerns, it seems to us inarguable that questions of ecology, of biology, of *vitality* itself need to be the central urban questions of our age.

NOTES

Introduction

1. We are grateful to the UK's Economic and Social Research Council and the other funders, listed in the acknowledgments, that supported this research. Our title was actually inspired by a paper by the microbiologist Carl Woese (see Woese, 2004).

2. Of course, there were 'biological' branches of many social sciences, for example biological anthropology, and some social theorists this many years ago pointed out that it was impossible to understand human sociality without reference to biological capacities and constraints (Hirst and Woolley, 1982). While the intellectual climate at that time was not very responsive to these arguments, now it has become routine to make reference to biological and neurobiological concepts, for example in relation to affect (Massumi, 2002; Blackman, 2012; Massumi, 2015), to vitalism (Greco, 2005; Braun, 2007), in 'non-representational theory' sometimes explicitly argued in relation to the urban (Thrift, 2004; Thrift, 2005), and in contemporary philosophy (Malabou, 2009). If our argument differs from the work of these scholars, it is because of our insistence that a genuine transformation of our disciplines requires a new relationship with biological and biomedical researchers themselves and close critical attention to the empirical research and conceptual development of the life sciences and neurosciences.

3. On the 'geosocial' in particular, see Clark and Yusoff, 2017.

4. To avoid cluttering the text, we have kept references to a minimum in this introduction; full references are contained in the substantive chapters that follow.

5. Of course, there is also the question of the empirical robustness of claims in this area, as the statistics are usually based on admission to mental hospitals, or diagnosis by specialists who are themselves more likely to occur in cities.

6. While we use the word neuroscience in the singular, in fact research in the brain sciences today takes place in a very large, rapidly growing, and highly heterogeneous field, publishing more than 100,000 academic papers a year, and divided into subdisciplines whose members attend different conferences, publish in different journals, use different and often incompatible bodies of evidence and experimental setups. So it is important to note here that we deliberately make use of some very specific parts of this domain for our purposes.

7. We thus ally ourselves with Jenny Reardon's argument for a new relation between science and justice that "resists any easy claim to the universal, and instead inquires after the specific practices and values that make it possible" (Reardon, 2013: 192).

8. See for example Rose, 2001; Fitzgerald, 2012; Rose, 2013; Fitzgerald and Callard, 2018.

9. Most excitement in the social sciences has concerned 'epigenetics,' which we discuss in a later chapter. For present purposes we can say that epigenetics refers to the shaping and modulation of gene expression—activation or de-activation—in different cells, tissues, and organs as a consequence of their interactions with their milieu—which range from other cells to the environment

exterior to the body. Environmental epigenetics refers to the effects of factors from chemical pollutants and diet to stress in this process. For a good review, see Landecker and Panofsky, 2013.

10. We phrase it in this way because to imply that 'the brain' is a single organ, like 'the liver,' is to homogenize what is, in reality, an assemblage of highly interconnected parts, often with distinct evolutionary histories: see, for example, Purves, 2010.

11. We write these words in the midst of the pandemic of SARS-CoV-2. However, we are not arguing that 'nature,' which once seemed to have been successfully banished, has now returned; our interest is rather in a style of thought which, for much of the last century and before, proceeded as if human life was in the process of somehow transcending ecological constraint—and which today has—sometimes painfully—learned to think otherwise.

12. Which is not to say that humans are the only creatures who construct their own habitats, or that cities are the only territories that humans have transformed: there is nothing natural about the 'wilderness' for which city dwellers are so often thought to pine (Cronon, 1996). And, indeed, from their earliest days, cities have not simply been ad hoc settlements where humans gather because they have evolved to inhabit such an environment. Cities have been constructed, organized, laid out, thought-through, built, leveled, made and re-made by politicians and planners, citizens, landlords, and squatters, in the light of particular knowledges, beliefs, and values about who should live in them, where, and how. Urban ecologies always embody calculated attempts to shape and manage the lives, bodies, and souls of the citizens that dwell in them through the organization of space, the spatialization of different activities and functions, the use of architectural forms and more (see Mumford, 1961).

13. In the years that followed, there has been an increasing attention to 'the nature of cities' among human geographers (Heynen, Kaika, et al., 2006a) and the emergence of a kind of 'ecological urbanism' (Hagan, 2014). In particular, the work of our colleague Ash Amin, writing with Nigel Thrift, has played a key role in proposing new ways of conceptualizing cities though attention to their material, biological, and ecological dynamics. We make no claims to be urban geographers, but our vitalistic approach resonates with theirs in many ways (Amin and Thrift, 2002; Amin and Thrift, 2016) as we explore the particular problem of space that is our concern in this book.

14. Our view here resonates with that of Ash Amin and Nigel Thrift, who see cities as "machines" whose surge comes from "the liveliness of various bodies, materials, symbols, and intelligences held in relation within specific networks of calculation and allocation, undergirded by diverse regimes and rituals of organization and operation" (Amin and Thrift, 2016: 8), although the metaphor of 'machine' and the use of the definite article—the city—seems to suggest that however "jerry-rigged" together, a kind of coherence emerges.

15. We do not share the current enthusiasm for the use of Gilles Deleuze's notion of 'assemblage' to capture this (see McFarlane, 2011; Blok and Farias, 2016). See also the work of Söderström and colleagues who think of the city as "a heterogeneous, non-deterministic and enabling milieu, rather than as an undifferentiated factor of psychic stress" (Söderström, Empson, et al., 2016).

16. As the United Nations points out in its World Migration Report 2018: "The great majority of people in the world do not migrate across borders; much larger numbers migrate within countries. https://publications.iom.int/system/files/pdf/wmr_2018_en.pdf, quoted from p. 2.

17. The Migration Observatory at the University of Oxford has a useful summary of the diverse meanings in law and policy that are given to the term 'migrant' in the UK. https://migrationobservatory.ox.ac.uk/resources/briefings/who-counts-as-a-migrant-definitions-and-their-consequences/

18. We are here paraphrasing a longer account of these studies in Fitzgerald, Rose, et al. (2016b).

19. For one recent compelling study, see the work of Elizabeth Case and Angus Deaton on increases in morbidity and mortality among white non-Hispanic Americans in midlife since the turn of the century and the role of changes in the US labor market (Case and Deaton, 2015).

20. Another area where there were close relations between the social sciences and the sciences of the brain—at least up to the dominance of behaviorism in US psychology—was that of 'habit' where sociologists made frequent references to the cerebral inscription of repeated behavior: because of the brain's plasticity, the sequence of movements that constitute repeated behavior, from minor (putting one's left sock on before one's right'—to major—smoking, drinking, style—gradually become ingrained in the circuits of the brain, and occur when in particular contexts, without the intervention of conscious decisions—a relationship described in great detail by Charles Camic (Camic, 1986).

21. While this is not the place for a detailed account of this mundane vitalism, or to defend it against critics, our view has been shaped, not just by the work of Georges Canguilhem on vitalism, but also by debates with Thomas Osborne (see especially Osborne, 2016).

Chapter 1: Modern Cities, Migrant Cities

1. No less was it at stake for Indigenous people whose dispossession and murder were often the precondition for these new forms of urban settlement. There is of course a whole series of counterhistories of the modern city and its 'vital' or necropolitical relationship to Indigeneity running alongside the neat story we are telling here, and to which we cannot at all do justice here. See for example Edmonds, 2010 or Dorries, Henry, et al., 2019.

2. For example, on Simmel's vitalism, see Kemple, 2018. We should of course remember that vitalism in the nineteenth and early twentieth centuries, especially in the German-speaking world, had a range of sociopolitical associations: for some, it was part of a holistic biology stressing the inseparability of body and mind, for others a turn to holism was an element in a racialized call for spiritual renewal that some commentators regard as paving the path for Nazism. The rise of mechanistic science, strongly opposed to the contemporary version of vitalism, aiming to identify causal modes of understanding living phenomena, including human life, was the target of most of these holistic vitalisms. Anne Harrington (Harrington, 1996) provides us with a compelling analysis of these intertwined yet conflicting styles of thought and their place in competing cultural and political movements. We can see residues of this conflict in the hostility of many biologists today to any trace of vitalism.

3. Steve Pile (Pile, 2005) also links Freud's thinking about dreams to the spaces of the city.

4. Characteristically, the phrase is attributed to W. I. Thomas, despite first appearing in this exact form under joint authorship with Dorothy Swaine Thomas, to whom he was then married. Nevertheless, the 'situation' is a central focus of Thomas's Methodological Note that introduces Volume One of *The Polish Peasant*, and the term 'definition of the situation' appears there several times (e.g., Thomas and Znaniecki, 1918: 68). It is worth pointing out that a key theme in the 1928 book with Dorothy Swaine Thomas, as indeed in W. I. Thomas's Introduction to *The Polish Peasant*, was the search for research methods that could illuminate techniques for the control of behavior.

5. The meaning of this term is contested, but broadly speaking it refers to illegitimately making inferences about the characteristics of individuals from evidence about the group to which they belong—ecology, in this way of thinking, being composed of analyses of the characteristics of groups.

6. Cited from Judith Flanders: https://www.bl.uk/romantics-and-victorians/articles/slums

7. 'Hopping' in the sense of picking hops, which was done by hand in the hop fields of Kent and elsewhere.

8. Hawking, at this time, referred to the practice of offering items for sale by calling out in the street.

9. Developments included the discovery of vitamins not long after Rowntree's volume was published.

10. Quotations from Thomas's memorandum in this section are from the extracts published in a useful review of 'The Early History of Migration Research' by Michael Greenwood and Gary Hunt (Greenwood and Hunt, 2003).

11. The original article was published as Walker FA (1896) Restriction of Immigration. *Atlantic Monthly* 77(464): 822–829. The argument for which Walker is best known is that immigration was a replacement of the native population by 'foreign elements' which was leading to a reduction in fertility in the native population, with the obvious detrimental consequences for the quality of the national population as a whole. It is worth noting that Walker's 1896 article was reprinted in 2004 by the Population Council; Mathew Connelly (2010) has argued that the focus of this organization on population control by family planning had distinctly eugenic origins.

12. The United States was not alone in trying to restrict the numbers of degenerate or defective migrants. In Canada, immigrants thought to be insane or feeble-minded were either screened out at the port of entry, or, if they had entered, actually deported (Menzies, 2014); the practice of deporting any immigrant diagnosed with a mental illness—including "idiots, imbeciles, morons, those who were insane, constitutionally psychopathic personalities, and those suffering from epilepsy"—continued under the 1952 Immigration Act at least up to 1956 (Scheinberg, 2016). Similar practices of deportation were deployed in New Zealand and Australia; see, for example, Philippa Martyr's study of deportation of lunatic migrants from Western Australia (Martyr, 2011).

13. As previously, this quotation is drawn from Greenwood and Hunt (2003: 15).

Chapter 2: Migration, the Metropolis, and Mental Disorder

1. http://www.un.org/en/development/desa/news/population/world-urbanization -prospects-2014.html. See also the 2018 UN world migration report, which has additional data on internal migration: https://publications.iom.int/system/files/pdf/wmr_2018_en.pdf

2. Michael Lipton (Lipton, 1977) provides one much cited version of the 'urban bias' thesis.

3. This absence of slums in China is a result of the specific process of managed migration that commenced in the 1980s (Gransow, 2010). For this reason, among others, we leave our discussion of mental health, migration, and megacities in China to the next chapter.

4. For a critical discussion of the concept of 'slum,' which also draws our attention to the increasing proportion of women migrants to the megacities of the Global South, see the introduction to Chant and McIlwaine, 2015.

5. Within the term 'slum,' Ezeh et al. include baladi, bandas de miseria, barraca, barrio marginal, barrio, bidonville, brarek, bustee, chalis, chereka bete, dagatan, estero, favela, galoos, gecekondu, ghetto, hrushebi, informal settlement, ishash, karyan, katras, looban, loteamento, medina achouaia, morro, mudun safi, musseque, shanty town, slum, solares, tanake, taudis, township, tugurio, udukku, umjondolo, watta, and zopadpattis (Ezeh, Oyebode, et al., 2016).

6. Some see Morel, who was born in Austria but grew up and practiced psychiatry in France, as a "progenitor of the current biological approach to psychiatric illnesses" (Schuster, Le Strat, et al., 2011). Of course, ideas of degeneracy were not limited to Euro-America, and there have been a number of good studies of the work of degeneracy outside the Global North, especially in regions subject to colonial rule (Chatterjee, 1989; Erasmus, 2011), in the eugenic arguments in Latin America (Stepan, 1991), and in China (Dikötter, 1998).

7. Johnson, a sociologist, was co-author of *Applied Eugenics* (Johnson and Popenoe, 1925), which became a popular textbook, and he founded the eugenics program at the University of Pittsburgh.

8. Other studies (e.g., Adair, Melling, et al., 1997) do not find an over-representation of migrants in asylum populations in Victorian England.

9. There have also been a number of studies of asylum populations in the colonies—in Canada, New Zealand, and Australia—in the late nineteenth and early twentieth centuries, with some

claiming that higher rates of incarceration arose, in part, because of the lack of social bonds among the migrant populations (Fairburn, 2013), while others have preferred to lay the blame on discrimination, marginalization, and exclusion (McCarthy and Coleborne, 2012; Coleborne, 2015). There are also many studies of exploring the proportions of long-distance migrants among inmates of colonial asylums (e.g., McCarthy, 2008).

10. David Rothman (Rothman, 1971) has shown that there were indeed a disproportionate number of foreign-born inmates in nineteenth-century asylums.

11. Some of what follows is derived directly from previous papers (Fitzgerald, Rose, et al., 2016b; Fitzgerald, Rose, et al., 2016a).

12. Ødegård trained under Adolf Meyer, and his influence is clear, for example when as late as 1975 he argued that "Mental disorders are reactions of the total personality to the total life situation, and cases in which a simple formulation is possible are rare" (Ødegård, 1975: 152). Nonetheless, his Wikipedia entry, drawing on the Norsk *Biografisk Keksikon* and the *Store Norsk Leksikon* (the Norwegian Biographical Encyclopedia and Great Norwegian Encyclopedia, both in Norwegian) tells us that he also conducted studies on the intelligence of women who fraternized with German soldiers during the occupation of Norway—he concluded that their level of intelligence was lower than average—and was apparently an enthusiast for lobotomizing inmates, though he was not alone in this.

13. The 'social defeat' paradigm was developed in experiments with rodents, where one animal, having been repeatedly defeated by another in experimentally staged bouts of aggression, demonstrates withdrawal and the symptoms of chronic stress when placed in visual or olfactory contact with others. Some psychologists argued that this paradigm could be extended to humans, with 'different terminology,' replacing the terms 'dominant' and 'subordinate' with terms such as 'bully' and 'victim' for humans (Björkqvist, 2001). Despite its widespread use in explanations of many forms of mental disorder, like all such extrapolations to humans from animal models, this explanatory model remains the subject of controversy.

14. This effect is much discussed in literature on immigration to Canada but has also been reported in the case of immigrants to Australia (Biddle, Kennedy, et al., 2007) and the United States (Singh and Siahpush, 2002).

15. This was a contribution to an edited collection arising from a Task Force set up by the World Psychiatric Association (Bhugra, Gupta, et al., 2011), its Action Plan 2008–2011 "identified mental health and mental healthcare in migrants as one of the priority issues to be addressed in its guidance" (Bhugra and Gupta, 2010: foreword).

16. This study preceded our collaboration, but led to it, and has led Andrade's group to further analysis of the data in relation to migration.

17. For an overview of the debate by one of the present authors, see chapter 4 of *Our Psychiatric Future* (Rose, 2018). For some sample contributions to the debate, see Wakefield, 1997; Rosenberg, 2002; Rosenberg, 2006; Conrad, 2007; Summerfield, 2008; Young, 2008; Frances and Widiger, 2012; Patel, 2014. For an overview of the key issues for contemporary anthropology, see a Special Issue on Genealogies and Anthropologies of Global Mental Health, in the journal *Culture, Medicine, and Psychiatry* 43(4): December 2019.

18. There are a number of papers that discuss suicidal ideation among street children and young slum dwellers in Sub-Saharan Africa, but we will not discuss those here. Most extrapolate mental health risk from more general evidence about slum living and mental health (e.g., Swahn, Palmier, et al., 2012). Atilola, making the case for better child mental health services in Sub-Saharan Africa, argues that "Bronfenbrenner's ecological model of childhood, the lack of opportunity for sharing quality time with children and the instability and unpredictability of family life that is created by precarious employment have been described as the most destructive force to child physical and mental wellbeing globally" (Atilola, 2014: 4–5).

19. We should note how infrequently epidemiological work in cities like Dhaka seems to include the work of local scholars, though Dhaka alone contains several highly prestigious universities; China is exceptional here in that much of the research on mental health in general, and mental health in relation to migration, is carried out by Chinese researchers.

20. https://www.psykiatri-regionh.dk/who-5/Pages/default.aspx. The WHO5, which was developed by researchers in Denmark, has been translated into more than 30 languages. It is considered to have "adequate validity both as a screening tool for depression and as an outcome measure in clinical trials and has been applied successfully across a wide range of study fields" (Topp, Østergaard, et al., 2015: 167). Respondents rate their feelings over the last two weeks to each of these statements on a scale of 1–5, where All of the time = 5; Most of the time = 4; More than half of the time = 3; Less than half of the time = 2; Some of the time = 1; At no time = 0. The total raw score, ranging from 0 to 25, is usually multiplied by 4 to give the final score, with 0 representing the worst imaginable well-being and 100 representing the best imaginable well-being.

Chapter 3: The Metropolis and Mental Life Today—Shanghai 2018

1. Our discussion of Shanghai has drawn extensively on our collaborative research cited in the introduction. Population data are for the whole of the Shanghai metropolitan area. Data from Shanghai Statistical Bureau, 2006–2015, were compiled by Ji Lie for the Mental Health, Migration and Megacities project. In China, individuals have residency permits (*hukou*): thus 88% of the net population growth in this period was made up of rural-urban migrants, without Shanghai *hukou*. For the purposes of this chapter, when we refer to rural-urban migrants in Shanghai, unless otherwise qualified, we are referring to those without Shanghai *hukou*. As we shall see, while those without a Shanghai *hukou* can live and work in Shanghai, their access to various benefits and services is limited.

2. As we say in note 1 above, when we refer to rural-to-urban migrants in China in this chapter, we refer to those who do not have urban *hukou*. However, Cindy Fan (Fan, 2007: 19) points out that many concepts are used for describing population movements in China (citing Zhou, 2002) and quotes comments by Jiao (2002) to the effect that the definitions of migrants in China are the most complex in the world. Michael Keith lists the following terms used to refer to migrants who come from the countryside to the city to find work: *qianyi renkou*: moving population; *liudong renkou*: floating population; *nongmingong*: peasant workers; *waichu wugongzhe/yuan*: people leaving to work for others; *jincheng wugongzhe/yuan*: people entering the city to work for others; *dagongmei/zai*: working girls/boys; *zanzhu renkou*: temporary population; *bianyuan ren*: marginal figure (Keith, Lash, et al., 2013: table 10.2). Each of these carries a different connotation.

3. In these next paragraphs, we draw on Solinger's account in chapter 5 of her book (whose subtitle is "The Floating Population Leaves Its Rural Origins") and the interviews she conducted in villages and with migrants in a number of Chinese cities: in the terms used by migration scholars, her argument is that rural-to-urban migration in China was a combination of push and pull, individual economically motivated rational choices and structural pressures, warped and constrained by State policies (Solinger, 1999: ch. 5).

4. We should note that the restrictions on family size under the 'one child policy' were usually not applied to families in the countryside, who often had two or three children; thus, it was usually the younger children who found that they had little to do at home: their parents and older siblings provided ample labor to work the land allocated to their family.

5. There is an old anthropological trope to the effect that people in China do not consider themselves to be individuals but members of kin groupings. Anyone who believes this is still the case should read the copious literature on the lives and aspirations of young migrants: as Lesley

Chang and Alec Ash among others show compellingly, while the young women and men who migrate to the cities often are linked into networks of others from their villages and towns, and maintain close links with their families in places of origin, their lives are shaped by aspirations for self-improvement (Chang, 2009; Ash, 2016).

6. In 1980, Shenzhen became the first of the Special Economic Zones established under the leadership of Deng Xiaoping as an early experiment in developing market capitalism with Chinese characteristics (Stoltenberg, 1984).

7. At the time of writing, Li Ziqui had 10.1 million subscribers to her YouTube channel, drawn by the tranquil beauty of the peasant life she portrays. An interview with her—also available on YouTube at https://www.youtube.com/watch?v=J9CfVcXoYh4, puts her Chinese fan base at 50 million; the interview suggests, unsurprisingly, that her videos show the life she would like to live, not the one she does actually live!

8. For another detailed study, see Biao Xiang's account of Zhejiangcun, a migrant village that grew up within Beijing (Xiang, 2004).

9. In our account of factory work in the new China, including the events at Foxconn, we have drawn extensively on the work of Jenny Chan and Pun Ngai (Chan and Pun, 2010; Pun and Lu, 2010b; Pun and Lu, 2010c; Pun and Lu, 2010a; Chan, 2013; Pun, 2017; Pun and Zhang, 2017; Pun, 2018). We do not share their class-based analysis, based on a particular view of the damage wrought by international capital seeking to benefit from China's low wage labor, and which sees the rise of a new Chinese proletariat in the making. But the picture painted by their empirical evidence is compelling.

10. For a journalistic account of the Foxconn factory in the Longhua Subdistrict of Shenzhen, see https://www.theguardian.com/technology/2017/jun/18/foxconn-life-death-forbidden-city -longhua-suicide-apple-iphone-brian-merchant-one-device-extract

11. Following these suicides, many international scholars signed a letter of concern calling for the implementation of human labor standards in such Chinese workplaces.

12. For a useful comparison, see Aihwa Ong's interpretation of episodes of 'hysteria' and 'spirit possession' as "tactics of resistance" to the discipline of the factory among Malayan women workers (Ong, 2010: 178). Note also that the Foxconn CEO was deploying the therapeutic language that was becoming common in the businesses employing the emerging Chinese middle class, but rarely in factories employing migrant labor.

13. *Dagong* was originally a Cantonese term for temporary wage labor, but now refers more generally to the movement of people from rural areas to the towns and cities to find work, and indeed for those migrants themselves; they are '*dagong* people.'

14. Karl Marx developed the 'reserve army of labour' thesis in *Capital*, Vol. 1, Ch. 25 (Marx, 1954 [1867]). On 'Taylorism,' see Harry Braverman's classic study of *Labor and Monopoly Capital: The Degradation of Work in the Twentieth Century* (Braverman, 1998).

15. We have drawn heavily on Kaxton Siu's account in this paragraph.

16. Michael Keith's chapter, 'Shenzhen dwelling: arrival and migrant urbanisms' (in Keith, Lash, et al., 2013) gives a good account of the ways that strange combinations of private capital and state funding have led to the growth of many gated communities around the perimeter of expanding megacities such as Shenzhen.

17. We are drawing here on our own visits to a number of such schools in Songjiang, Shanghai.

18. Our account in this section is entirely indebted to the work of Lisa Richaud, and the ethnographic account that she has written with Ash Amin. We thank them for permission to draw extensively upon their work here.

19. A 2009 headline in the *British Daily Telegraph*, quoting the Director of China's National Centre for Mental Health which was established in 2002, proclaimed "China has 100 million people with mental illness"; http://www.telegraph.co.uk/news/worldnews/asia/china/5235487/China -has-100-million-people-with-mental-illness.html

20. https://news.gallup.com/poll/189077/worry-stress-rise-china.aspx . As this article is in English, it is not clear what Chinese word was translated as 'stress.'

21. *Yali* in this context is usually translated as 'pressure.'

22. Similar arguments were made by Anne Thurston on the basis of her interviews with participants in the Cultural Revolution (Thurston, 1987) and by Ralph Thaxton (Thaxton, 2008) in his study of Da Fo Village in the famine during Mao's Great Leap Forward.

23. The first edition was published in 1979.

24. Note that some studies suggest that, among elderly Chinese, levels of depression as measured by standard depression scales are higher among those 'empty-nest' elderly who have been left behind in the countryside when their child has moved to the city (see, for example, Su, Wu, et al., 2012).

25. They refer to speculations by Shen et al.: "methodological problems that cause downward bias in estimates, such as stigma related under-reporting and diagnostic incongruity with a somatopsychic mode of symptom presentation" (Shen, Zhang, et al., 2006: 257).

26. http://www.prnewswire.com/news-releases/research-report-on-chinas-antidepressant -market-2013-2017-211159091.html. They may find a ready market: as anyone who has visited a pharmacy in a major Chinese city can confirm, there is a healthy appetite for pharmaceuticals in contemporary China, with one recent study reporting that the "average Chinese citizen consumes ten times as many antibiotics as the average American" (Burki, 2017: 353).

27. Over the last five years, this growth has raised concerns among psy professionals in China and there are attempts to require those who provide them to have some professional credentials, as, for instance, in the so- called Wuhan declaration issued in 2016 from a meeting hosted by Chinese National Applied Psychology Graduate Education Steering Committee, which is authorized and charged by The Chinese Ministry of Education to promote the construction of applied psychology as a discipline (Lin, Jiang, et al., 2016) and also in concerns expressed by CAPA (the Chinese American Psychoanalytic Alliance) (Fishkin and Levine, 2020).

28. This recognition—that not all institutions, authorities, or strategies for the conduct of conduct have their point of origin in the formal political apparatus of the State was, of course, the central argument of Michel Foucault's conception of 'government' (see the discussion in Rose, 1999; Miller and Rose, 2008).

29. Presenteeism is the situation where someone attends work though feeling ill, and as a result does not work at full capacity (see, for example, Yang, Guo, et al., 2017).

30. These studies, by colleagues in the School of Public Health, Fudan University, arising from our research in Shanghai, were published in a Special Supplement of the journal *International Health* (see Fitzgerald, Manning, et al., 2019).

31. The researchers used a self-administered questionnaire, with depression measured by the Patient Health Questionnaire-9 (PHQ-9) scale and poor mental health measured by the World Health Organization Five-Item Well-Being Index (WHO-5) scale.

32. This study used the Chinese Version of Patient Health Questionnaire (PHQ-9) and Personal Well-Being Index scale (PWI).

33. One of the four case studies in Emily Ng's study of changing ideas of agency among hospitalized patients in Shenzhen is of a 24-year-old migrant laborer referred to psychiatric hospital by his employer after concerns were raised by his co-workers and after consultation with his parents in rural Henan (Ng, 2009); it is not clear how many employers of migrant labor would behave in such a 'caring' manner.

34. Chlorpromazine, known as Thorazine in the United States and Largactil in Europe, is a first-generation antipsychotic, highly sedating, and now rarely used because of severe adverse effects.

35. This was part of a global study called WAVE (Well-being of Adolescents in Vulnerable Environments) which included Baltimore, Ibadan, Johannesburg, New Delhi, as well as Shanghai;

it used interviews with key informants, in-depth interviews with adolescents between 15 and 19 years old, community mapping, focus group discussions, and photovoice methods. According to the authors of this paper, the main theoretical framework was Bronfenbrenner's ecological systems theory (Bronfenbrenner and Morris, 1998) supplemented by acculturation theory.

36. These policies have attracted much discussion in the British Press; see https://www .theguardian.com/world/2017/dec/08/beijing-gentrification-china-migrant-villages-destroyed; https://www.theguardian.com/cities/2018/mar/19/plan-big-city-disease-populations-fall-beijing -shanghai; and more generally Saskia Sassen's study of 'expulsions' (Sassen, 2014).

Chapter 4: Everyone Knows What Stress Is and No One Knows What Stress Is

1. https://www.nytimes.com/2019/04/25/us/americans-stressful.html.

2. https://www.mentalhealth.org.uk/news/stressed-nation-74-uk-overwhelmed-or-unable -cope-some-point-past-year

3. This book was written before the Covid-19 pandemic, which is in its third—or possibly fourth—wave in the UK as we review the proofs. Clearly it would take more than a note to consider the issue of 'stress' in relation to contagion, sickness, and death, including experiences of chronic illness, and the consequences of restrictive measures such as "lockdown," isolation. Here we restrict ourselves to making just three points. First, in the light of repeated surveys during the pandemic that have reported high levels of Covid-related mental health problems in Europe and North America, it is relevant to point out the continuity with the high levels of self-reported mental health problems in the pre-pandemic years that we note here—clearly, when asked how they are feeling, a lot of people have been reporting high levels of distress and unhappiness for many years. Second, evidence from previous crises—war, disaster, political transformation, and pandemics—does not show enduring negative consequences for mental health. While those directly exposed to devastating events do, unsurprisingly, experience sadness, severe distress, and heightened anxiety, the elevated rates of anxiety and depression in the general population seldom persist. 'Recovery' in these situations is thus not a result of interventions by psy professionals, but comes rather from the reduction in the disruptions that have caused stress, and especially because of positive support from community and religious leaders and others in local communities. Of course, those who are hardest hit are those who were already experiencing systematic racism and structural violence (see Lees-Manning, et al., 2021). Third, while there are currently few studies of migrant mental health and Covid-19, it would be most surprising if the feelings of distress and insecurity that we noted in the previous chapter were not exacerbated over this period for obvious reasons. In particular it is striking how much of the political and epidemiological response to Covid has been about fixing people in place, not just through "lockdown" but also by restricting movement across national boundaries, and often between different regions of one country. For those migrants making their lives far from their families, who have constructed personal and working lives across distance, these interventions have made life incredibly difficult. We await epidemiological research that assesses the toll of such restricted mobility on mental and physical health.

4. The Poll shows that the 'top ten' stressed nations are Greece, Philippines, Tanzania, Albania, Iran, Sri Lanka, United States, Uganda, Costa Rica, and Rwanda: the United States comes in seventh—see https://www.gallup.com/analytics/248906/gallup-global-emotions-report-2019 .aspx–.

5. Mark Jackson's excellent study *The Age of Stress: Science and the Search for Stability* has been an invaluable source of references to primary materials, as well as insights on their interpretation (Jackson, 2013). As Jackson notes in relation to this point, this was linked to a longer tradition of concerns about the impact of the conduct of life on neurasthenia and frank insanity.

6. In his book *The Wisdom of the Body*, first published in 1932 (Cannon, 1939).

7. He is drawing on Cannon's classic papers published in the 1920s (Cannon, 1922a; Cannon, 1922b; Cannon 1928; Cannon, 1929).

8. In this account of Selye's work, in addition to his original papers, we have drawn on the analyses by John Mason and Mark Jackson (Mason, 1975a; Mason, 1975b; Jackson, 2013).

9. It is now known that from the late 1950s, Selye accepted funding from major US tobacco companies, and by the late 1960s he was explicitly arguing against anti-smoking messages and in favor of the stress-reducing benefits of smoking tobacco (Petticrew and Lee, 2011).

10. Stress was also central in Moran's classic *The Anatomy of Courage* (Moran, 1945): as Charles Wilson, Lord John Moran was in service as a doctor with the Royal Fusiliers for two and a half years in the First World War (see also Long, 2014).

11. According to Virginia Berridge, Jerry Morris's "association with the social statistician and pioneer of the post-war welfare state, Richard Titmuss began when he made contact with Titmuss, after reading the latter's *Poverty and Population*, published the year before the war broke out. Thus began what Titmuss's daughter, Ann Oakley, calls 'an unusually vital working partnership' which lasted until Titmuss's death in the early 1970s and which fueled research and policy activity. During the war, despite Morris's absence in India, the two produced three papers hailed by the social medicine pioneer John Ryle as the 'first example of a practical social medicine'" (Berridge, 2001: 1141).

12. We have drawn extensively on Ramsden's work in the paragraphs that follow, and his guidance as to further sources has been invaluable.

13. The problem of American urban rats is a recurrent one. As we write, a new strategy is being adopted to control the rat population in New York—this uses traps imported from Italy by Rat Trap Inc. that ply the rodents with alcohol and then drown them: https://www.theguardian .com/us-news/2019/sep/06/new-yorks-new-rat-plan-ply-rodents-with-alcohol-and-then-drown -them?CMP=Share_iOSApp_Other

14. We have drawn here both on Richter's own account of his involvement in the memoir cited earlier and on Christine Keiner's study of this episode (Keiner, 2005).

15. Ramsden also discusses the influence of Christian's work. Robert Sullivan, in his memoir of "A Year with New York's Most Unwanted Inhabitants," calls Davis "the founder of modern rat studies" (Sullivan, 2006): his group was of the view that what was involved in the limit on population growth in mammals such as rats was not habitat factors, such as food or shelter, but aggressive social behavior having effects on the physiological system, especially the hormones. However, in his 1987 article, Davis did not speculate on the implications for humans.

16. See https://mcharg.upenn.edu/ian-l-mcharg

17. Adams and Ramsden suggest that those who claimed evidence of the pathological consequences of high population density were drawing on a long tradition of concern about the anti-social nature and consequences of human crowds, enabling all sorts of vicious acts to take place in relative secrecy and anonymity, a tradition that goes back at least to Le Bon (Le Bon, 1982 [1896]).

18. According to Ramsden, those involved included "the psychiatrist Eric Lindemann; sociologists Herbert Gans, Erving Goffman, August B. Hollingshead, and John Seely; planners Catherine Bauer, Richard Meier, Richard Poston, and Melvin Webber; ecologists, ethologists, and comparative psychologists such as T. C. Schneirla and Edward Deevey; the systems theorists Nicolas Rashevsky and John Q. Stewart; social psychologists Marie Jahoda, Daniel Wilner, and Marc Fried; anthropologist Thomas Gladwin; health planner Henrik Blum; and the economist Harvey Perloff. By the time of their conclusion, they had included Ernest Caspari, Albert Deutsch, Joel Elkes, Ian McHarg, Eugene Rostow, Geoffrey Vickers, Michael Young, and even Robert C. Weaver . . . [who] served as the first United States secretary of Housing and Urban Development (HUD) from 1966" (Ramsden, 2014: 294).

19. Kirk is quoting from an article on stress and mental disorder in *The Lancet* (Atkin, 1957). Kirk's own focus, as the title of his article makes clear, is the way in which the work of Selye on the general adaptation syndrome and in particular on 'adrenal stress' was used to debate the causes of suffering and death in both experimental and farmed animals.

20. See his partial biography and bibliography at http://cohen.socialpsychology.org/

21. http://www.psy.cmu.edu/~scohen/

Chapter 5: The Urban Brain

1. The lead author on this publication, Mazda Adli, was a participant in our Urban Brain workshops in 2013; see https://urbanbrainlab.com/urban-brain-lab-about/

2. This is, of course, a generalization. Neurobiology and neuroscience are themselves very heterogeneous fields: around 100,000 peer-reviewed papers are published across the neurosciences every year, and the annual meetings of the Society for Neuroscience now attract more than 30,000 attendees from over 80 countries, pursuing hundreds of different research programs, with different objects, problems, methods, bodies of literature, and so forth. Nonetheless, this way of thinking persists in some of the major neuroscientific endeavors, for example the European Union's multimillion-euro Human Brain Project in which one of the present authors was involved for many years, and where, despite many criticisms, these key conceptual issues have been relegated to a largely rhetorical concern with 'social and ethical implications': https://www.humanbrainproject.eu/en/

3. This way of thinking has become increasingly significant in the 'neurodevelopmental' approach to mental disorders (Gałecki and Talarowska, 2018; Lima-Ojeda, Rupprecht, et al., 2018).

4. The idea is not restricted to urban issues. It has also been central to the genre of research termed 'DOHaD'—the Developmental Origins of Health and Disease—specifically focusing on the role of social capital in protecting against stress experienced by children in their earliest years of life, and hence more generally, has been important in 'neurodevelopmental approaches' emphasizing the importance of experiences in the early years to mental ill health across one's whole life. We discuss the weaknesses of this approach later in the book.

5. For example, see the 'caps' enabling "precise multichannel EEG and brain stimulation (tDCS, tACS, tRNS)" developed by Neuroelectrics: http://www.neuroelectrics.com/products/caps/

6. For one example of a NIRS cap, see http://www.brainproducts.com/files/public/products/brochures_material/pr_articles/1304_EEG-NIRS.pdf

7. This section is derived from Fitzgerald, Rose, et al., 2016a.

8. There is now a considerable literature examining the health effects of 'forest bathing'—for example: (Park, Tsunetsugu, et al., 2009; Hansen, Jones, et al., 2017; Antonelli, Barbieri, et al., 2019; Farrow and Washburn, 2019; Furuyashiki, Tabuchi, et al., 2019)—as well as media discussions of how forest bathing can make us feel better, such as https://www.theguardian.com/environment/2019/jun/08/forest-bathing-japanese-practice-in-west-wellbeing

9. The work of Ole Söderström and his group exemplifies this very clearly: see for example Söderström, 2016; Söderström, Empson, et al., 2016; Söderström, Söderström, et al., 2017.

10. http://www.sciencemag.org/news/2011/06/mental-hazards-city-living

11. http://www.nature.com/news/2011/110622/full/474429a.html

12. http://www.wired.com/2011/06/city-brains/

13. Internal references have been omitted for clarity.

14. https://richardcoyne.com/list-of-blog-posts/

15. Inflammation is normally a protective response to an infection, but here it is activated over a long period without the presence of infection. This thesis is popularly known as 'the inflamed brain' or sometimes 'the inflamed mind' hypothesis: see, for example, http://bebrainfit.com/brain

-inflammation-depression/; http://www.bbc.co.uk/news/health-37166293. It is now the subject of a somewhat evangelical book oddly called, not 'the inflamed brain,' but 'the inflamed mind' (Bullmore, 2018).

16. They cite this from the website of Shonkoff's Centre on the Developing Child, at Harvard: http://developingchild.harvard.edu/science/key-concepts/toxic-stress/

17. It is important to note that, in their report, Shonkoff and colleagues are setting out the official position adopted by the Committee on Psychosocial Aspects of Child and Family Health and the Committee on Early Childhood, Adoption, and Dependent Care, and its Section on Developmental and Behavioral Pediatrics. They not only argue that their "ecobiodevelopmental framework . . . illustrates how early experiences and environmental influences can leave a lasting signature on the genetic predispositions that affect emerging brain architecture and long-term health." They argue that an "ecobiodevelopmental framework also underscores the need for new thinking about the focus and boundaries of pediatric practice. It calls for pediatricians to serve as both front-line guardians of healthy child development and strategically positioned, community leaders to inform new science-based strategies that build strong foundations for educational achievement, economic productivity, responsible citizenship, and lifelong health" (Shonkoff, Garner, et al., 2012: e232). While we disagree with their exclusive focus on the early years, we too argue that a 'neuroecosocial' approach underscores the need for a radically new role for those wishing to transform urban mental health.

18. Sadly, Bruce McEwen died in January 2020 as we were preparing the final manuscript of this book. Despite our criticisms of some aspects of his work, he was a powerful advocate for non-reductionist accounts of the impact of social adversity on the lives of the most disadvantaged.

19. We should note that the methods used in this paper, which rely heavily on neuroimaging, have been subject to devastating criticism by Monica Ellwood Lowe and colleagues on the grounds of the problems of reverse inference, the confounding of SES with cultural language use, bilingualism, and first language, and the problems with the use of cognitive tests in this context (Ellwood-Lowe, Sacchet, et al., 2016).

20. Indeed, McEwen and Shonkoff and colleagues co-wrote a much-cited article (Shonkoff, Boyce, et al., 2009) arguing that neuroscience and molecular biology were beginning to understand the childhood roots of health disparities and could provide the basis for a "New Framework for Health Promotion and Disease Prevention."

21. See how UNICEF frames this as "The first 1,000 days of life: The brain's window of opportunity": https://www.unicef-irc.org/article/958-the-first-1000-days-of-life-the-brains-window-of-opportunity.html

22. The problematic uses of animal models and model animals in neurobiology are discussed extensively in chapter 3 of *Neuro: The New Brain Sciences and the Management of the Mind* (Rose and Abi-Rached, 2013).

23. See our earlier discussion of debates over the role of rodent evidence in debating the supposed pathogenic consequences of urban density. Note that some papers, including this one, refer to neuroimaging studies claiming volumetric changes in the hippocampus of humans diagnosed with various mental disorders; however, "a significant number of studies have failed to find evidence of hippocampus atrophy in depressed patients" and in general, except in elderly patients, finding are inconsistent and show considerable heterogeneity (Krishnan, 2012). It is likely that volumetric changes in adult patients with a diagnosis of schizophrenia are due to lifestyle changes and the psychiatric medication itself (Murray, Quattrone, et al., 2016).

24. We can note the same unreflective extrapolation from animal experiments to support the lifelong significance of a damaging human caretaking environment in Allan Schore's much praised 'integration' of 'brain research' with John Bowlby that inspired quasi-psychoanalytic emphasis on the lasting consequences of attachment in the early years for later psychiatric disorders, especially

those related to stress (Schore, 2001). At the time we write, this paper had been cited over 1,600 times. Eva Rass (Rass, 2017) provides an enthusiastic and uncritical overview and appraisal of Schore's work.

25. Dysbiosis, here, is used to refer to 'difficult living' or 'lives in distress' shaped by the ecoscial location of some, not as a result of choice but arising from socioeconomic and sociopolitical forces.

26. This, for example, was the fate of the much publicized claim by Egeland and colleagues (Egeland, Gerhard, et al., 1987) to have discovered the gene for bipolar disorder among the Old Amish, which failed tests of replication; http://www.nytimes.com/1989/11/07/science/scientists-now-doubt-they-found-faulty-gene-linked-to-mental-illness.html?pagewanted=all&mcubz=1

27. Of course, this conclusion is disputed by proponents of psychiatric genetics (Collins and Sullivan, 2013), but it remains the case that despite thousands of studies, and dozens of claims and counterclaims, there exists no genetic marker or combination of genetic markers that unequivocally distinguishes diagnosed cases from normal controls, or that any genetic marker of clinical utility has been identified for any psychiatric disorder (Rose, 2018).

28. We are not going to discuss the belief that epigenetic changes can be inherited, for which there is rather limited evidence in some highly specific regions of the genome. The transgenerational pathways identified, for example, by Michael Meany and his group, do not work through the inheritance of epigenetic marks, but by maternal shaping of the neural pathways that regulate the behavior of the animals who rear the next generation of pups.

29. It remains the case that cell differentiation is a complex process involving gene activation and inactivation by chemical gradients, cell contiguity, and signaling pathways, and ill understood processes of morphogenesis (Davies, 2013). Nowhere in human anatomy is this more true than in brain.

30. Researchers at the Allen Institute are trying to map gene expression in the brain: https://portal.brain-map.org/

31. We have put 'the brain' in scare quotes here for the one and only time, as of course it would be unwise to assume that this was a unified organ: the mammalian brain has evolved over millennia and is heterogeneous, with regions that have evolved at different times and in relation to different evolutionary pressures; the extent to which 'the brain' is a unified whole is questionable, although undoubtedly there are very complex interactions between these different regions and between each of them and the nervous and sensory systems of the body, and hence with their milieu. It would be tedious to keep pointing this out, but our use of the term 'the brain' would be misleading if it was taken to imply a unified organic system.

32. Of course, 'adolescence' is itself a relatively recent cultural phenomenon, so the link is more accurately made with puberty (Sisk and Zehr, 2005).

33. Paul Bach-y-Rita, working with patients who had lost sight or other sensory capacities, showed that stimulation of highly innervated areas of the body—notably the tongue—could, with training, be recognized by the brain: 'sensory plasticity' in the brain meant that one could learn to 'see' with one's tongue (Bach-y-Rita, 1967). Other research showed that the mapping of sensory functions such as vision onto the cortex could be 'redrawn' even into adulthood (Wall, Kaas, et al., 1986; Merzenich, Recanzone, et al., 1988; Jenkins, Merzenich, et al., 1990; Buonomano and Merzenich, 2003). Controversial research on monkeys by Edward Taub and others demonstrated use-dependent cortical reorganization—increases in the area of the cortex involved in the innervation of movement of the affected limb—which could be used in therapy for humans who had suffered cerebrovascular accidents (Taub, Uswatte, et al., 1999).

34. The identification of neurogenesis is a highly technical task, and there are controversies over methods and interpretation as well as any implications. See, for instance, Jason Snyder's blog from his neuroscience lab at the University of British Columbia entitled "WTF! No neurogenesis

in humans??" at http://snyderlab.com/2018/03/07/wtf-no-neurogenesis-in-humans/ "So, some things are still not clear . . . and with neurogenesis we often can't even agree on the interpretation of neuroanatomical and immunohistochemical images. And the question about humans is important because we know from rodent work that adult neurogenesis plays a significant role in hippocampal physiology and behavior. There is a lot of evidence in favor of adult human hippocampal neurogenesis. But human studies are challenging. The tissue is rare, you don't have control over how it was prepared and preserved, the subjects may be ill, histological techniques that work in nicely-prepared animal tissue may not work the same in humans, the brain is different so it may be hard to even know what to look for etc." Nonetheless, citing a range of studies, he concludes, "Individually, none of these studies are entirely convincing of adult neurogenesis in humans but, collectively, they provide strong converging evidence. They convinced me."

35. Like so many current sociological concepts, the idea of 'atmosphere' is enmeshed in a host of often arcane theoretical and metaphysical debates (Gandy, 2017) which we will not discuss here. It bears some relationship to the ideas about spheres, bubbles, foams, and globes in the speculative philosophy of Peter Sloterdijk (Sloterdijk, 2011).

36. We have drawn here on John Urry's brief but brilliant essay on this topic (Urry, 2003). John Urry, who is sorely missed, was a participant in the early workshops on the urban brain that inspired this book.

37. Hence the signs reading "beware of gropers'—see for example: http://www.abc.net.au/news/2017-01-07/women-subjected-to-daily-trauma-on-tokyo-subway-gropers/8166672

38. Research on the amazing discriminatory characteristics of the olfactory system led to the award of a Nobel Prize to Linda Buck and Richard Axel; see (Buck and Axel, 1991).

39. Drawing on 'non-representational' social theory, it is possible to imagine 'marketing the city of smells,' using smell to build an urban identity and in 'place marketing,' "identifying ways in which smell might be used in future urban place marketing activities, and in particular to more explicitly communicate the experiential attributes of being in a particular city" (Henshaw, Medway, et al., 2016: 153).

Chapter 6: Another Urban Biopolitics Is Possible

1. Let alone the location within the city of hospitals, prisons, factories, and other institutions and indeed their internal organization. And, of course, we have already remarked on the concern of early urban reformers from Mayhew onward with the internal organization of living quarters and their separation of persons—males, females, children, animals, and of the vital functions of sleeping, eating, washing, defecating.

2. This is despite the fact that geographers have returned frequently to the works of Michel Foucault, notably Huxley, 2008 and Elden, 2016.

3. Harvey is intervening in a 1960s debate within urban design and planning about the extent to which spatial form shapes people and their behavior, and whether buildings or people should be the object of the planner's art (see, for example, Gans, 1969).

4. The essay derived from a radio talk that Foucault gave on the topic of utopias. The essay he developed from this was entitled "Des Espaces Autres'—'of other spaces': the first English translation in *Diacritics* is of a text that formed the basis of a lecture that Foucault gave in March 1967 (Foucault, 1986).

5. We have corrected the translation, which has "suspect" instead of "suspend." In his reflections on Foucault's essay, Peter Johnson reminds us that heterotopia was "originally a medical term referring to a particular tissue that develops at a place other than is usual. The tissue is not diseased or particularly dangerous but merely placed elsewhere, a dislocation" (Johnson, 2006: 76).

6. Perhaps we are in danger of reading too much into it. Peter Johnson begins his reflections on the essay by referring to the account given by Foucault's partner Daniel Defert who quotes a letter he received from a seemingly rather bewildered Foucault: "Do you remember the telegram that gave us such a laugh, where an architect said he glimpsed a new conception of urbanism? But it wasn't in the book; it was in a talk on the radio about utopia. They want me to give it again" (Defert, 1997: 274, quoted in Johnson, 2006: 76).

7. We are drawing on Peter Johnson's excellent article of 2012, "The Changing Face of the Modern Cemetery: Loudon's Design for Life and Death," available at https://www.berfrois.com /2012/06/foucault-and-the-cemetery/

8. We are quoting from the 2014 translation by Richard A. Lynch from the version published in *Dits et Ecrits*, vol. 3, pp. 725–742. As the note to that translation points out, this is the second of two texts that Michel Foucault published under the title "The Politics of Health in the Eighteenth Century"; the first appeared in a volume published in Paris in 1976 by the *Institut de l'environnement* and was translated into English by Colin Gordon for his collection *Power/Knowledge* (Gordon, 1980). This version served as the introduction to a collection of writings by Foucault and others on the origins of modern hospitals as 'machines for curing' (Foucault, Barret-Kriegel, et al., 1979).

9. Here, Foucault refers to these as dimensions of 'police,' noting that police had among its major objectives "the adjustment of a population to an economic apparatus of production and exchange." George Rosen and Pasquale Pasquino give different but informative accounts of the meaning of this notion of police in the eighteenth century (Rosen, 1974; Pasquino, 1978). However, Foucault also remarks that its concern was "the management of the social body in its materiality including the biological phenomena proper to a 'population'" (p.117), prefiguring his remarks in his lecture on governmentality in his course at the College de France on *Naissance de la biopolitique* (Foucault, 2004), translated as 'On Governmentality' (Foucault, 1979).

10. We can find such an approach in many cities, for example the city we are studying in Canada—Toronto; see the 'Vital Signs' Report at https://torontofoundation.ca/wp-content /uploads/2018/01/TF-VS-web-FINAL-4MB.pdf, or the Well Being Report compiled by Toronto's Urban Health Institute and the YWCA: https://ymcagta.org/-/media/pdfs/about_us /ymcalifeinthegtaonline.pdf?la=en&hash=78DA2D0AEFAE95FAC63FE08D880943594FB91E61

11. Space does not permit a full exploration of Lynch's powerful, but somewhat neglected, discussion, in appendix A of his book, for example his examples of those who have lost the ability to orient themselves in their surroundings because of brain injuries.

12. There were several other elements of the methods Lynch used, all well described in appendix B of his book, but we will not describe those here.

13. NR thanks the members of his 'thought collective' and co-authors of this paper—Rasmus Birk and Nick Manning—for their agreement and encouragement to draw heavily on the arguments in what follows.

14. We should note that Rietveld and colleagues propose their own ways of using their approach in psychiatry "to understand the changes that patients suffering with obsessive compulsive disorder (OCD) undergo when undergoing treatment with deep brain stimulation" (Rietveld and Kiverstein, 2014: 347). We do not engage with this argument here.

15. The work of this group runs parallel with our own writing of this book, and although there are considerable similarities in our arguments, we encountered their work at a late stage in the development of this manuscript, and since then have had many very productive discussions with them in the development of our ecosocial, or 'neuroecosocial,' approach.

16. Note that our approach draws together what have often been framed as opposing ways of framing the embeddedness of living creatures in their *Umwelt*: what Baggs and Chemero (2018) call the 'ecological' and the 'enactive approach': our approach stresses that human beings actively

create (enact) their *Umwelten* under the constraints and opportunities afforded them, reshaping and reconstructing these in the process.

17. This paragraph draws heavily on the account provided in Rose, Birk, et al., 2021. Note that while we have drawn in some detail on Downey's excellent description, for reasons explicated in more detail in that paper, we do not follow him in his speculations on the potential evolutionary conditions and consequences of the variety of urban niches that humans have constructed.

18. https://www.urbantransformations.ox.ac.uk/debate/the-neurosocial-city/

Conclusion: Toward a Sociology of Inhabitation

1. See, for example, Ella Braidwood's (2017) feature in the *Architects Journal* entitled 'Are Architects Doing Enough to Tackle Dementia?'; https://www.architectsjournal.co.uk/news/news-feature-are-architects-doing-enough-to-tackle-dementia

2. The centers are named for Maggie Keswick, who died of cancer in 1995; the charity that builds the centers was founded by Keswick's husband, the landscape designer and architectural historian, Charles Jencks. See https://www.maggies.org/

3. This leaflet, *Putting Health into Place: Introducing NHS England's Healthy New Towns Programme* produced by NHS England, is available at https://www.england.nhs.uk/wp-content/uploads/2018/09/putting-health-into-place-v4.pdf. For the results of the program, see https://www.england.nhs.uk/ourwork/innovation/healthy-new-towns/

4. See also, for South Africa, https://www.unicef.org/southafrica/media/551/file/ZAF-First-1000-days-brief-2017.pdf, and more generally, https://www.unicef-irc.org/article/958-the-first-1000-days-of-life-the-brains-window-of-opportunity.html

5. https://thrivenyc.cityofnewyork.us/

6. https://thriveldn.co.uk/

7. http://thriveto.ca/

8. Some questioned the value of the $850 million allocated to it, the value of its initiatives, raised issues of financial probity: https://www.politico.com/states/new-york/albany/story/2019/02/26/with-obscure-budget-and-elusive-metrics-850m-thrivenyc-program-attempts-a-reset-873945, and claimed that it failed to help those who were most in need; https://nypost.com/2020/05/04/child-advocates-slam-chirlane-mccrays-1b-thrivenyc-program/.

9. The earlier versions of the ThriveNYC website are no longer available, but for the most recent, updated to try to meet the criticisms noted above, see https://thrivenyc.cityofnewyork.us/

10. We should note, however, that the authors are fully aware of the ways that social and economic policies are fundamental to addressing issues of mental health, in increasing economic opportunity, housing, and income stability, attacking structural racism and so forth. However, these macro-social challenges are not the direct focus of the strategy of Thrive. In making these points, we are not allying ourselves with the criticisms noted earlier; indeed, it may well be that the strategy that we propose, which focuses not on immediate needs but on urban transformations whose beneficial effects are unlikely to be evident in the short term, would appeal even less to the critics who, understandably given the dire state of mental health services, prioritize immediate access to services.

11. Indeed, the one sentence they include on this issue is supported by some 15 references.

BIBLIOGRAPHY

Abbott, A. (1999) *Department and Discipline: Chicago Sociology at One Hundred*, Chicago: Chicago University Press.

Abbott, A. (2012) 'Stress and the City: Urban Decay', *Nature* 490(7419): 162.

Adair, R., Melling, J., and Forsythe, B. (1997) 'Migration, Family Structure and Pauper Lunacy in Victorian England: Admissions to the Devon County Pauper Lunatic Asylum, 1845–1900', *Continuity and Change* 12(3): 373–401.

Adams, J. and Ramsden, E. (2011) 'Rat Cities and Beehive Worlds: Density and Design in the Modern City', *Comparative Studies in Society and History* 53(04): 722–756.

Adli, M., Berger, M., Brakemeier, E.-L., Engel, L., et al. (2017) 'Neurourbanism: Towards a New Discipline', *The Lancet Psychiatry* 4(3): 183–185.

Ahmed, M. (2020) 'Health and Well-Being of Climate Migrants in Slum Areas of Dhaka', pp. 277–293 in W. Leal Filho, et al. (eds.) *Good Health and Well-Being. Encyclopedia of the UN Sustainable Development Goals*, New York: Springer.

Aiello, A. E., Dowd, J. B., Jayabalasingham, B., Feinstein, L., et al. (2016) 'PTSD Is Associated with an Increase in Aged T Cell Phenotypes in Adults Living in Detroit', *Psychoneuroendocrinology* 67: 133–141.

Alaimo, S. (2010) *Bodily Natures: Science, Environment, and the Material Self*, Bloomington: Indiana University Press.

Allen, J., Balfour, R., Bell, R., and Marmot, M. (2014) 'Social Determinants of Mental Health', *International Review of Psychiatry* 26(4): 392–407.

Almedom, A. M. (2005) 'Social Capital and Mental Health: An Interdisciplinary Review of Primary Evidence', *Social Science & Medicine* 61(5): 943–964.

Amin, A. (2013) 'Telescopic Urbanism and the Poor', *City* 17(4): 476–492.

Amin, A. and Thrift, N. (2002) *Cities: Reimagining the Urban*, Cambridge: Polity.

Amin, A. and Thrift, N. (2016) *Seeing Like a City*, London: John Wiley & Sons.

Anderson, B. (2009) 'Affective Atmospheres', *Emotion, Space and Society* 2: 77–81.

Anderson, B. (2019) 'New Directions in Migration Studies: Towards Methodological De-Nationalism', *Comparative Migration Studies* 7(1): 1–13.

Anderson, E. (1996) 'Introduction to the 1996 Edition of *The Philadelphia Negro*', *The Philadelphia Negro: A Social Study*, Philadelphia: University of Pennsylvania Press.

Andrade, L. H., Wang, Y.-P., Andreoni, S., Silveira, C. M., et al. (2012) 'Mental Disorders in Megacities: Findings from the Sao Paulo Megacity Mental Health Survey, Brazil', *PloS One* 7(2): e31879.

Antonelli, M., Barbieri, G., and Donelli, D. (2019) 'Effects of Forest Bathing (Shinrin-Yoku) on Levels of Cortisol as a Stress Biomarker: A Systematic Review and Meta-Analysis', *International Journal of Biometeorology* 2019 63(8): 1117–1134.

Appadurai, A. (2001) 'Deep Democracy: Urban Governmentality and the Horizon of Politics', *Environment and Urbanization* 13(2): 23–43.

Arden, J. B. (2010) *Rewire Your Brain: Think Your Way to a Better Life*, London: John Wiley.

Ash, A. (2016) *Wish Lanterns: Young Lives in New China*, London: Picador.

Aspinall, P., Mavros, P., Coyne, R., and Roe, J. (2013) 'The Urban Brain: Analysing Outdoor Physical Activity with Mobile EEG', *British Journal of Sports Medicine*, EPub: doi: 10.1136/bjsports-2012-091877.

Atilola, O. (2014) 'Where Lies the Risk? An Ecological Approach to Understanding Child Mental Health Risk and Vulnerabilities in Sub-Saharan Africa', *Psychiatry Journal* 2014: 698348.

Atkin, I. (1957) '"Stress" and Mental Disorders', *The Lancet* 270(6984): 43–44.

Atwater, W. O. and Rosa, E. B. (1899) 'Description of a New Respiration Calorimeter and Experiments on the Conservation of Energy in the Human Body', *Experiment Station Bulletin* (United States Office of Experiment Stations): no. 63.

Bach-y-Rita, P. (1967) 'Sensory Plasticity', *Acta Neurologica Scandinavica* 43(4): 417–426.

Baggs, E. and Chemero, A. (2018) 'Radical Embodiment in Two Directions', *Synthese 198 (Suppl 9): 2175–2190.*

Bahn, A. K., Chandler, C. A., and Eisenberg, L. (1961) 'Diagnostic and Demographic Characteristics of Patients Seen in Outpatient Psychiatric Clinics for an Entire State (Maryland): Implications for the Psychiatrist and the Mental Health Program Planner', *American Journal of Psychiatry* 117(9): 769–778.

Bakolis, I., Hammoud, R., Smythe, M., Gibbons, J., et al. (2018) 'Urban Mind: Using Smartphone Technologies to Investigate the Impact of Nature on Mental Well-Being in Real Time', *BioScience* 68(2): 134–145.

Bakolis, I., Hammoud, R., Stewart, R., Beevers, S., et al. (2020) 'Mental Health Consequences of Urban Air Pollution: Prospective Population-Based Longitudinal Survey', *Social Psychiatry and Psychiatric Epidemiology*: 1–13. doi: https://doi.org/10.1007/s00127-020-01966-x

Ball, M. and Sunderland, D. T. (2002) *An Economic History of London 1800–1914*, London: Routledge.

Barker, D. J. (2007) 'The Origins of the Developmental Origins Theory', *Journal of Internal Medicine* 261(5): 412–417.

Barles, S. (2007) 'Feeding the City: Food Consumption and Flow of Nitrogen, Paris, 1801–1914', *Science of the Total Environment* 375(1–3): 48–58.

Barwich, A. (2020) *Smellosophy: What the Nose Tells the Mind*, Cambridge, MA: Harvard University Press.

Baudelaire, C. (2010) *The Painter of Modern Life*, London: Penguin.

Bay, M. (1998) '"The World Was Thinking Wrong About Race": *The Philadelphia Negro* and Nineteenth-Century Science', in M. B. Katz and T. J. Sugrue (eds.) *W.E.B. Dubois, Race and the City: The Philadelphia Negro and Its Legacy*, Philadelphia: University of Pennsylvania Press.

Beard, G. (1869) 'Neurasthenia, or Nervous Exhaustion', *The Boston Medical and Surgical Journal* 80(13): 217–221.

Beaulieu, A. (2000) 'The Space inside the Skull: Digital Representations, Brain Mapping and Cognitive Neuroscience in the Decade of the Brain', Ph.D. Dissertation, University of Amsterdam.

Begley, S. (2009) *The Plastic Mind*, London: Constable and Robinson Limited.

Béhague, D. P. (2009) 'Psychiatry and Politics in Pelotas, Brazil', *Medical Anthropology Quarterly* 23(4): 455–482.

Belkin, G. and McCray, C. (2019) 'ThriveNYC: Delivering on Mental Health', *American Journal of Public Health* 109(S3): S156–S163.

Bellet, S., Roman, L., and Kostis, J. (1969) 'The Effect of Automobile Driving on Catecholamine and Adrenocortical Excretion', *The American Journal of Cardiology* 24(3): 365–368.

Benjamin, W. (2010) 'The Arcades Project', in G. Bridge and S. Watson (eds.) *The Blackwell City Reader*, London: Wiley-Blackwell.

Bernard, C. (1878) *Principes de médecine experimentale, ou de l'expérimentation appliquée à la physiologie, à la pathologie et à la thérapeutique*, Paris: Baillière.

Berridge, V. (2001) 'Jerry Morris', *International Journal of Epidemiology* 30(5): 1141–1145.

Berry, J. W. and Annis, R. C. (1974) 'Acculturative Stress: The Role of Ecology, Culture and Differentiation', *Journal of Cross-Cultural Psychology* 5(4): 382–406.

Berry, J. W., Kim, U., Minde, T., and Mok, D. (1987) 'Comparative Studies of Acculturative Stress', *International Migration Review* 21(3): 491–511.

Bhugra, D. (2004a) 'Migration and Mental Health', *Acta Psychiatrica Scandinavica* 109(4): 243–258.

Bhugra, D. (2004b) 'Migration, Distress and Cultural Identity', *British Medical Bulletin* 69(1): 129–141.

Bhugra, D. and Gupta, S. (2010) *Migration and Mental Health*, Cambridge: Cambridge University Press.

Bhugra, D., Gupta, S., Bhui, K., Craig, T., et al. (2011) 'WPA Guidance on Mental Health and Mental Health Care in Migrants', *World Psychiatry* 10(1): 2–10.

Biddle, N., Kennedy, S., and McDonald, J. T. (2007) 'Health Assimilation Patterns Amongst Australian Immigrants', *Economic Record* 83(260): 16–30.

Biehl, J. (2013) *Vita: Life in a Zone of Social Abandonment*, Oakland: University of California Press.

Bieler, P. and Klausner, M. (2019) 'Niching in Cities under Pressure. Tracing the Reconfiguration of Community Psychiatric Care and the Housing Market in Berlin', *Geoforum*, 101: 202–21.

Bister, M. D., Klausner, M., and Niewöhner, J. (2016) 'The Cosmopolitics of 'Niching'. Rendering the City Habitable Along Infrastructures of Mental Health Care', in A. Blok and I. U. Farias (eds.) *Urban Cosmopolitics. Agencements, Assemblies, Atmospheres*, London: Routledge.

Björkqvist, K. (2001) 'Social Defeat as a Stressor in Humans', *Physiology & Behavior* 73(3): 435–442.

Blackman, L. (2012) *Immaterial Bodies: Affect, Embodiment, Mediation*, London: Sage.

Blakemore, S. J. and Choudhury, S. (2006) 'Brain Development During Puberty: State of the Science', *Developmental Science* 9(1): 11–14.

Blok, A. and Farias, I. (2016) *Urban Cosmopolitics: Agencements, Assemblies, Atmospheres*, London: Routledge.

Bloom, B. L. (1968) 'An Ecological Analysis of Psychiatric Hospitalizations', *Multivariate Behavioral Research* 3(4): 423–463.

Booth, C. (1889) *Labour and Life of the People (1st Series), Vol. 1*, London: Williams and Norgate.

Booth, C. (1891) *Labour and Life of the People, Volume II (2nd Edition): London, Continued*, London: Williams and Norgate.

Booth, C. (1893) 'Life and Labour of the People in London: First Results of an Inquiry Based on the 1891 Census. Opening Address of Charles Booth, Esq., President of the Royal Statistical Society. Session 1893–94', *Journal of the Royal Statistical Society* 56(4): 557–595.

Borrell-Carrió, F., Suchman, A. L., and Epstein, R. M. (2004) 'The Biopsychosocial Model 25 Years Later: Principles, Practice, and Scientific Inquiry', *The Annals of Family Medicine* 2(6): 576–582.

Boughton, J. (2018) *Municipal Dreams: The Rise and Fall of Council Housing*, London: Verso.

Bourdieu, P. and Wacquant, L. J. (1992) *An Invitation to Reflexive Sociology*, Chicago: University of Chicago Press.

Braun, B. (2007) 'Biopolitics and the Molecularization of Life', *Cultural Geographies* 14(1): 6–28.

Braverman, H. (1998) *Labor and Monopoly Capital: The Degradation of Work in the Twentieth Century*, New York: NYU Press.

Brenner, N. and Schmid, C. (2014) 'The "Urban Age" in Question', *International Journal of Urban and Regional Research* 38(3): 731–755.

Brenner, N. and Schmid, C. (2015) 'Towards a New Epistemology of the Urban?', *City* 19(2–3): 151–182.

Brettell, C. B. and Hollifield, J. F. (2013) 'Theorizing Migration in Anthropology: The Social Construction of Networks, Identities, Communities, and Globalscapes', *Migration Theory*, London: Routledge.

Briggs, A. (1961) *Social Thought and Social Action: A Study of the Work of Seebohm Rowntree, 1871–1954*, London: Longmans.

Bronfenbrenner, U. and Morris, P. A. (1998) 'The Ecology of Developmental Processes', in R. M. Lerner (ed.) *Handbook of Child Psychology: Volume 1. Theoretical Models of Human Development*, 5th edition, New York: Wiley.

Brown, G. W. and Harris, T. (1978) *Social Origins of Depression: A Study of Psychiatric Disorder in Women*, London: Tavistock.

Buchen, L. (2010) 'Neuroscience: In Their Nurture', *Nature* 467(7312): 146–148.

Buck, L. and Axel, R. (1991) 'A Novel Multigene Family May Encode Odorant Receptors: A Molecular Basis for Odor Recognition', *Cell* 65(1): 175–187.

Bullmore, E. (2018) *The Inflamed Mind: A Radical New Approach to Depression*, London: Short Books.

Bulmer, M. (1984) *The Chicago School of Sociology: Institutionalization, Diversity, and the Rise of Sociological Research*, Chicago; London: University of Chicago Press.

Bunce, S. C., Izzetoglu, M., Izzetoglu, K., Onaral, B., et al. (2006) 'Functional Near-Infrared Spectroscopy', *Engineering in Medicine and Biology Magazine, IEEE* 25(4): 54–62.

Buonomano, D. and Merzenich, M. (2003) 'Cortical Plasticity: From Synapses to Maps', *Annual Review of Neuroscience* 21: 149–186.

Burgess, E. W. (1925) 'Can Neighborhood Work Have a Scientific Basis', *The City*: 142–155.

Burki, T. (2017) 'China Faces Challenges to Fix Its Pharmaceutical System', *The Lancet* 389(10067): 353–354.

Burr, R. H. (1903) 'A Statistical Study of Patients Admitted at the Connecticut Hospital for Insane from the Years 1868 to 1901', *Publications of the American Statistical Association* 8(62): 305–343.

Bustamante, A. C., Aiello, A. E., Koenen, K. C., Galea, S., et al. (2013) 'Childhood Maltreatment Is Associated with Epigenetic Differences in Hypothalamic-Pituitary-Adrenal (HPA) Axis Genes in the Detroit Neighborhood Health Study', *Comprehensive Psychiatry* 54(8): e17.

Cacioppo, J. T. and Patrick, W. (2008) *Loneliness: Human Nature and the Need for Social Connection*, 1st edition, New York: W.W. Norton.

Calhoun, J. B. (1950) 'The Study of Wild Animals under Controlled Conditions', *Annals of the New York Academy of Sciences* 51(6): 1113–1122.

Cameron, H. A. and Gould, E. (1994) 'Adult Neurogenesis Is Regulated by Adrenal-Steroids in the Dentate Gyrus', *Neuroscience* 61(2): 203–209.

Cameron, H. A., McEwen, B. S., and Gould, E. (1995) 'Regulation of Adult Neurogenesis by Excitatory Input and NMDA Receptor Activation in the Dentate Gyrus', *Journal of Neuroscience* 15(6): 4687–4692.

Cameron, N. M., Champagne, F. A., Fish, C., Ozaki-Kuroda, K., et al. (2005) 'The Programming of Individual Differences in Defensive Responses and Reproductive Strategies in the Rat through Variations in Maternal Care', *Neuroscience and Biobehavioral Reviews* 29(4–5): 843–865.

Camic, C. (1986) 'The Matter of Habit', *American Journal of Sociology* 91(5): 1039–1087.

Campion, J., Bhugra, D., Bailey, S., and Marmot, M. (2013) 'Inequality and Mental Disorders: Opportunities for Action', *The Lancet* 382(9888): 183.

Cannon, W. B. (1914) 'The Emergency Function of the Adrenal Medulla in Pain and the Major Emotions', *American Journal of Physiology* 33(2): 356–372.

Cannon, W. B. (1922a) 'New Evidence for Sympathetic Control of Some Internal Secretions', *American Journal of Psychiatry* 79(1): 15–30.

Cannon, W. B. (1922b) 'Some Conditions Controlling Internal Secretion', *Journal of the American Medical Association* 79(2): 92–95.

Cannon, W. B. (1928) 'The Mechanism of Emotional Disturbance of Bodily Functions', *New England Journal of Medicine* 198(17): 877–884.

Cannon, W. B. (1929) *Bodily Changes in Pain, Hunger, Fear and Pain*, Boston: Charles T. Branford.

Cannon, W. B. (1939) *The Wisdom of the Body*, New York: Norton.

Cannon, W. B. (1942) '"Voodoo" Death', *American Anthropologist* 44: 169–181.

Cantor, D. and Ramsden, E. (2014) *Stress, Shock, and Adaptation in the Twentieth Century*, Rochester, NY: University of Rochester Press.

Cantor-Graae, E. and Selten, J.-P. (2005) 'Schizophrenia and Migration: A Meta-Analysis and Review', *American Journal of Psychiatry* 162(1): 12–24.

Carey, N. (2012) *The Epigenetics Revolution: How Modern Biology Is Rewriting Our Understanding of Genetics, Disease, and Inheritance*, New York: Columbia University Press.

Case, A. and Deaton, A. (2015) 'Rising Morbidity and Mortality in Midlife among White Non-Hispanic Americans in the 21st Century', *Proceedings of the National Academy of Sciences* 112(49): 15078–15083.

Casey, B. J., Giedd, J. N., and Thomas, K. M. (2000) 'Structural and Functional Brain Development and Its Relation to Cognitive Development', *Biological Psychology* 54(1): 241–257.

Caspi, A., McClay, J., Moffitt, T. E., Mill, J., et al. (2002) 'Role of Genotype in the Cycle of Violence in Maltreated Children', *Science* 297(5582): 851–854.

Caspi, A. and Moffitt, T. E. (2006) 'Gene–Environment Interactions in Psychiatry: Joining Forces with Neuroscience', *Nature Reviews Neuroscience* 7: 583–590.

Caspi, A., Sugden, K., Moffitt, T., Taylor, A., et al. (2003) 'Influence of Life Stress on Depression: Moderation by a Polymorphism in the 5-HTT Gene', *Science* 301: 386–389.

Champagne, F. A., Chretien, P., Stevenson, C. W., Zhang, T. Y., et al. (2004) 'Variations in Nucleus Accumbens Dopamine Associated with Individual Differences in Maternal Behavior in the Rat', *Journal of Neuroscience* 24(17): 4113–4123.

Champagne, F. A. and Meaney, M. J. (2006) 'Stress During Gestation Alters Postpartum Maternal Care and the Development of the Offspring in a Rodent Model', *Biological Psychiatry* 59(12): 1227–1235.

Chan, J. (2013) 'A Suicide Survivor: The Life of a Chinese Worker', *New Technology, Work and Employment* 28(2): 84–99.

Chan, J. and Pun, N. (2010) 'Suicide as Protest for the New Generation of Chinese Migrant Workers: Foxconn, Global Capital, and the State', *Asia-Pacific Journal: Japan Focus* 8(37, 2): n.p.

Chang, D. F., Tong, H., Shi, Q., and Zeng, Q. (2005) 'Letting a Hundred Flowers Bloom: Counseling and Psychotherapy in the People's Republic of China', *Journal of Mental Health Counseling* 27(2): 104–116.

Chang, L. T. (2009) *Factory Girls: Voices from the Heart of Modern China*, London: Picador.

Chant, S. and McIlwaine, C. (2015) *Cities, Slums and Gender in the Global South: Towards a Feminised Urban Future*, London: Routledge.

Charlson, F. J., Baxter, A. J., Cheng, H. G., Shidhaye, R., et al. (2016) 'The Burden of Mental, Neurological, and Substance Use Disorders in China and India: A Systematic Analysis of Community Representative Epidemiological Studies', *The Lancet* 388(10042): 376–389.

Chatterjee, P. (1989) 'Colonialism, Nationalism, and Colonialized Women: The Contest in India', *American Ethnologist* 16(4): 622–633.

Chen, C., Nakagawa, S., An, Y., Ito, K., et al. (2017) 'The Exercise-Glucocorticoid Paradox: How Exercise Is Beneficial to Cognition, Mood, and the Brain While Increasing Glucocorticoid Levels', *Frontiers in Neuroendocrinology* 44(Supplement C): 83–102.

Chen, Y. F. (2002) 'Chinese Classification of Mental Disorders (CCMD-3): Towards Integration in International Classification', *Psychopathology* 35(2–3): 171–175.

Chiang, H. (2015) *Psychiatry and Chinese History*, London: Routledge.

Christian, J. J. (1950) 'The Adreno-Pituitary System and Population Cycles in Mammals', *Journal of Mammalogy* 31(3): 247–259.

Chua, J. L. (2014) *In Pursuit of the Good Life: Aspiration and Suicide in Globalizing South India*, Oakland: University of California Press.

Clark, N. and Yusoff, K. (2017) 'Geosocial Formations and the Anthropocene', *Theory, Culture & Society* 34(2–3): 3–23.

Classen, C. (2005) *The Book of Touch*, Oxford: Berg.

Classen, C. (2012) *The Deepest Sense: A Cultural History of Touch*, Urbana: University of Illinois Press.

Classen, C., Howes, D., and Synnott, A. (1994) *Aroma: The Cultural History of Smell*, London: Routledge.

Cohen, M. (2004) 'Benjamin's Phantasmagoria: The Arcades Project', in D. S. Ferris (ed.) *The Cambridge Companion to Walter Benjamin*, Cambridge: Cambridge University Press.

Cohen, M. E. and White, P. D. (1953) 'Life Situations, Emotions and Neurocirculatory Asthenia (Anxiety Neurosis, Neurasthenia, Effort Syndrome)', *Association for Research in Nervous and Mental Disease* 29: 832–869.

Cohen, S. and Lezak, A. (1977) 'Noise and Inattentiveness to Social Cues', *Environment and Behavior* 9(4): 559–572.

Coleborne, C. (2015) *Insanity, Identity and Empire: Immigrants and Institutional Confinement in Australia and New Zealand, 1873–1910*, Oxford: Oxford University Press.

Coleman, J. S. (1988) 'Social Capital in the Creation of Human Capital', *American Journal of Sociology* 94: S95–S120.

Collier, S. J. and Lakoff, A. (2007) 'On Regimes of Living', in A. Ong and S. J. Collier (eds.) *Global Assemblages: Technology, Politics, and Ethics as Anthropological Problems*, New York: Wiley.

Collins, A. L. and Sullivan, P. F. (2013) 'Genome-Wide Association Studies in Psychiatry: What Have We Learned?', *British Journal of Psychiatry* 202(1): 1–4.

Collins, R. (2004) *Interaction Ritual Chains*, Princeton, NJ; Oxford: Princeton University Press.

Connelly, M. (2010) *Fatal Misconceptions: The Struggle to Control World Populations*, Cambridge, MA: Harvard University Press.

Conrad, P. (2007) *The Medicalization of Society: On the Transformation of Human Conditions into Treatable Disorders*, Baltimore, MD: Johns Hopkins University Press.

Cooper, C. (2013) 'David Barker (1938–2013)', *Nature* 502: 304.

Cox, C., Marland, H., and York, S. (2012) 'Emaciated, Exhausted, and Excited: The Bodies and Minds of the Irish in Late Nineteenth-Century Lancashire Asylums', *Journal of Social History* 46(2): 500–524.

Cressey, P. F. (1938) 'Population Succession in Chicago: 1898–1930', *American Journal of Sociology* 44(1): 59–69.

Cressy, P. G. (1932) *The Taxi-Dance Hall*, Chicago: University of Chicago Press.

Crile, G. W. (1915) *The Origin and Nature of the Emotions; Miscellaneous Papers*, Philadelphia, PA: Saunders.

Cronon, W. (1996) *Uncommon Ground: Rethinking the Human Place in Nature*, New York: W.W. Norton.

Dantzer, R., O'Connor, J. C., Freund, G. G., Johnson, R. W., et al. (2008) 'From Inflammation to Sickness and Depression: When the Immune System Subjugates the Brain', *Nature Reviews Neuroscience* 9(1): 46–56.

Das, V. (2015) *Affliction: Health, Disease, Poverty*, New York: Fordham University Press.

Das-Munshi, J., Leavey, G., Stansfeld, S., and Prince, M. (2012) 'Migration, Social Mobility and Common Mental Disorders: Critical Review of the Literature and Meta-Analysis', *Ethnicity & Health* 17(1–2): 17–53.

Davidson, R. J. and McEwen, B. S. (2012) 'Social Influences on Neuroplasticity: Stress and Interventions to Promote Well-Being', *Nature Neuroscience* 15(5): 689–695.

Davies, J. A. (2013) *Mechanisms of Morphogenesis*, 2nd edition, London: Academic Press.

Davis, D. E. (1987) 'Early Behavioral Research on Populations', *American Zoologist* 27(3): 825–837.

Davis, M. (2006) *Planet of Slums*, London: Verso.

Davis, S. W. (1956) 'Stress in Combat', *Scientific American* 194(3): 31–35.

Davis, S. W., Elmadjian, F., Hanson, L. F., Liddell, H. S., et al. (1953) 'A Study of Combat Stress, Korea', Baltimore, MD: Johns Hopkins University Operations Research Office.

De Boeck, F. and Baloji, S. (2016) *Suturing the City. Living Together in Congo's Urban Worlds*, London: Autograph ABP.

DeBord, D. G., Carreón, T., Lentz, T. J., Middendorf, P. J., et al. (2016) 'Use of the "Exposome" in the Practice of Epidemiology: A Primer on -Omic Technologies', *American Journal of Epidemiology* 184(4): 302–314.

Deleuze, G. (1992) 'Postscript on the Societies of Control', *October* 59: 3–7.

Deleuze, G. (1993) *The Fold: Leibniz and the Baroque*, Minneapolis: University of Minnesota Press.

Denault, A., Shaaban-Ali, M., Cournoyer, A., Aymen Benkreira, A., et al. (2018) 'Near-Infrared Spectroscopy', in H. Prabhakar (ed.) *Neuromonitoring Techniques*, New York: Academic Press.

Deng, L., Lin, X., Lan, J., and Fang, X. (2013) 'Family Therapy in China', *Contemporary Family Therapy* 35(2): 420–436.

Dennis, R. (2008) *Cities in Modernity: Representations and Productions of Metropolitan Space, 1840–1930*, Cambridge: Cambridge University Press.

Devlin, J. T. and Poldrack, R. A. (2007) 'In Praise of Tedious Anatomy', *Neuroimage* 37(4): 1033–1041.

Dickens, C. (1838) *Oliver Twist*, London: Lacy.

Dikötter, F. (1998) *Imperfect Conceptions: Medical Knowledge, Birth Defects, and Eugenics in China*, New York: Columbia University Press.

Doidge, N. (2007) *The Brain That Changes Itself: Stories of Personal Triumph from the Frontiers of Brain Science*, London: Penguin.

Dokumaci, A. (2020) 'People as Affordances: Building Disability Worlds through Care Intimacy', *Current Anthropology* 61(S21): S97–S108.

Dorries, H., Henry, R., Hugill, D., McCreary, T., et al. (2019) *Settler City Limits: Indigenous Resurgence and Colonial Violence in the Urban Prairie West*, Winnipeg: University of Manitoba Press.

Downey, G. (2016) 'Being Human in Cities: Phenotypic Bias from Urban Niche Construction', *Current Anthropology* 57(S13): S52–S64.

Driver, F. (1988) 'Moral Geographies: Social Science and the Urban Environment in Mid-Nineteenth Century England', *Transactions of the Institute of British Geographers* 13(3): 275–287.

Du Bois, W. E. B. (1899) *The Philadelphia Negro: A Social Study . . . Together with a Special Report on Domestic Service, by Isabel Eaton*, New York: Benjamin Blom.

Du Bois, W. E. B. (1996 [1899]) *The Philadelphia Negro: A Social Study*, Philadelphia: University of Pennsylvania Press.

Duhl, L. (1963) *The Urban Condition: People and Policy in the Metropolis*, New York: Basic Books.

Dumit, J. (2003) *Picturing Personhood: Brain Scans and Biomedical Identity*, Princeton, NJ: Princeton University Press.

Dunham, H. W. (1966) 'Epidemiology of Psychiatric Disorders as a Contribution to Medical Ecology', *Archives of General Psychiatry* 14(1): 1–19.

Edmonds, P. (2010) 'Unpacking Settler Colonialism's Urban Strategies: Indigenous Peoples in Victoria, British Columbia, and the Transition to a Settler-Colonial City', *Urban History Review/ Revue d'histoire urbaine* 38(2): 4–20.

Egeland, J. A., Gerhard, D. S., Pauls, D. L., Sussex, J. N., et al. (1987) 'Bipolar Affective Disorders Linked to DNA Markers on Chromosome 11', *Nature* 325(6107): 783–787.

Ehsan, A. M. and De Silva, M. J. (2015) 'Social Capital and Common Mental Disorder: A Systematic Review', *Journal of Epidemiology and Community Health* 69(10): 1021–1028.

Eisenberger, N. I. and Moieni, M. (2020) 'Inflammation Affects Social Experience: Implications for Mental Health', *World Psychiatry* 19(1): 109.

Elden, S. (2016) *Space, Knowledge and Power: Foucault and Geography*, London: Routledge.

Elland, H. and Jennings, M. W. (2014) *Walter Benjamin: A Critical Life*, Cambridge, MA: Harvard University Press.

Ellwood-Lowe, M. E., Sacchet, M. D., and Gotlib, I. H. (2016) 'The Application of Neuroimaging to Social Inequity and Language Disparity: A Cautionary Examination', *Developmental Cognitive Neuroscience* 22: 1–8.

Engel, G. L. (1977) 'The Need for a New Medical Model: A Challenge for Biomedicine', *Science* 196(4286): 129–136.

Engels, F. (2010 [1844]) 'The Great Towns', in G. Bridge and S. Watson (eds.) *The Blackwell City Reader*, London: Blackwell.

Epel, E. S., Crosswell, A. D., Mayer, S. E., Prather, A. A., et al. (2018) 'More Than a Feeling: A Unified View of Stress Measurement for Population Science', *Frontiers in Neuroendocrinology* 49: 146–169.

Erasmus, Z. (2011) 'Creolization, Colonial Citizenship(S) and Degeneracy: A Critique of Selected Histories of Sierra Leone and South Africa', *Current Sociology* 59(5): 635–654.

Erhan, L., Ndubuaku, M., Ferrara, E., Richardson, M., et al. (2019) 'Analyzing Objective and Subjective Data in Social Sciences: Implications for Smart Cities', *IEEE Access* 7: 19890–19906.

Evans, J. and Jones, P. (2011) 'The Walking Interview: Methodology, Mobility and Place', *Applied Geography* 31(2): 849–858.

Ezeh, A., Oyebode, O., Satterthwaite, D., Chen, Y.-F., et al. (2016) 'The History, Geography, and Sociology of Slums and the Health Problems of People Who Live in Slums', *The Lancet* 389(10068): 547–558.

Fairburn, M. (2013) *The Ideal Society and Its Enemies: Foundations of Modern New Zealand Society, 1850–1900*, Auckland: Auckland University Press.

Fan, C. C. (2007) *China on the Move: Migration, the State, and the Household*, London: Routledge.

Farah, M. J. (2018) 'Socioeconomic Status and the Brain: Prospects for Neuroscience-Informed Policy', *Nature Reviews Neuroscience* 19(7): 428–438.

Faris, R. E. L. (1970) *Chicago Sociology, 1920–1932, Etc*, Chicago; London: University of Chicago Press.

Faris, R. E. L. and Dunham, H. W. (1939) *Mental Disorders in Urban Areas: An Ecological Study of Schizophrenia and Other Psychoses*, Chicago: University of Chicago Press.

Farmer, P. E., Nizeye, B., Stulac, S., and Keshavjee, S. (2006) 'Structural Violence and Clinical Medicine', *PLoS Medicine* 3(10): e449.

Farrow, M. R. and Washburn, K. (2019) 'A Review of Field Experiments on the Effect of Forest Bathing on Anxiety and Heart Rate Variability', *Global Advances in Health and Medicine* 8: 2164956119848654.

Fett, A.-K. J., Lemmers-Jansen, I. L. J., and Krabbendam, L. (2019) 'Psychosis and Urbanicity: A Review of the Recent Literature from Epidemiology to Neurourbanism', *Current Opinion in Psychiatry* 32(3): 232–241.

Finnegan, R. (2005) 'Tactile Communication', pp. 18–25 in Classen, C. (ed.) *The Book of Touch*, Oxford: Berg.

Firdaus, G. (2017) 'Mental Well-Being of Migrants in Urban Center of India: Analyzing the Role of Social Environment', *Indian Journal of Psychiatry* 59(2): 164.

Fishkin, R. E. and Levine, F. J. (2020) 'Ethical Issues in Psychotherapy Training in China', *Psychoanalytic Inquiry* 40(1): 50–55.

Fitzgerald, D. (2012) *Tracing Autism: Ambiguity and Difference in a Neuroscientific Research Practice*, Ph.D. Thesis, London: The London School of Economics and Political Science (LSE).

Fitzgerald, D. and Callard, F. (2018) 'Experimental Entanglements: Social Science and Neuroscience Beyond Interdisciplinarity', *The Palgrave Handbook of Biology and Society*, NewYork: Springer.

Fitzgerald, D., Manning, N., Rose, N., and Fu, H. (2019) 'Mental Health, Migration and the Megacity', *International Health* 11(Supplement-1): S1–S6.

Fitzgerald, D., Rose, N., and Singh, I. (2016a) 'Living Well in the Neuropolis', *The Sociological Review Monographs* 64(1): 221–237.

Fitzgerald, D., Rose, N., and Singh, I. (2016b) 'Revitalizing Sociology: Urban Life and Mental Illness between History and the Present', *The British Journal of Sociology* 67(1): 138–160.

Foucault, M. (1967) 'Des espaces autres', in M. Foucault *Dits Et Écrits*, Vol. 4, Paris: Gallimard.

Foucault, M. (1977 [1975]) *Discipline and Punish: The Birth of the Prison*, London: Allen Lane.

Foucault, M. (1979) 'On Governmentality', *Ideology & Consciousness* (6): 5–21.

Foucault, M. (1984) 'Space, Knowledge and Power', in P. Rabinow (ed.) *The Foucault Reader*, New York: Pantheon.

Foucault, M. (1986 [1967]) 'Of Other Spaces, Translated by Jay Miskowiec', *diacritics* 16(1): 22–27.

Foucault, M. (1999) 'The Politics of Health in the Eighteenth Century', in J. D. Faubion (ed.) *Michel Foucault: The Essential Works, Volume 3: Power*, New York: New Press.

Foucault, M. (2004) *Naissance de la biopolitique: cours au collège de france (1978–1979)*, Paris: Gallimard, Seuil.

Foucault, M., Barret-Kriegel, B., Thalamy, A., Beguin, F., et al. (1979) *Les Machines À Guérir: Aux Origines De L'hôpital Moderne*, Bruxelles: Pierre Mardaga.

Frances, A. J. and Widiger, T. (2012) 'Psychiatric Diagnosis: Lessons from the DSM-IV Past and Cautions for the DSM-5 Future', *Annual Review of Clinical Psychology* 8: 109–130.

Franklin, V. P. (1998) 'Operation Street Corner the Wharton Centre and the Juvenile Gang Problem in Philadelphia, 1945–1958', in M. B. Katz and T. J. Sugrue (eds.) *W.E.B. Du Bois, Race, and the City: The Philadelphia Negro and Its Legacy*, Philadelphia: Penn Press.

Fraser, M., Kember, S., and Lury, C. (2005) 'Inventive Life: Approaches to the New Vitalism', Thousand Oaks, CA: Sage.

Freedman, J. L. (1975) *Crowding and Behavior*, New York: W.H. Freeman.

Fried, A. and Elman, R. M. (1969) 'Introduction', in A. Fried and R. M. Elman (eds.) *Charles Booth's London: A Portrait of the Poor at the Turn of the Century, Drawn from His 'Life and Labour of the People in London'*, London: Hutchinson.

Frisby, D. (2001) *Cityscapes of Modernity: Critical Explorations*, Cambridge: Polity.

Fritz, A. (2018) '"I Was a Sociological Stranger": Ethnographic Fieldwork and Undercover Performance in the Publication of the Taxi-Dance Hall, 1925-1932', *Gender & History* 30(1): 131–152.

Fuchs, E. and Flügge, G. (2014) 'Adult Neuroplasticity: More Than 40 Years of Research', *Neural Plasticity*, https://doi.org/10.1155/2014/541870.

Fuchs, R. G. and Moch, L. P. (1990) 'Pregnant, Single, and Far from Home: Migrant Women in Nineteenth-Century Paris', *American Historical Review* 95(4): 1007–1031.

Furuyashiki, A., Tabuchi, K., Norikoshi, K., Kobayashi, T., et al. (2019) 'A Comparative Study of the Physiological and Psychological Effects of Forest Bathing (Shinrin-Yoku) on Working Age People with and without Depressive Tendencies', *Environmental Health and Preventive Medicine* 24(1): 46.

Galea, S. and Link, B. G. (2013) 'Six Paths for the Future of Social Epidemiology', *American Journal of Epidemiology* 178(6): 843–849.

Galea, S., Uddin, M., and Koenen, K. (2011) 'The Urban Environment and Mental Disorders: Epigenetic Links', *Epigenetics* 6(4): 400–404.

Galea, S. and Vlahov, D. (2005) 'Urban Health: Evidence, Challenges, and Directions', *Annual Review of Public Health* 26: 341–365.

Gałecki, P. and Talarowska, M. (2018) 'Neurodevelopmental Theory of Depression', *Progress in Neuro-Psychopharmacology and Biological Psychiatry* 80: 267–272.

Galle, O. R., Gove, W. R., and McPherson, J. M. (1972) 'Population Density and Pathology: What Are the Relations for Man?', *Science* 176(4030): 23–30.

Galton, F. (1904) 'Eugenics: Its Definition, Scope, and Aims', *American Journal of Sociology* 10(1): 1–25.

Galtung, J. and Höivik, T. (1971) 'Structural and Direct Violence: A Note on Operationalization', *Journal of Peace Research* 8(1): 73–76.

Gandy, M. (2017) 'Urban Atmospheres', *Cultural Geographies* 24(3): 353–374.

Gans, H. J. (1969) 'Planning for People, Not Buildings', *Environment and Planning A* 1(1): 33–46.

Gibson, J. J. (1979) *The Ecological Approach to Visual Perception*, Boston: Houghton Mifflin.

Glass, D. C. and Singer, J. E. (1972) *Urban Stress: Experiments on Noise and Social Stressors*, New York: Academic Press.

Goffman, E. (1961) *Asylums: Essays on the Social Situation of Mental Patients and Other Inmates*, New York: Anchor Books.

Goffman, E. (1963) *Behavior in Public Places. Notes on the Social Organization of Gatherings*, New York: Free Press of Glencoe.

Goffman, E. (1967) *Interaction Ritual: Essays on Face-to-Face Behavior*, New York: Doubleday.

Goffman, E. (1983) 'The Interaction Order: American Sociological Association, 1982 Presidential Address', *American Sociological Review* 48(1): 1–17.

Goldmann, E., Aiello, A., Uddin, M., Delva, J., et al. (2011) 'Pervasive Exposure to Violence and Posttraumatic Stress Disorder in a Predominantly African American Urban Community: The Detroit Neighborhood Health Study', *Journal of Traumatic Stress* 24(6): 747–751.

Goldsmith, W. and Blakely, E. (2010) *Separate Societies: Poverty and Inequality in US Cities*, Philadelphia, PA: Temple University Press.

Gonzalez, A., Guffanti, G., Ratanatharathorn, A., Kotov, R., et al. (2014) 'Epigenetic Findings for PTSD and Lower Respiratory Symptoms in Male WTC Responders', *Comprehensive Psychiatry* 55(8): e49.

Goodman, N. (1978) *Ways of Worldmaking*, Hassocks: Harvester Press.

Goodrich, C. (1936) *Migration and Economic Opportunity*, Philadelphia: University of Pennsylvania Press.

Gordon, C. (1980) *Power/Knowledge: Selected Interviews and Other Writings by Michel Foucault, 1972–1977*, New York: Pantheon.

Gould, E. and McEwen, B. S. (1993) 'Neuronal Birth and Death', *Current Opinion in Neurobiology* 3(5): 676–682.

Gould, E., Reeves, A. J., Graziano, M. S. A., and Gross, C. G. (1999) 'Neurogenesis in the Neocortex of Adult Primates', *Science* 286(5439): 548–552.

Gould, E., Tanapat, P., Hastings, N. B., and Shors, T. J. (1999) 'Neurogenesis in Adulthood: A Possible Role in Learning', *Trends in Cognitive Sciences* 3(5): 186–192.

Gove, W. R., Hughes, M., and Galle, O. R. (1979) 'Overcrowding in the Home: An Empirical Investigation of Its Possible Pathological Consequences', *American Sociological Review* 44(February): 59–80.

Gransow, B. (2010) 'Slum Formation or Urban Innovation? Migrant Communities and Social Change in Chinese Megacities', *Proceeding from Rural-Urban Migrations in Mega Cities and Mega-Slums 'Our Common Future'*, Essen, Germany.

Greco, M. (2005) 'On the Vitality of Vitalism', *Theory Culture & Society* 22(1): 15–27.

Greenwood, M. J. and Hunt, G. L. (2003) 'The Early History of Migration Research', *International Regional Science Review* 26(1): 3–37.

Grinker, R. and Spiegel, J. (1945) 'The Neurotic Reactions to Severe Combat Stress', *Men under Stress*, Philadelphia: Blackiston.

Grob, G. N. (1985) 'The Origins of American Psychiatric Epidemiology', *American Journal of Public Health* 75(3): 229–236.

Grosz, E. (2001) *Architecture from the Outside: Essays on Virtual and Real Space*, Cambridge, MA: MIT Press.

Gruebner, O., Khan, M. M. H., Lautenbach, S., Müller, D., et al. (2012) 'Mental Health in the Slums of Dhaka—a Geoepidemiological Study', *BMC Public Health* 12(1): 177.

Gulas, C. S. and Bloch, P. H. (1995) 'Right under Our Noses: Ambient Scent and Consumer Responses', *Journal of Business and Psychology* 10(1): 87–98.

Guloksuz, S., Rutten, B. P., Pries, L.-K., Ten Have, M., et al. (2018) 'The Complexities of Evaluating the Exposome in Psychiatry: A Data-Driven Illustration of Challenges and Some Propositions for Amendments', *Schizophrenia Bulletin* 44(6): 1175–1179.

Guxens, M., Lubczyńska, M. J., Muetzel, R. L., Dalmau-Bueno, A., et al. (2018) 'Air Pollution Exposure During Fetal Life, Brain Morphology, and Cognitive Function in School-Age Children', *Biological Psychiatry* 84(4): 295–303.

Hacking, I. (2004) 'Between Michel Foucault and Erving Goffman: Between Discourse in the Abstract and Face-to-Face Interaction', *Economy and Society* 33(3): 277–302.

Hackman, D. A. and Farah, M. J. (2009) 'Socioeconomic Status and the Developing Brain', *Trends in Cognitive Sciences* 13(2): 65–73.

Haerle Jr., R. K. (1991) 'William Isaac Thomas and the Helen Culver Fund for Race Psychology: The Beginnings of Scientific Sociology at the University of Chicago, 1910–1913', *Journal of the History of the Behavioral Sciences* 27(1): 21–41.

Hagan, S. (2014) *Ecological Urbanism: The Nature of the City*, London: Routledge.

Hagner, M. (1997) *Homo Cerebralis: Der Wandel Vom Seelenorgan Zum Gehirn*, Berlin: Berlin Verlag.

Hagner, M. (2001) 'Cultivating the Cortex in German Neuroanatomy', *Science in Context* 14(4): 541–563.

Hagner, M. and Borck, C. (2001) 'Mindful Practices: On the Neurosciences in the Twentieth Century', *Science in Context* 14(4): 507–510.

Han, C. (2012) *Life in Debt: Times of Care and Violence in Neoliberal Chile*, Chicago: University of California Press.

Haney, M. J., Zhao, Y., Harrison, E. B., Mahajan, V., et al. (2013) 'Specific Transfection of Inflamed Brain by Macrophages: A New Therapeutic Strategy for Neurodegenerative Diseases', *PloS One* 8(4): e61852.

Hansen, M. M., Jones, R., and Tocchini, K. (2017) 'Shinrin-Yoku (Forest Bathing) and Nature Therapy: A State-of-the-Art Review. 2017, 14, 851.', *International Journal of Environmental Research and Public Health* 14: 851–899.

Hanssen, B. (2006) *Walter Benjamin and the Arcades Project*, London: Continuum.

Hare, E. (1952) 'The Ecology of Mental Disease', *The British Journal of Psychiatry* 98(413): 579–594.

Hare, E. (1955) 'Mental Illness and Social Class in Bristol', *British Journal of Preventive & Social Medicine* 9(4): 191.

Harrington, A. (1996) *Reenchanted Science: Holism in German Culture from Wilhelm II to Hitler*, Princeton, NJ: Princeton University Press.

Harvey, D. (1996) 'The Environment of Justice', pp. 366–402 in S. Vanderheide (ed.) *Justice, Nature and the Geography of Difference*, Malden, MA: Blackwell.

Harvey, D. (2009 [1973]) *Social Justice and the City* (Rev. Ed.), Athens: University of Georgia Press.

Hatton, T. J. and Williamson, J. G. (1992) *What Drove the Mass Migrations from Europe in the Late Nineteenth Century?*, Cambridge, MA: National Bureau of Economic Research.

Hebb, D. O. (1949) *The Organization of Behavior. A Neuropsychological Theory*, pp. xix, 335. New York: John Wiley & Sons.

Hecht, J. M. (2003) *The End of the Soul: Scientific Modernity, Atheism, and Anthropology in France*, New York: Columbia University Press.

Hedlund, M. (2012) 'Epigenetic Responsibility', *Medicine Studies* 3(3): 171–183.

Henshaw, V., Medway, D., Warnaby, G., and Perkins, C. (2016) 'Marketing the "City of Smells"', *Marketing Theory* 16(2): 153–170.

Herd, P., Palloni, A., Rey, F., and Dowd, J. B. (2018) 'Social and Population Health Science Approaches to Understand the Human Microbiome', *Nature Human Behaviour* 2(11): 808–815.

Hesketh, T., Jun, Y. X., Lu, L., and Mei, W. H. (2008) 'Health Status and Access to Health Care of Migrant Workers in China', *Public Health Reports* 123(2): 189–197.

Heynen, N., Kaika, M., and Swyngedouw, E. (2006a) *In the Nature of Cities: Urban Political Ecology and the Politics of Urban Metabolism*, London; New York: Routledge.

Heynen, N., Kaika, M., and Swyngedouw, E. (2006b) *In the Nature of Cities: Urban Political Ecology and the Politics of Urban Metabolism*, London: Taylor & Francis.

Hill, O. (1970 [1883]) *Homes of the London Poor*, London: Frank Cass & Company.

Hinkle, L. E. and Plummer, N. (1952) 'Life Stress and Industrial Absenteeism; the Concentration of Illness and Absenteeism in One Segment of a Working Population', *Industrial Medicine & Surgery* 21(8): 363–375.

Hirst, P. Q. and Woolley, P. (1982) *Social Relations and Human Attributes*, London: Tavistock.

Hizi, G. (2017) '"Developmental" Therapy for a "Modernised" Society: The Sociopolitical Meanings of Psychology in Urban China', *China: An International Journal* 15(2): 98–119.

Hoare, E., Jacka, F., and Berk, M. (2019) 'The Impact of Urbanization on Mood Disorders: An Update of Recent Evidence', *Current Opinion in Psychiatry* 32(3): 198–203.

Hochstadt, S. (1986) 'Urban Migration in Imperial Germany: Towards a Quantitative Model', *Historical Papers / Communications historiques* 21(1): 197–210.

Hoek, G., Brunekreef, B., Goldbohm, S., Fischer, P., et al. (2002) 'Association between Mortality and Indicators of Traffic-Related Air Pollution in the Netherlands: A Cohort Study', *The Lancet* 360(9341): 1203–1209.

Hoffman, D. J., Reynolds, R. M., and Hardy, D. B. (2017) 'Developmental Origins of Health and Disease: Current Knowledge and Potential Mechanisms', *Nutrition Reviews* 75(12): 951–970.

Horwitz, A. V. and Grob, G. N. (2011) 'The Checkered History of American Psychiatric Epidemiology', *The Milbank Quarterly* 89(4): 628–657.

Howard, J. M., Olney, J. M., Frawley, J. P., Peterson, R. E., et al. (1955) 'Studies of Adrenal Function in Combat and Wounded Soldiers: A Study in the Korean Theatre', *Annals of Surgery* 141(3): 314.

Hsuan-Ying, H. (2015) 'From Psychotherapy to Psycho-Boom: A Historical Overview of Psychotherapy in China', *Psychoanalysis & Psychotherapy in China* 1: 1–30.

Human Microbiome Project Consortium (2012) 'A Framework for Human Microbiome Research', *Nature* 486(7402): 215–221.

Huxley, M. (2008) 'Space and Government: Governmentality and Geography', *Geography Compass* 2(5): 1635–1658.

Jablonka, E. and Lamb, M. J. (2014) *Evolution in Four Dimensions, Revised Edition: Genetic, Epigenetic, Behavioral, and Symbolic Variation in the History of Life*, Cambridge, MA: MIT Press.

Jackson, M. (2013) *The Age of Stress: Science and the Search for Stability*, Oxford: Oxford University Press.

Jacob, F. and Monod, J. (1961) 'Genetic Regulatory Mechanisms in the Synthesis of Proteins', *Journal of Molecular Biology* 3: 318–356.

Jacobs, J. (1972) *The Death and Life of Great American Cities*, Harmondsworth: Penguin.

Jenkins, W., Merzenich, M., Ochs, M., Allard, T., et al. (1990) 'Functional Reorganization of Primary Somatosensory Cortex in Adult Owl Monkeys after Behaviorally Controlled Tactile Stimulation', *Journal of Neurophysiology* 63(1): 82.

Jiao, J. (2002) 'A Study on Floating Population from Rights Point of View', *Renkou Yu Jingji (Population and Economics)* 3: 73–75.

Jo Cox Commission on Loneliness (2017) 'Combatting Loneliness One Conversation at a Time: A Call to Action'. London: Jo Cox Commission.

Johnson, P. (2006) 'Unravelling Foucault's "Different Spaces"', *History of the Human Sciences* 19(4): 75–90.

Johnson, P. (2012) 'The Changing Face of the Modern Cemetery: Loudon's Design for Life and Death', *Heterotopian Studies*, http://www.heterotopiastudies.com

Johnson, R. B. and Popenoe, P. (1925) *Applied Eugenics*, New York: Macmillan.

Johnson, R. H. (1926) 'The Eugenics of the City', *Journal of Heredity* 17(4): 146–146.

Kasinitz, P. (2012) 'The Sociology of International Migration: Where We Have Been; Where Do We Go from Here?', *Sociological Forum* 27(3): 579–590.

Katukiza, A., Ronteltap, M., Niwagaba, C., Kansiime, F., et al. (2015) 'Grey Water Characterisation and Pollutant Loads in an Urban Slum', *International Journal of Environmental Science and Technology* 12(2): 423–436.

Kawachi, I. and Berkman, L. F. (2001) 'Social Ties and Mental Health', *Journal of Urban Health* 78(3): 458–467.

Keiner, C. (2005) 'Wartime Rat Control, Rodent Ecology, and the Rise and Fall of Chemical Rodenticides', *Endeavour* 29(3): 119–125.

Keith, M. (2005) *After the Cosmopolitan?: Multicultural Cities and the Future of Racism*, London: Routledge.

Keith, M., Lash, S., Arnoldi, J., and Rooker, T. (2013) *China Constructing Capitalism: Economic Life and Urban Change*, London: Routledge.

Kelly, J. R., Kennedy, P. J., Cryan, J. F., Dinan, T. G., et al. (2015) 'Breaking Down the Barriers: The Gut Microbiome, Intestinal Permeability and Stress-Related Psychiatric Disorders', *Frontiers in Cellular Neuroscience* 9: 392.

Kelly-Irving, M. and Delpierre, C. (2019) 'A Critique of the Adverse Childhood Experiences Framework in Epidemiology and Public Health: Uses and Misuses', *Social Policy and Society* 18(3): 445–456.

Kempermann, G., Gage, F. H., Aigner, L., Song, H., et al. (2018) 'Human Adult Neurogenesis: Evidence and Remaining Questions', *Cell Stem Cell* 23(1): 25–30.

Kemple, T. (2018) *Simmel*, Cambridge: Polity Press.

Kevles, B. (1997) *Naked to the Bone: Medical Imaging in the Twentieth Century*, New Brunswick, NJ: Rutgers University Press.

Keyes, K. M. and Galea, S. (2017) 'Commentary: The Limits of Risk Factors Revisited: Is It Time for a Causal Architecture Approach?', *Epidemiology* 28(1): 1–5.

Kiechle, M. A. (2017) *Smell Detectives: An Olfactory History of Nineteenth-Century Urban America*, Seattle: University of Washington Press.

Kim, T.-H., Jeong, G.-W., Baek, H.-S., Kim, G.-W., et al. (2010) 'Human Brain Activation in Response to Visual Stimulation with Rural and Urban Scenery Pictures: A Functional Magnetic Resonance Imaging Study', *Science of the Total Environment* 408(12): 2600–2607.

Kim, G.-W., Jeong, G.-W., Kim, T.-H., Baek, H.-S., et al. (2010) 'Functional Neuroanatomy Associated with Natural and Urban Scenic Views in the Human Brain: 3.0 T Functional MR Imaging', *Korean Journal of Radiology* 11(5): 507–513.

Kinver, M. (2014) 'Green Spaces Have Lasting Positive Effect on Well-Being', *BBC News*, http://www.bbc. com/news/scienceenvironment-25682368.

Kirk, R. G. W. (2014) 'The Invention of the "Stressed Animal" and the Development of a Science of Animal Welfare, 1947–86', in D. Cantor and E. Ramsden (eds.) *Stress, Shock, and Adaptation in the Twentieth Century*, Rochester, NY: University of Rochester Press.

Kirkbride, J. B. and Jones, P. B. (2010) 'Epidemiological Aspects of Migration and Mental Illness', in D. Bhugra (ed.) *Migration and Mental Health*, Cambridge: Cambridge University Press.

Kirmayer, L. J., Narasiah, L., Munoz, M., Rashid, M., et al. (2011) 'Common Mental Health Problems in Immigrants and Refugees: General Approach in Primary Care', *Canadian Medical Association Journal* 183(12): E959–E967.

Kitanaka, J. (2016) 'Depression as a Problem of Labor: Japanese Debates About Work, Stress, and a New Therapeutic Ethos', in J. Wakefield and S. Demazeux (eds.) *Sadness or Depression?. History, Philosophy and Theory of the Life Sciences*, vol 15. Dordrecht: Springer.

Kleinman, A. (1982) 'Neurasthenia and Depression: A Study of Somatization and Culture in China', *Culture, Medicine and Psychiatry* 6(2): 117–190.

Kleinman, A. (1986) *Social Origins of Distress and Disease: Depression, Neurasthenia, and Pain in Modern China*, New Haven, CT: Yale University Press.

Kleinman, A. (2010) 'Remaking the Moral Person in China: Implications for Health', *The Lancet* 375(9720): 1074–1075.

Kleinman, A., Das, V., and Lock, M. M. (1997) *Social Suffering*, Berkeley: University of California Press.

Knipscheer, J. W. and Kleber, R. J. (2006) 'The Relative Contribution of Posttraumatic and Acculturative Stress to Subjective Mental Health among Bosnian Refugees', *Journal of Clinical Psychology* 62(3): 339–353.

Knowles, C. (2010) 'Theorising Race and Ethnicity: Contemporary Paradigms and Perspectives', pp. 23–42 in P. Hill Collins and J. Solomos (eds.) *The Sage Handbook of Race and Ethnic Studies*, London: Sage

Kondo, M. C., Jacoby, S. F., and South, E. C. (2018) 'Does Spending Time Outdoors Reduce Stress? A Review of Real-Time Stress Response to Outdoor Environments', *Health & Place* 51: 136–150.

Krabbendam, L. and Van Os, J. (2005) 'Schizophrenia and Urbanicity: A Major Environmental Influence—Conditional on Genetic Risk', *Schizophrenia Bulletin* 31(4): 795–799.

Krabbendam, L., van Vugt, M., Conus, P., Söderström, O., et al. (2021) 'Understanding Urbanicity: How Interdisciplinary Methods Help to Unravel the Effects of the City on Mental Health', *Psychological Medicine* 51(7): 1099–1110.

Krieger, N. (1994) 'Epidemiology and the Web of Causation: Has Anyone Seen the Spider?', *Social Science & Medicine* 39(7): 887–903.

Krieger, N. (2001) 'Theories for Social Epidemiology in the 21st Century: An Ecosocial Perspective', *International Journal of Epidemiology* 30(4): 668–677.

Krieger, N. (2014) 'Got Theory? On the 21st Century CE Rise of Explicit Use of Epidemiologic Theories of Disease Distribution: A Review and Ecosocial Analysis', *Current Epidemiology Reports* 1(1): 45–56.

Krishna, A. (2011) *Sensory Marketing: Research on the Sensuality of Products*, London: Routledge.

Krishnan, K. R. R. (2012) 'Structural Imaging in Psychiatic Disorders', in T. E. Schlepfer and C. B. Nemeroff (eds.) *Handbook of Clinical Neurology*, Vol. 306, Philadelphia, PA: Elsevier.

Kull, K. (1999) 'Biosemiotics in the Twentieth Century: A View from Biology', *Semiotica* 127(1–4): 385–414.

Kull, K. (2003) 'Thomas A. Sebeok and Biology: Building Biosemiotics', *Cybernetics & Human Knowing* 10(1): 47–60.

Kuznets, S. S. and Thomas, D. S. T. (1957) *Population Redistribution and Economic Growth: United States, 1870–1950*, Vol. 1, Philadephia, PA: American Philosophical Society.

Landecker, H. (2019) 'A Metabolic History of Manufacturing Waste: Food Commodities and Their Outsides', *Food, Culture & Society* 22(5): 530–547.

Landecker, H. and Panofsky, A. (2013) 'From Social Structure to Gene Regulation, and Back: A Critical Introduction to Environmental Epigenetics for Sociology', *Annual Review of Sociology* 39(1): 333–357.

Lappé, M. and Landecker, H. (2015) 'How the Genome Got a Life Span', *New Genetics and Society* 34(2): 152–176.

Laurencin, C. T. and McClinton, A. (2020) 'The Covid-19 Pandemic: A Call to Action to Identify and Address Racial and Ethnic Disparities', *Journal of Racial and Ethnic Health Disparities* 7: 398–402

Lazarus, R. S. (1966) *Psychological Stress and the Coping Process*, New York: McGraw Hill.

Lazarus, R. S. (1998) *The Life and Work of an Eminent Psychologist*, Berlin: Springer.

Lazarus, R. S. (2013) *Fifty Years of the Research and Theory of RS Lazarus: An Analysis of Historical and Perennial Issues*, New York: Psychology Press.

Lazarus, R. S. and Folkman, S. (1984) *Stress, Appraisal, and Coping,* New York: Springer.

Le Bon, G. (1982 [1896]) *The Crowd, a Study of the Popular Mind*, Marietta, GA: Cherokee Publishing.

Lederbogen, F., Kirsch, P., Haddad, L., Streit, F., et al. (2011) 'City Living and Urban Upbringing Affect Neural Social Stress Processing in Humans', *Nature* 474(7352): 498–501.

Lee, S. (2011) 'Depression Coming of Age in China', in A. E. Kleinman (ed.) *Deep China: The Moral Life of the Person*, Berkeley: University of California Press.

Lee, S., Tsang, A., Huang, Y.-Q., He, Y.-L., et al. (2009) 'The Epidemiology of Depression in Metropolitan China', *Psychological Medicine* 39(5): 735–747.

Lees-Manning, E., Kienzler, H., Manning, N., Morgan, C., et al. (2021) *Crises and Mental Life: Implications for COVID 19*, London: King's Centre for Society and Mental Health.

Lefebvre, H. (1996 [1968]) 'The Right to the City', in E. Kofman and E. Lebas (eds.) *Writings on Cities: Henri Lefebvre*, Oxford: Blackwell.

Leslie, E. (2006) 'Ruin and Rubble in the Arcades', in B. Hanssen (ed.) *Walter Benjamin and the Arcades Project*, London: Continuum.

Leuner, B., Glasper, E. R., and Gould, E. (2010) 'Parenting and Plasticity', *Trends in Neurosciences* 33(10): 465–473.

Lewis, D. L. (1993) *W.E.B. Du Bois: Biography of a Race, 1868–1919*, New York: Henry Holt.

Lewis, G., David, A., Andréassson, S., and Allebeck, P. (1992) 'Schizophrenia and City Life', *The Lancet* 340(8812): 137–140.

Li, J. and Rose, N. (2017) 'Urban Social Exclusion and Mental Health of China's Rural-Urban Migrants—a Review and Call for Research', *Health & Place* 48: 20–30.

Li, Z., Dai, J., Wu, N., Gao, J., et al. (2019) 'The Mental Health and Depression of Rural-to-Urban Migrant Workers Compared to Non-Migrant Workers in Shanghai: A Cross-Sectional Study', *International Health* 11(Supplement_1): S55–S63.

Lima-Ojeda, J. M., Rupprecht, R., and Baghai, T. C. (2018) 'Neurobiology of Depression: A Neurodevelopmental Approach', *The World Journal of Biological Psychiatry* 19(5): 349–359.

Lin, X., Jiang, G., and Duan, C. (2016) 'Necessity and Urgency of Increasing Graduate Training in Chinese Clinical and Counseling Psychology: Wuhan Declaration', *Psychotherapy Bulletin* 51(4): 26–29.

Lindert, J., von Ehrenstein, O. S., Priebe, S., Mielck, A., et al. (2009) 'Depression and Anxiety in Labor Migrants and Refugees—a Systematic Review and Meta-Analysis', *Social Science & Medicine* 69(2): 246–257.

Link, B. G. and Phelan, J. (1995) 'Social Conditions as Fundamental Causes of Disease', *Journal of Health and Social Behavior*. Extra Issue: Forty Years of Medical Sociology: The State of the Art and Directions for the Future: 80–94.

Lipina, S. J. and Evers, K. (2017) 'Neuroscience of Childhood Poverty: Evidence of Impacts and Mechanisms as Vehicles of Dialog with Ethics', *Frontiers in Psychology* 8: 61.

Lipowski, Z. (1971) 'Surfeit of Attractive Information Inputs: A Hallmark of Our Environment', *Behavioral Science* 16(5): 467–471.

Lipowski, Z. (1977) 'Psychosomatic Medicine in the Seventies', *Psychosomatic Medicine and Liaison Psychiatry*, New York: Springer.

Lipowski, Z. J. (1985) *Psychosomatic Medicine and Liaison Psychiatry: Selected Papers*, New York: Plenum.

Lipton, M. (1977) *Why Poor People Stay Poor: A Study of Urban Bias in World Development*: Canberra: Australian National University Press.

Liu, Y., He, S., Wu, F., and Webster, C. (2010) 'Urban Villages under China's Rapid Urbanization: Unregulated Assets and Transitional Neighbourhoods', *Habitat International* 34(2): 135–144.

Liu, Z., Wang, Y., and Chen, S. (2017) 'Does Formal Housing Encourage Settlement Intention of Rural Migrants in Chinese Cities? A Structural Equation Model Analysis', *Urban Studies* 54(8): 1834–1850.

Lock, M. (2013) 'The Epigenome and Nature/Nurture Reunification: A Challenge for Anthropology', *Medical Anthropology* 32(4): 291–308.

Lock, M., Burke, W., Dupré, J., Landecker, H., et al. (2015) 'Comprehending the Body in the Era of the Epigenome', *Current Anthropology* 56(2): 163–164.

Lock, M. and Kaufert, P. (2001) 'Menopause, Local Biologies, and Cultures of Aging', *American Journal of Human Biology* 13(4): 494–504.

Lock, M. M. (1993) *Encounters with Aging: Mythologies of Menopause in Japan and North America*, Berkeley: University of California Press.

Long, T. (2014) 'The Machinery and the Morale: Physiological Approaches to Military Stress Research in the Early Cold War Era', in D. Cantor and E. Ramsden (eds.) *Stress, Shock, and Adaptation in the Twentieth Century*, Rochester, NY: Unversity of Rochester Press.

Lorimer, J. (2016) 'Gut Buddies: Multispecies Studies and the Microbiome', *Environmental Humanities* 8(1): 57–76.

Lu, Y. W., Lee, S., Liu, M. L., Wing, Y. K., et al. (1999) 'Too Costly to Be Ill: Psychiatric Disorders among Hospitalized Migrant Workers in Shenzhen', *Transcultural Psychiatry* 36(1): 95–109.

Lund, C., Breen, A., Flisher, A. J., Kakuma, R., et al. (2010) 'Poverty and Common Mental Disorders in Low and Middle Income Countries: A Systematic Review', *Social Science & Medicine* 71(3): 517–528.

Lundberg, U. (1976) 'Urban Commuting: Crowdedness and Catecholamine Excretion', *Journal of Human Stress* 2(3): 26–32.

Lupien, S. J., McEwen, B. S., Gunnar, M. R., and Heim, C. (2009) 'Effects of Stress Throughout the Lifespan on the Brain, Behaviour and Cognition', *Nature Reviews Neuroscience* 10: 434.

Lynch, K. (1960) *The Image of the City*, Cambridge, MA: Technology Press.

Mahfoud, T., McLean, S., and Rose, N. (eds.) (2017) *Vital Models: The Making and Use of Models in the Brain Sciences*, Vol. 233, Cambridge, MA: Academic Press.

Malabou, C. (2009) *What Should We Do with Our Brain?* New York: Fordham University Press.

Mann, F., Bone, J., Ma, R., Pinfold, V., et al. (2017) 'Loneliness and Mental Health: A State of the Art Review', *Social Psychiatry and Psychiatric Epidemiology* 52: 627–638.

Marcuse, P. (2009) 'From Critical Urban Theory to the Right to the City', *City* 13(2–3): 185–197.

Marmot, M. (2015) *The Health Gap: The Challenge of an Unequal World*, London: Bloomsbury.

Marmot, M., Allen, J., Boyce, B. Goldblatt, P., and Morrison, J. (2020) *Health Equity in England: The Marmot Review 10 Years On*, London: The Health Foundation.

Marmot, M. and Bell, R. (2012) 'Fair Society, Healthy Lives', *Public Health* 126: S4–S10.

Martyr, P. (2011) 'Having a Clean Up? Deporting Lunatic Migrants from Western Australia, 1924–1939', *History Compass* 9(3): 171–199.

Marx, K. (1954 [1867]) *Capital: A Critical Analysis of Capitalist Production. Volume 1*, London: Lawrence and Wishart.

Mason, J. W. (1975a) 'A Historical View of the Stress Field—Part One', *Journal of Human Stress* 1(1): 6–12.

Mason, J. W. (1975b) 'A Historical View of the Stress Field—Part Two', *Journal of Human Stress* 1(2): 22–36.

Massumi, B. (2002) *Parables for the Virtual: Movement, Affect, Sensation*, Durham, NC: Duke University Press Books.

Massumi, B. (2015) *Politics of Affect*. New York: John Wiley.

Mayer, E. A., Tillisch, K., and Gupta, A. (2015) 'Gut/Brain Axis and the Microbiota', *The Journal of Clinical Investigation* 125(3): 926–938.

Mbembe, A. (2019) *Necropolitics*, Durham, NC: Duke University Press.

McCarthy, A. (2008) 'Ethnicity, Migration and the Lunatic Asylum in Early Twentieth-Century Auckland, New Zealand', *Social History of Medicine* 21(1): 47–65.

McCarthy, A. and Coleborne, C. (2012) *Migration, Ethnicity, and Mental Health: International Perspectives, 1840–2010*, London: Routledge.

McEwan, K., Richardson, M., Brindley, P., Sheffield, D., et al. (2020) 'Shmapped: Development of an App to Record and Promote the Well-Being Benefits of Noticing Urban Nature', *Translational Behavioral Medicine* 10(3): 723–733.

McEwen, B. S. (1998) 'Protective and Damaging Effects of Stress Mediators', *New England Journal of Medicine* 338(3): 171–179.

McEwen, B. S. (2012) 'Brain on Stress: How the Social Environment Gets under the Skin', *Proceedings of the National Academy of Sciences* 109 (Supplement 2): 17180–17185.

McEwen, B. S. (2013) 'The Brain on Stress: Toward an Integrative Approach to Brain, Body, and Behavior', *Perspectives on Psychological Science* 8(6): 673–675.

McEwen, B. S., Bowles, N. P., Gray, J. D., Hill, M. N., et al. (2015) 'Mechanisms of Stress in the Brain', *Nature Neuroscience* 18(10): 1353.

McEwen, B. S. and Lasley, E. N. (2002) *The End of Stress as We Know It*, Washington, DC: Joseph Henry Press.

McEwen, Bruce S. and Morrison, John H. (2013) 'The Brain on Stress: Vulnerability and Plasticity of the Prefrontal Cortex over the Life Course', *Neuron* 79(1): 16–29.

McEwen, C. A. and McEwen, B. S. (2017) 'Social Structure, Adversity, Toxic Stress, and Intergenerational Poverty: An Early Childhood Model', *Annual Review of Sociology* 43: 445–472.

McFarlane, C. (2011) 'Assemblage and Critical Urbanism', *City* 15(2): 204–224.

McGowan, P., Sasaki, A., D'Alessio, A., Dymov, S., et al. (2009) 'Epigenetic Regulation of the Glucocorticoid Receptor in Human Brain Associates with Childhood Abuse', *Nature Neuroscience* 12: 342–348.

McKenzie, K., Fearon, P., and Hutchinson, G. (2008) 'Migration, Ethnicity and Psychosis', pp. 143–160 in C. Morgan, K. McKenzie, and P. Fearon (eds.) *Society and Psychosis*, Cambridge: Cambridge University Press.

McKenzie, R. D. (1924) 'The Ecological Approach to the Study of the Human Community', *American Journal of Sociology* 30(3): 287–301.

Meaney, M. J., Aitken, D. H., Bodnoff, S. R., Iny, L. J., et al. (1985) 'The Effects of Postnatal Handling on the Development of the Glucocorticoid Receptor Systems and Stress Recovery in the Rat', *Progress in Neuro-Psychopharmacology & Biological Psychiatry* 9(5–6): 731–734.

Meaney, M. J. and Ferguson-Smith, A. C. (2010) 'Epigenetic Regulation of the Neural Transcriptome: The Meaning of the Marks', *Nature Neuroscience* 13(11): 1313–1318.

Meaney, M. J. and Stewart, J. (1979) 'Environmental Factors Influencing the Affiliative Behavior of Male and Female Rats (Rattus-Norvegicus)', *Animal Learning & Behavior* 7(3): 397–405.

Meloni, M. (2014) 'The Social Brain Meets the Reactive Genome: Neuroscience, Epigenetics and the New Social Biology', *Frontiers in Human Neuroscience* 8. doi: 10.3389/fnhum.2014.00309.

Melosi, M. V. (1993) 'The Place of the City in Environmental History', *Environmental History Review* 17(1): 1–23.

Menzies, R. (2014) 'Governing Mentalities: The Deportation of "Insane" and "Feebleminded" Immigrants Out of British Columbia from Confederation to World War II', *Canadian Journal of Law and Society* 13(2): 135–173.

Merzenich, M., Recanzone, G., Jenkins, W., Allard, T., et al. (1988) *Cortical Representational Plasticity*, New York: John Wiley.

Milgram, S. (1974) 'The Experience of Living in Cities', *Crowding and Behavior* 167: 41.

Milgram, S. (1992) 'A Psychological Map of New York City; Psychological Maps of Paris', in J. Sabini and M. Silver (eds.) *The Individual in a Social World: Essays and Experiments*, New York: McGraw-Hill.

Milgram, S. and Gudehus, C. (1978) *Obedience to Authority*, Chicago: Ziff-Davis.

Miller, P. and Rose, N. (1995) 'Production, Identity, and Democracy', *Theory and Society* 24(3): 427–467.

Miller, P. and Rose, N. (2008) *Governing the Present: Administering Economic, Social and Personal Life*, Oxford: Polity Press.

Minton, A. (2017) *Big Capital: Who Is London For?* London: Penguin.

Mintz, N. L. and Schwartz, D. T. (1964) 'Urban Ecology and Psychosis: Community Factors in the Incidence of Schizophrenia and Manic-Depression among Italians in Greater Boston', *International Journal of Social Psychiatry* 10(2): 101–118.

Mirescu, C., Peters, J. D., and Gould, E. (2004) 'Early Life Experience Alters Response of Adult Neurogenesis to Stress', *Nature Neuroscience* 7(8): 841–846.

Mitman, G., Murphy, M., and Sellers, C. (2004) 'Introduction: A Cloud over History', *Osiris* (19):1–17.

Moch, L. (1995) 'Moving Europeans: Historical Migration Practices in Western Europe', in R. Cohen (ed.) *The Cambridge Survey of World Migration*, Cambridge: Cambridge University Press.

Moch, L. P. (2003) *Moving Europeans: Migration in Western Europe since 1650*, Bloomington: Indiana University Press.

Montesquieu, Charles de Secondat (1773) *Persian Letters*, London: Alexander Donaldson.

Moore, S. and Kawachi, I. (2017) 'Twenty Years of Social Capital and Health Research: A Glossary', *Journal of Epidemiology & Community Health* 71: 513–517.

Moran, J. (1945) *The Anatomy of Courage*, London: Constable.

Morel, B. A. (1857) *Traité des dégénérescences physiques, intellectuelles et morales de l'espèce humaine et des causes qui produisent ces variétés maladives*, Paris: Baillière.

Morel, B. A. (1860) 'Traitsé Des Maladies Mentales', *American Journal of Psychiatry* 17(2): 199–211.

Morgan, C., Burns, T., Fitzpatrick, R., Pinfold, V., et al. (2007) 'Social Exclusion and Mental Health', *The British Journal of Psychiatry* 191(6): 477–483.

Morgan, C., Charalambides, M., Hutchinson, G., and Murray, R. M. (2010) 'Migration, Ethnicity, and Psychosis: Toward a Sociodevelopmental Model', *Schizophrenia Bulletin* 36(4): 655–664.

Morris, A. D. (2015) *The Scholar Denied: W.E.B. Du Bois and the Birth of Modern Sociology*. Berkeley: University of California Press.

Morris, J. N. (1957) *Uses of Epidemiology*, Edinburgh and London: Livingstone.

Morris, J. N. and Titmuss, R. (1944) 'Epidemiology of Peptic Ulcer', *The Lancet* 244(6331): 841–845.

Mueller, J. H. (1940) 'Review of the Book *Mental Disorders in Urban Areas: An Ecological Study of Schizophrenia and Other Psychoses*, by R. E. L. Faris and H. W. Dunham'. *The Journal of Abnormal and Social Psychology*, 35(4), 593–594.

Mumford, L. (1961) *The City in History: Its Origins, Its Transformations, and Its Prospects*, Vol. 67, Boston, MA: Houghton Mifflin Harcourt.

Murphy, M. (2006) *Sick Building Syndrome and the Problem of Uncertainty*, Durham, NC: Duke University Press.

Murray, R. M., Quattrone, D., Natesan, S., van Os, J., et al. (2016) 'Should Psychiatrists Be More Cautious About the Long-Term Prophylactic Use of Antipsychotics?', *The British Journal of Psychiatry* 209(5): 361–365.

Myerson, A. (1940) 'Mental Disorders in Urban Areas. An Ecological Study of Schhizophrenia and Other Psychoses', *American Journal of Psychiatry* 96(4): 995–997.

Nash, L. (2006) *Inescapable Ecologies: A History of Environment, Disease, and Knowledge*, Berkeley: University of California Press.

Needles, W. (1945) 'A Statistical Study of One Hundred Neuropsychiatric Casualties from the Normandy Campaign (with Control Material)', *American Journal of Psychiatry* 102(2): 214–221.

Ng, E. (2009) 'Heartache of the State, Enemy of the Self: Bipolar Disorder and Cultural Change in Urban China', *Culture, Medicine, and Psychiatry* 33(3): 421.

Niedzwiecki, M. M., Walker, D. I., Vermeulen, R., Chadeau-Hyam, M., et al. (2019) 'The Exposome: Molecules to Populations', *Annual Review of Pharmacology and Toxicology* 59: 107–127.

Niewöhner, J. and Lock, M. (2018) 'Situating Local Biologies: Anthropological Perspectives on Environment/Human Entanglements', *BioSocieties* 13(4), 681–669.

Norris, N. C. (2018) 'Squatters, Shanties, and Technocratic Professionals: Urban Migration and Housing Shortages in Twentieth-Century Chile', MA Thesis, City University of New York (CUNY).

O'Day, R. and Englander, D. (1993) *Mr Charles Booth's Inquiry: Life and Labour of the People in London Reconsidered*, London: Hambledon.

Oakley, A. (2007) 'Fifty Years of JN Morris's Uses of Epidemiology', *International Journal of Epidemiology* 36(6): 1184–1185.

Ødegård, O. (1932) 'Emigration and Insanity', *Acta Psychiatrica et Neurologica* 4(1): 1–206.

Ødegård, Ø. (1975) 'Social and Ecological Factors in the Etiology, Outcome, Treatment and Prevention of Mental Disorders', in H. Argelander et al. (eds.) *Soziale und Angewandte Psychiatrie. Psychiatrie der Gegenwart (Forschung und Praxis)*, vol 3. Berlin: Springer.

Office for National Statistics (UK) (2020) 'Coronavirus (Covid-19) Related Deaths by Ethnic Group, England and Wales: 2 March 2020 to 10 April 2020', London: Office for National Statistics.

Oh, Y., Koeske, G. F., and Sales, E. (2002) 'Acculturation, Stress, and Depressive Symptoms among Korean Immigrants in the United States', *Journal of Social Psychology* 142(4): 511–526.

Ong, A. (2010) *Spirits of Resistance and Capitalist Discipline: Factory Women in Malaysia*, Albany: SUNY Press.

Opendak, M., Briones, B. A., and Gould, E. (2016) 'Social Behavior, Hormones and Adult Neurogenesis', *Frontiers in Neuroendocrinology* 41: 71–86.

Osborne, T. (2016) 'Vitalism as Pathos', *Biosemiotics* 9(2): 185–205.

Osborne, T. and Rose, N. (1999) 'Governing Cities: Notes on the Spatialisation of Virtue', *Environment and Planning D-Society & Space* 17(6): 737–760.

Palm, K., Schmitz, S., and Mangelsdorf, M. (2013) 'Embodiment and Ecosocial Theory—Interview with Nancy Krieger', *FZG–Freiburger Zeitschrift für GeschlechterStudien* 19(2): 109–120.

Pariante, C. M. (2017) 'Why Are Depressed Patients Inflamed? A Reflection on 20 Years of Research on Depression, Glucocorticoid Resistance and Inflammation', *European Neuropsychopharmacology* 27(6): 554–559.

Pariante, C. M. and Lightman, S. L. (2008) 'The HPA Axis in Major Depression: Classical Theories and New Developments', *Trends in Neurosciences* 31(9): 464–468.

Park, B. J., Tsunetsugu, Y., Kasetani, T., Kagawa, T., et al. (2009) 'The Physiological Effects of Shinrin-Yoku (Taking in the Forest Atmosphere or Forest Bathing): Evidence from Field Experiments in 24 Forests across Japan', *Environmental Health and Preventive Medicine* 15(1): 18.

Park, R. E., Burgess, E. W., and Mackenzie, R. D. (1967) *The City*, Chicago: University of Chicago Press.

Parkar, S. R., Fernandes, J., and Weiss, M. G. (2003) 'Contextualizing Mental Health: Gendered Experiences in a Mumbai Slum', *Anthropology & Medicine* 10(3): 291–308.

Pasquino, P. (1978) 'Theatrum Politicum: The Genealogy of Capital—Police and the State of Prosperity', *Ideology and Consciousness* 4: 41–54.

Patel, V. (2014) 'Rethinking Mental Health Care: Bridging the Credibility Gap', *Intervention* 12: 15–20.

Pedersen, C. and Mortensen, P. (2001) 'Evidence of a Dose-Response Relationship between Urbanicity During Upbringing and Schizophrenia Risk', *Archives of General Psychiatry* 58(11): 1039–1046.

Pentecost, M. (2018) 'The First Thousand Days: Epigenetics in the Age of Global Health', pp. 269–294 in M. Meloni, et al. (eds.) *The Palgrave Handbook of Biology and Society*, New York: Springer.

Pentecost, M. and Meloni, M. (2020) '"It's Never Too Early": Preconception Care and Postgenomic Models of Life', *Frontiers in Sociology* 5: 21.

Petticrew, M. P. and Lee, K. (2011) 'The "Father of Stress" Meets "Big Tobacco": Hans Selye and the Tobacco Industry', *American Journal of Public Health* 101(3): 411–418.

Pfautz, H. W. (1967) 'Introduction', *Charles Booth on the City: Physical Pattern and Social Structure*, Chicago: University of Chicago Press.

Phelan, J. C. and Link, B. G. (2010) 'Fundamental Social Causes of Health Inequalities', in C. Morgan and D. Bhugra (eds.) *Principles of Social Psychiatry*, London: Wiley.

Phelan, J. C. and Link, B. G. (2013) 'Fundamental Cause Theory', in W. C. Cockerham (ed.) *Medical Sociology on the Move*, New York: Springer.

Phillips, M. R., Zhang, J., Shi, Q., Song, Z., et al. (2009) 'Prevalence, Treatment, and Associated Disability of Mental Disorders in Four Provinces in China During 2001–05: An Epidemiological Survey', *The Lancet* 373(9680): 2041–2053.

Pick, D. (1989) *Faces of Degeneration: A European Disorder C.1848–C.1918*, Cambridge: Cambridge University Press.

Picot, G. and Sweetman, A. (2012) *Making It in Canada: Immigration Outcomes and Policies*, Montreal: Institute for Reseach on Public Policy.

Pile, S. (2005) *Real Cities: Modernity, Space and the Phantasmagorias of City Life*, London: SAGE.

Pinto, S. (2014) *Daughters of Parvati: Women and Madness in Contemporary India*, Philadephia: University of Pennsylvania Press.

Pisarevskaya, A., Levy, N., Scholten, P., and Jansen, J. (2019) 'Mapping Migration Studies: An Empirical Analysis of the Coming of Age of a Research Field', *Migration Studies* 8(3): 455–481.

Plomin, R. and McGuffin, P. (2003) 'Psychopathology in the Postgenomic Era', *Annual Review of Psychology* 54: 205–228.

Pollock, H. M. (1925) 'Mental Disease in the United States in Relation to Environment, Sex and Age, 1922', *American Journal of Psychiatry* 82(2): 219–232.

Pollock, K. (1988) 'On the Nature of Social Stress: Production of a Modern Mythology', *Social Science & Medicine* 26(3): 381–392.

Pooley, C. and Turnbull, J. (2005) *Migration and Mobility in Britain since the Eighteenth Century*, London: Routledge.

Portes, A. (2010) 'Migration and Social Change: Some Conceptual Reflections', *Journal of Ethnic and Migration Studies* 36(10): 1537–1563.

Portes, A. and Fernández-Kelly, P. (2008) 'No Margin for Error: Educational and Occupational Achievement among Disadvantaged Children of Immigrants', *Annals of the American Academy of Political and Social Science* 620(1): 12–36.

Portes, A. and Zhou, M. (1993) 'The New Second Generation: Segmented Assimilation and Its Variants', *Annals of the American Academy of Political and Social Science* 530(1): 74–96.

Porzionato, N., Mantiñan, M., Bussi, E., Grinberg, S., et al. (2015) 'Accumulation of Pollutants, Self-Purification and Impact on Peripheral Urban Areas: A Case Study in Shantytowns in Argentina', *Journal of Environmental, Ecological, Geological and Mining Engineering* 9(5): 296–300.

Povinelli, E. A. (2011) *Economies of Abandonment: Social Belonging and Endurance in Late Liberalism*, Durham, NC: Duke University Press.

Prato, G. B. (2016) *Beyond Multiculturalism: Views from Anthropology*, London: Routledge.

Prescott, S. and Logan, A. (2016) 'Transforming Life: A Broad View of the Developmental Origins of Health and Disease Concept from an Ecological Justice Perspective', *International Journal of Environmental Research and Public Health* 13(11): 1075.

Pronko, N. H. and Leith, W. R. (1956) 'Behavior under Stress: A Study of Its Disintegration', *Psychological Reports* 2(3): 205–222.

Pruessner, J. C., Champagne, F., Meaney, M. J., and Dagher, A. (2004) 'Dopamine Release in Response to a Psychological Stress in Humans and Its Relationship to Early Life Maternal Care: A Positron Emission Tomography Study Using [C-11]Raclopride', *Journal of Neuroscience* 24(11): 2825–2831.

Pun, N. (2000) 'Opening a Minor Genre of Resistance in Reform China: Scream, Dream, and Transgression in a Workplace', *Positions: East Asia Cultures Critique* 8(2): 531–555.

Pun, N. (2002) 'Am I the Only Survivor? Global Capital, Local Gaze, and Social Trauma in China', *Public Culture* 14(2): 341–347.

Pun, N. (2017) *Migrant Labor in China. Post-Socialist Transformations*, Cambridge: Polity.

Pun, N. (2018) 'The Making of the Migrant Working Class in China', in H. Veltmeyer and P. Bowles (eds.) *The Essential Guide to Critical Development Studies*, London: Routledge.

Pun, N. and Lu, H. (2010a) 'A Culture of Violence: The Labor Subcontracting System and Collective Action by Construction Workers in Post-Socialist China', *The China Journal* (64): 143–158.

Pun, N. and Lu, H. (2010b) 'Neoliberalism, Urbanism and the Plight of Construction Workers in China', *World Review of Political Economy* 1(1): 127–141.

Pun, N. and Lu, H. (2010c) 'Unfinished Proletarianization: Self, Anger, and Class Action among the Second Generation of Peasant-Workers in Present-Day China', *Modern China* 36(5): 493–519.

Pun, N. and Zhang, H. (2017) 'Injury of Class: Compressed Modernity and the Struggle of Foxconn Workers', *Temporalités. Revue de sciences sociales et humaines* (26).

Purves, D. (2010) *Brains: How They Seem to Work*, Upper Saddle River, NJ: Financial Times/Prentice Hall.

Rabinow, P. and Rose, N. (2006) 'Biopower Today', *BioSocieties* 1(2): 195–218.

Rader, K. A. (1998) '"The Mouse People": Murine Genetics Work at the Bussey Institution, 1909–1936', *Journal of the History of Biology* 31: 327–354.

Rader, K. A. (2004) *Making Mice: Standardizing Animals for American Biomedical Research, 1900–1955*, Princeton, NJ: Princeton University Press.

Rakic, P. (1985) 'Limits of Neurogenesis in Primates', *Science* 227(4690): 1054–1056.

Ramsden, E. (2011) 'From Rodent Utopia to Urban Hell: Population, Pathology, and the Crowded Rats of NIMH', *Isis* 102(4): 659–688.

Ramsden, E. (2014) 'Stress in the City: Mental Health, Urban Planning and the Social Sciences in the Postwar United States', in D. Cantor and E. Ramsden (eds.) *Stress, Shock and Adaptation in the Twentieth Century*, Suffolk: Boyden and Brewer.

Ranney, M. (1850) 'On Insane Foreigners', *American Journal of Psychiatry* 7(1): 53–63.

Rapoport, A. (1978) 'Culture and the Subjective Effects of Stress', *Urban Ecology* 3(3): 241–261.

Rass, E. (2017) *The Allan Schore Reader: Setting the Course of Development*, London: Routledge.

Reardon, J. (2013) 'On the Emergence of Science and Justice', *Science, Technology, & Human Values* 38(2): 176–200.

Redfield, R., Linton, R., and Herskovits, M. J. (1936) 'Memorandum for the Study of Acculturation', *American Anthropologist* 38(1): 149–152.

Reichert, M., Braun, U., Lautenbach, S., Zipf, A., et al. (2020) 'Studying the Impact of Built Environments on Human Mental Health in Everyday Life: Methodological Developments, State-of-the-Art and Technological Frontiers', *Current Opinion in Psychology* 32: 158–164.

Renson, A., Herd, P., and Dowd, J. B. (2020) 'Sick Individuals and Sick (Microbial) Populations: Challenges in Epidemiology and the Microbiome', *Annual Review of Public Health* 41: 63–80.

Rex, J. and Moore, R. S. (1969) *Race, Community and Conflict: A Study of Sparkbrook*, London: Institute of Race Relations.

Rhys-Taylor, A. (2013) 'The Essences of Multiculture: A Sensory Exploration of an Inner-City Street Market', *Identities* 20(4): 393–406.

Richaud, L. and Amin, A. (2019) 'Mental Health, Subjectivity and the City: An Ethnography of Migrant Stress in Shanghai', *International Health* 11: S7–S13.

Richaud, L. and Amin, A. (2020) 'Life Amidst Rubble: Migrant Mental Health and the Management of Subjectivity in Urban China', *Public Culture* 32(1): 77–106.

Richter, C. P. (1952) 'Domestication of the Norway Rat and Its Implications for the Problem of Stress', in H. G. Wolff (ed.) *Life Stress and Bodily Disease*, New York: Harper.

Richter, C. P. (1968) 'Experiences of a Reluctant Rat-Catcher: The Common Norway Rat—Friend or Enemy?', *Proceedings of the American Philosophical Society* 112(6): 403–415.

Rietveld, E. and Kiverstein, J. (2014) 'A Rich Landscape of Affordances', *Ecological Psychology* 26(4): 325–352.

Robbins, R. N., Scott, T., Joska, J. A., and Gouse, H. (2019) 'Impact of Urbanization on Cognitive Disorders', *Current Opinion in Psychiatry* 32(3): 210–217.

Roberts, F. (1950) 'Stress and the General Adaptation Syndrome', *British Medical Journal* 2(4670): 104.

Robinson, J. (2006) *Ordinary Cities: Between Modernity and Development*, London: Routledge.

Robinson, W. S. (1950) 'Ecological Correlations and the Behavior of Individuals,' *American Sociological Review* 15: 351–357.

Rose, N. (1985) *The Psychological Complex: Psychology, Politics and Society in England, 1869–1939*, London: Routledge and Kegan Paul.

Rose, N. (1989) *Governing the Soul: The Shaping of the Private Self*, London: Routledge.

Rose, N. (1996) *Inventing Our Selves: Psychology, Power, and Personhood*, New York: Cambridge University Press.

Rose, N. (1999) *Powers of Freedom: Reframing Political Thought*, New York: Cambridge University Press.

Rose, N. (2001) 'The Politics of Life Itself', *Theory, Culture & Society* 18(6): 1–30.

Rose, N. (2013) 'The Human Sciences in a Biological Age', *Theory, Culture & Society* 30(1): 3–34.

Rose, N. (2018) *Our Psychiatric Future: The Politics of Mental Health*, London: Polity.

Rose, N. and Abi-Rached, J. M. (2013) *Neuro: The New Brain Sciences and the Management of the Mind*, Princeton, NJ: Princeton University Press.

Rose, N., Birk, R., and Manning, N. (2021) 'Towards Neuroecosociality: Mental Health in Adversity', *Theory, Culture and Society*, January 2021. doi:10.1177/0263276420981614.

Rose, N., Manning, N., Bentall, R., Bhui, K., et al. (2020) 'The Social Underpinnings of Mental Distress in the Time of Covid-19—Time for Urgent Action', *Wellcome Open Research* 5:166. doi: 10.12688/wellcomeopenres.16123.1. eCollection 2020.

Rosen, G. (1974) *From Medical Police to Social Medicine: Essays on the History of Health Care*, New York: Science History Publications.

Rosenberg, C. E. (2002) 'The Tyranny of Diagnosis: Specific Entities and Individual Experience', *The Milbank Quarterly* 80(2): 237–260.

Rosenberg, C. E. (2006) 'Contested Boundaries—Psychiatry, Disease, and Diagnosis', *Perspectives in Biology and Medicine* 49(3): 407–424.

Rosenblat, J. D., Cha, D. S., Mansur, R. B., and McIntyre, R. S. (2014) 'Inflamed Moods: A Review of the Interactions between Inflammation and Mood Disorders', *Progress in Neuro-Psychopharmacology and Biological Psychiatry* 53: 23–34.

Rosenborg, J. D. (1968) 'Introduction to the Dover Edition of Mayhew's "London Labour and the London Poor"' *London Labour and the London Poor*, New York: Dover.

Rothman, D. J. (1971) *The Discovery of the Asylum; Social Order and Disorder in the New Republic*, Boston MA: Little.

Rowitz, L. and Levy, L. (1968) 'Ecological Analysis of Treated Mental Disorders in Chicago', *Archives of General Psychiatry* 19(5): 571–579.

Rowntree, S. (1922) *Poverty, a Study of Town Life. New Edition*, New York: Longmans, Green.

Rowntree, S. (2000 [1901]) *Poverty: A Study of Town Life*, Bristol: Policy Press.

Roy, D. (2018) *Molecular Feminisms: Biology, Becomings, and Life in the Lab*. Seattle: University of Washington Press.

Rutter, M. (2002) 'Nature, Nurture, and Development: From Evangelism through Science toward Policy and Practice', *Child Development* 73(1): 1–21.

Rutter, M., Beckett, C., Castle, J. et al. (2007) 'Effects of Profound Early Institutional Deprivation: An Overview of Findings from a UK Longitudinal Study of Romanian Adoptees', *European Journal of Developmental Psychology* 4(3): 332–350.

Ryu, J. K. and McLarnon, J. G. (2009) 'A Leaky Blood–Brain Barrier, Fibrinogen Infiltration and Microglial Reactivity in Inflamed Alzheimer's Disease Brain', *Journal of Cellular and Molecular Medicine* 13(9a): 2911–2925.

Saito, K. (2017) *Capital, Nature, and the Unfinished Critique of Political Economy. Karl Marx's Ecosocialism*, New York: Monthly Review Press.

Sampson, L., Ettman, C. K., and Galea, S. (2020) 'Urbanization, Urbanicity, and Depression: A Review of the Recent Global Literature', *Current Opinion in Psychiatry* 33(3): 233–244.

Sampson, R. J. (2012) *Great American City: Chicago and the Enduring Neighborhood Effect*, Chicago: University of Chicago Press.

Sandi, C. and Haller, J. (2015) 'Stress and the Social Brain: Behavioural Effects and Neurobiological Mechanisms', *Nature Reviews Neuroscience* 16(5): 290–304.

Sassen, S. (2014) *Expulsions*, Cambridge, MA: Harvard University Press.

Saunders, D. (2010) *Arrival City: How the Largest Migration in History Is Reshaping Our World*, London: William Heinemann.

Savage, M. and Warde, A. (1993) *Urban Sociology, Capitalism and Modernity*, New York: Continuum.

Schaeffer, M. H., Street, S. W., Singer, J. E., and Baum, A. (1988) 'Effects of Control on the Stress Reactions of Commuters: 1', *Journal of Applied Social Psychology* 18(11): 944–957.

Schatzman, L. and Strauss, A. (1966) 'A Sociology of Psychiatry: A Perspective and Some Organizing Foci', *Social Problems* 14(1): 3–16.

Scheinberg, E. (2016) 'Canada's Deportation of "Mentally and Morally Defective" Female Immigrants after the Second World War', in M. Harper (ed.) *Migration and Mental Health*, London: Palgrave Macmillan.

Schofield, P., Das-Munshi, J., Bécares, L., Morgan, C., et al. (2016) 'Minority Status and Mental Distress: A Comparison of Group Density Effects', *Psychological Medicine* 46(14): 3051.

Schofield, P., Thygesen, M., Das-Munshi, J., Becares, L., et al. (2017) 'Ethnic Density, Urbanicity and Psychosis Risk for Migrant Groups—a Population Cohort Study', *Schizophrenia Research* 190: 82–87.

Schopler, J. and Stockdale, J. E. (1977) 'An Interference Analysis of Crowding', *Environmental Psychology and Nonverbal Behavior* 1(2): 81–88.

Schore, A. N. (2001) 'The Effects of Early Relational Trauma on Right Brain Development, Affect Regulation, and Infant Mental Health', *Infant Mental Health Journal* 22(1): 201–269.

Schroeder, C. W. (1942) 'Mental Disorders in Cities', *American Journal of Sociology* 48(1): 40–47.

Schulkin, J. (2005) *Curt Richter: A Life in the Laboratory*, Baltimore, MD: Johns Hopkins University Press.

Schuster, J.-P., Le Strat, Y., Krichevski, V., Bardikoff, N., et al. (2011) 'Benedict Augustin Morel (1809–1873)', *Acta Neuropsychiatrica* 23(1): 35–36.

Scull, A. (2005) *Most Solitary of Afflictions: Madness and Society in Britain 1700–1900*, New Haven, CT: Yale University Press.

Scull, A. and Schulkin, J. (2009) 'Psychobiology, Psychiatry, and Psychoanalysis: The Intersecting Careers of Adolf Meyer, Phyllis Greenacre, and Curt Richter', *Medical History* 53(01): 5–36.

See, J. J. and Mustian, R. D. (1976) 'The Emerging Role of Sociological Consultation in the Field of Community Mental Health', *Community Mental Health Journal* 12(3): 267–274.

Segretin, M. S., et al. (2016) 'Childhood Poverty and Cognitive Development in Latin America in the 21st Century', *New Directions for Child and Adolescent Development*, 2016(152): 9–29.

Selye, H. (1936) 'A Syndrome Produced by Diverse Nocuous Agents', *Nature* 138(3479): 32.

Selye, H. (1956) *The Stress of Life*, New York: McGraw Hill.

Selye, H. (1973) 'The Evolution of the Stress Concept: The Originator of the Concept Traces Its Development from the Discovery in 1936 of the Alarm Reaction to Modern Therapeutic Applications of Syntoxic and Catatoxic Hormones', *American Scientist* 61(6): 692–699.

Selye, H. (1979) *The Stress of My Life: A Scientist's Memoirs*, 2nd edition, New York: Van Nostrand Reinhold.

Senst, L. and Bains, J. (2014) 'Neuromodulators, Stress and Plasticity: A Role for Endocannabinoid Signalling', *The Journal of Experimental Biology* 217(1): 102–108.

Sharp, G. C., Lawlor, D. A., and Richardson, S. S. (2018) 'It's the Mother!: How Assumptions About the Causal Primacy of Maternal Effects Influence Research on the Developmental Origins of Health and Disease', *Social Science & Medicine* 213: 20–27.

Shen, Y.-C., Zhang, M.-Y., Huang, Y.-Q., He, Y.-L., et al. (2006) 'Twelve-Month Prevalence, Severity, and Unmet Need for Treatment of Mental Disorders in Metropolitan China', *Psychological Medicine* 36(2): 257–267.

Shonkoff, J. P. (2012) 'Leveraging the Biology of Adversity to Address the Roots of Disparities in Health and Development', *Proceedings of the National Academy of Sciences* 109 (Supplement 2): 17302.

Shonkoff, J. P., Boyce, W. T., and McEwen, B. S. (2009) 'Neuroscience, Molecular Biology, and the Childhood Roots of Health Disparities: Building a New Framework for Health Promotion and Disease Prevention', *Journal of the American Medical Association* 301(21): 2252–2259.

Shonkoff, J. P., Garner, A. S., Siegel, B. S., Dobbins, M. I., et al. (2012) 'The Lifelong Effects of Early Childhood Adversity and Toxic Stress', *Pediatrics* 129(1): e232–e246.

Simmel, G. ([1903] 2002) 'The Metropolis and Mental Life', in G. Bridges and S. Watson (eds.) *The Blackwell City Reader*, Oxford ; Malden, MA: Blackwell.

Simone, A. (2010) *City Life from Jakarta to Dakar: Movements at the Crossroads*, London: Routledge.

Singer, J. E., Lundberg, U., and Frankenhaeuser, M. (1974) *Stress on the Train: A Study of Urban Commuting*, Stockholm: Psychological Laboratories, University of Stockholm.

Singh, G. K. and Siahpush, M. (2002) 'Ethnic-Immigrant Differentials in Health Behaviors, Morbidity, and Cause-Specific Mortality in the United States: An Analysis of Two National Data Bases', *Human Biology* 74(1): 83–109.

Sipahi, L., Aiello, A., Galea, S., Koenen, K. C., et al. (2013) 'Longitudinal Epigenetic Variation at DNA Methyltransferase Genes Is Associated with Risk For and Resilience to PTSD', *Comprehensive Psychiatry* 54(8): e36.

Sisk, C. L. and Zehr, J. L. (2005) 'Pubertal Hormones Organize the Adolescent Brain and Behavior', *Frontiers in Neuroendocrinology* 26(3–4): 163–174.

Siu, K. (2015) 'Continuity and Change in the Everyday Lives of Chinese Migrant Factory Workers', *The China Journal* (74): 43–65.

Sleiman, S. F., Henry, J., Al-Haddad, R., El Hayek, L., et al. (2016) 'Exercise Promotes the Expression of Brain Derived Neurotrophic Factor (BDNF) through the Action of the Ketone Body B-Hydroxybutyrate', *Elife* 5: e15092.

Sloterdijk, P. (2011) *Bubbles: Spheres Volume I: Microspherology*, Los Angeles, CA: Semiotext(e).

Smith, B. (2009) 'Toward a Realistic Science of Environments', *Ecological Psychology* 21(2): 121–130.

Smith, D. (1988) *The Chicago School: A Liberal Critique of Capitalism*, Basingstoke: Macmillan Education.

Smith, D. A. (1995) 'The New Urban Sociology Meets the Old: Rereading Some Classical Human Ecology', *Urban Affairs Quarterly* 30(3): 432–457.

Smith, M. P. (1980) *The City and Social Theory*, Oxford: Blackwell.

Söderström, O. (2016) '"I Don't Care About Places": The Whereabouts of Design in Mental Health Care', in C. Bates, R. Imrie, and K. Kullman (eds.) *Care and Design: Bodies, Buildings*, New York: Wiley.

Söderström, O., Empson, L. A., Codeluppi, Z., Söderström, D., et al. (2016) 'Unpacking "the City": An Experience-Based Approach to the Role of Urban Living in Psychosis', *Health & Place* 42: 104–110.

Söderström, O., Söderström, D., Codeluppi, Z., Empson, L. A., et al. (2017) 'Emplacing Recovery: How Persons Diagnosed with Psychosis Handle Stress in Cities', *Psychosis*, 9(4): 322–329.

Solinger, D. J. (1997) 'The Impact of the Floating Population on the Danwei: Shifts in the Pattern of Labor Mobility Control and Entitlement Provision', in X. Lü and E. J. Perry (eds.) *Danwei: The Changing Chinese Workplace in Historical and Comparative Perspective*, London: Routledge.

Solinger, D. J. (1999) *Contesting Citizenship in Urban China: Peasant Migrants, the State, and the Logic of the Market*, Berkeley: University of California Press.

Sorrells, S. F., Paredes, M. F., Cebrian-Silla, A., Sandoval, K., et al. (2018) 'Human Hippocampal Neurogenesis Drops Sharply in Children to Undetectable Levels in Adults', *Nature* 555: 377.

Spence, C. (2015) 'Leading the Consumer by the Nose: On the Commercialization of Olfactory Design for the Food and Beverage Sector', *Flavour* 4(1): 31.

Stepan, N. (1991) *"The Hour of Eugenics": Race, Gender and Nation in Latin America*, Ithaca, NY: Cornell University Press.

Sterling, P. and Eyer, J. (1988) 'Allostasis: A New Paradigm to Explain Arousal Pathology', in S. Fisher and J. Reason (eds.) *Handbook of Life Stress, Cognition and Health*, New York: John Wiley.

Stoltenberg, C. D. (1984) 'China's Special Economic Zones: Their Development and Prospects', *Asian Survey* 24(6): 637–654.

Stranahan, A. M., Khalil, D., and Gould, E. (2006) 'Social Isolation Delays the Positive Effects of Running on Adult Neurogenesis', *Nature Neuroscience* 9(4): 526–533.

Su, D., Wu, X.-N., Zhang, Y.-X., Li, H.-P., et al. (2012) 'Depression and Social Support between China's Rural and Urban Empty-Nest Elderly', *Archives of Gerontology and Geriatrics* 55(3): 564–569.

Subbaraman, R., Nolan, L., Shitole, T., Sawant, K., et al. (2014) 'The Psychological Toll of Slum Living in Mumbai, India: A Mixed Methods Study', *Social Science & Medicine* 119: 155–169.

Sugrue, T. J. and Katz, M. B. (1998) *W.E.B. Dubois, Race, and the City: The Philadelphia Negro and Its Legacy*, Philadelphia: University of Pennsylvania Press.

Sullivan, R. (2006) *Rats: A Year with New York's Most Unwanted Inhabitants*, London: Granta.

Summerfield, D. (2008) 'How Scientifically Valid Is the Knowledge Base of Global Mental Health?', *British Medical Journal* 336(7651): 992–994.

Suskind, P. (1986) *Perfume: The Story of a Murderer*, London: Hamilton.

Swahn, M. H., Palmier, J. B., Kasirye, R., and Yao, H. (2012) 'Correlates of Suicide Ideation and Attempt among Youth Living in the Slums of Kampala', *International Journal of Environmental Research and Public Health* 9(2): 596–609.

Swider, S. (2016) *Building China: Informal Work and the New Precariat*, Ithaca, NY: Cornell University Press.

Szabo, C. P. (2019) 'Editorial: Urbanization and Mental Health: Toward a Disorder-Based Understanding', *Current Opinion in Psychiatry* 32(3): 196–197.

Szyf, M., McGowan, P., and Meaney, M. J. (2008) 'The Social Environment and the Epigenome', *Environmental and Molecular Mutagenesis* 49: 46–60.

Szyf, M., Weaver, I. C. G., Provencal, N., McGowan, P., et al. (2007) 'How Does Early Life Social Environment Sculpt Our Genes?', *Biology of Reproduction*, 77(Suppl_1): 64–64.

Tabery, J. and Griffiths, P. E. (2010) 'Perspectives on Behavioral Genetics and Developmental Science', in K. E. Hood, C. T. Halpern, G. Greenberg, and R. M. Lerner (eds.) *Handbook of Developmental Science, Behavior, and Genetics*, Oxford: Blackwell.

Tai, D. B. G., Shah, A., Doubeni, C. A., Sia, I. G., et al. (2020) 'The Disproportionate Impact of Covid-19 on Racial and Ethnic Minorities in the United States', *Clinical Infectious Diseases*, ciaa815, https://doi.org/10.1093/cid/ciaa815.

Tang, S. and Feng, J. (2015) 'Cohort Differences in the Urban Settlement Intentions of Rural Migrants: A Case Study in Jiangsu Province, China', *Habitat International* 49: 357–365.

Targum, S. D. and Kitanaka, J. (2012) 'Overwork Suicide in Japan: A National Crisis', *Innovations in Clinical Neuroscience* 9(2): 35.

Taub, E., Uswatte, G., and Pidikiti, R. (1999) 'Constraint-Induced Movement Therapy: A New Family of Techniques with Broad Application to Physical Rehabilitation—a Clinical Review', *Journal of Rehabilitation Research and Development* 36(3): 237.

Thaxton, R. (2008) *Catastrophe and Contention in Rural China: Mao's Great Leap Forward: Famine and the Origins of Righteous Resistance in Da Fo Village*, Cambridge: Cambridge University Press.

Thoman, L. V. and Surís, A. (2004) 'Acculturation and Acculturative Stress as Predictors of Psychological Distress and Quality-of-Life Functioning in Hispanic Psychiatric Patients', *Hispanic Journal of Behavioral Sciences* 26(3): 293–311.

Thomas, D. S. (1936) 'Internal Migrations in Sweden: A Note on Their Extensiveness as Compared with Net Migration Gain or Loss', *American Journal of Sociology* 42(3): 345–357.

Thomas, D. S. (1938) *Research Memorandum on Migration Differentials*, New York: Social Science Research Council.

Thomas, D. S. (1941) *Social and Economic Aspects of Swedish Population Movements: 1750–1933*, New York: Macmillan.

Thomas, F. (2016) *Handbook of Migration and Health*, Cheltenham: Edward Elgar Publishing.

Thomas, W. I. and Thomas, D. S. (1928) *The Child in America: Behavior Problems and Programs*, New York: Knopf.

Thomas, W. I. and Znaniecki, F. (1918) *The Polish Peasant in Europe and America. Volume One*, Chicago: University of Chicago Press.

Thompson, E. P. (1963) *The Making of the English Working Class*, London: Gollanzz.

Thornthwaite, C. W. and Slentz, H. I. (1934) *Internal Migration in the United States*, Philadelphia: University of Pennsylvania Press.

Thrift, N. (2004) 'Intensities of Feeling: Towards a Spatial Politics of Affect', *Geografiska Annaler: Series B, Human Geography* 86(1): 57–78.

Thrift, N. (2005) 'From Born to Made: Technology, Biology and Space', *Transactions of The Institute of British Geographers* 30(4): 463–476.

Thrive NYC (2019) 'Roadmap for Mental Health for All', New York: Mayor's Office, City of New York.

Thurston, A. F. (1987) *Enemies of the People*, New York: Alfred Knopf.

Tillott, P. M. (1961) *The Victoria History of the County of York: The City of York*, Oxford: Oxford University Press.

Tilly, C. (1978) 'Migration in Modern Europe History', in W. H. McNeill and R. S. Adams (eds.) *Human Migration: Patterns and Policies*, Bloomington: Indiana University Press.

Topp, C. W., Østergaard, S. D., Søndergaard, S., and Bech, P. (2015) 'The WHO-5 Well-Being Index: A Systematic Review of the Literature', *Psychotherapy and Psychosomatics* 84(3): 167–176.

Toyokawa, S., Uddin, M., Koenen, K. C., and Galea, S. (2012) 'How Does the Social Environment "Get into the Mind"? Epigenetics at the Intersection of Social and Psychiatric Epidemiology', *Social Science & Medicine* 74(1): 67–74.

Tsunetsugu, Y. and Miyazaki, Y. (2005) 'Measurement of Absolute Hemoglobin Concentrations of Prefrontal Region by Near-Infrared Time-Resolved Spectroscopy: Examples of Experiments and Prospects', *Journal of Physiological Anthropology and Applied Human Science* 24(4): 469–472.

Turnbaugh, P. J., Ley, R. E., Hamady, M., Fraser-Liggett, C., et al. (2007) 'The Human Microbiome Project: Exploring the Microbial Part of Ourselves in a Changing World', *Nature* 449(7164): 804–810.

UN-Habitat (2003) *Slums of the World: The Face of Urban Poverty in the New Millennium*, Nairobi: United Nations Human Settlements Programme.

United Nations Department of Economic and Social Affairs Population Division (2014) *World Urbanization Prospects 2014 Revision*, New York: United Nations.

United Nations Development Programme (2010) *Human Development Report 2010: The Real Wealth of Nations: Pathways to Human Development*, New York: Palgrave.

United States Bureau of the Census (1914) *Special Reports: Insane and Feeble-Minded in Institutions*, New York: US Government Printing Office.

Urry, J. (2003) 'City Life and the Senses', in G. Bridge and S. Watson (eds.) *A Companion to the City*, Oxford: Blackwell.

Valencia, P. M., Richard, M., Brock, J., and Boglioli, E. (2017) 'The Human Microbiome: Opportunity or Hype?', *Nature Reviews Drug Discovery* 16: 823.

van der Kooij, M. A., Fantin, M., Rejmak, E., Grosse, J., et al. (2014) 'Role for MMP-9 in Stress-Induced Downregulation of Nectin-3 in Hippocampal CA1 and Associated Behavioural Alterations', *Nature Communications* 5, 4995, https://doi.org/10.1038/ncomms5995

Van Essen, D. C. (1997) 'A Tension-Based Theory of Morphogenesis and Compact Wiring in the Central Nervous System', *Nature* 385(6614): 313.

Ventimiglia, I. and Seedat, S. (2019) 'Current Evidence on Urbanicity and the Impact of Neighbour-hoods on Anxiety and Stress-Related Disorders', *Current Opinion in Psychiatry* 32(3): 248–253.

Vertovec, S. (2013) *Anthropology of Migration and Multiculturalism: New Directions*, London: Routledge.

von Uexküll, J. ([1934] 2010) *A Foray into the Worlds of Animals and Humans*, Minneapolis: Minnesota University Press.

Wacquant, L. (2008) *Urban Outcasts: A Comparative Sociology of Advanced Marginality*, Cambridge: Polity.

Wahlberg, A. (2016) 'Serious Disease as Kinds of Living', in A. Wahlberg and S. Bauer (eds.) *Contested Categories*, London: Routledge.

Wakefield, J. C. (1997) 'Diagnosing DSM IV: DSM IV and the Concept of Disorder', *Behaviour Research and Therapy* 35(7): 633–649.

Walker, F. A. (2004 [1896]) 'Restriction of Immigration into the United States', *Population and Development Review* 30(4): 743–754.

Walkowitz, J. R. (2013) *City of Dreadful Delight: Narratives of Sexual Danger in Late-Victorian London*. Chicago: University of Chicago Press.

Wall, J., Kaas, J., Sur, M., Nelson, R., et al. (1986) 'Functional Reorganization in Somatosensory Cortical Areas 3b and 1 of Adult Monkeys after Median Nerve Repair: Possible Relationships to Sensory Recovery in Humans', *Journal of Neuroscience* 6(1): 218.

Walton, J. K. (1979) 'Lunacy in the Industrial Revolution: A Study of Asylum Admissions in Lancashire, 1848–50', *Journal of Social History* 13(1): 1–22.

Wang, F., Lan, Y., Li, J., Dai, J., et al. (2019) 'Patterns, Influencing Factors and Mediating Effects of Smartphone Use and Problematic Smartphone Use among Migrant Workers in Shanghai, China', *International Health* 11(Supplement_1): S33–S44.

Wang, L., Chen, H., Ye, B., Gao, J., et al. (2019) 'Mental Health and Self-Rated Health Status of Internal Migrant Workers and the Correlated Factors Analysis in Shanghai, China: A Cross-Sectional Epidemiological Study', *International Health* 11(Supplement_1): S45–S54.

Wang, M. and Ning, Y. (2016) 'The Social Integration of Migrants in Shanghai's Urban Villages', *The China Review* 16(3): 93–120.

Wang, W.-J. (2016) 'Neurasthenia and the Rise of Psy Disciplines in Republican China', *East Asian Science, Technology and Society* 10(2): 141–160.

Weaver, I. C. G., Cervoni, N., Champagne, F. A., D'Alessio, A. C., et al. (2004) 'Epigenetic Programming by Maternal Behavior', *Nature Neuroscience* 7(8): 847–854.

Webb, B. (1926) *My Apprenticeship*, London: Longmans.

Webb, S. D. and Collette, J. (1979) 'Rural-Urban Stress: New Data and New Conclusions', *American Journal of Sociology* 84(6): 1446–1452.

Wheaton, B., Young, M., Montazer, S., and Stuart-Lahman, K. (2013) 'Social Stress in the Twenty-First Century', in C. Aneshensel, J. Phelan, and A. Bierman (eds.) *Handbook of the Sociology of Mental Health* ,Netherlands: Springer.

Whyte, W. H. (1980) *The Social Life of Small Urban Spaces. Project for Public Spaces*, New York: Municipal Art Society of New York.

Whyte, W. H. (1988) *City: Rediscovering the Center*, Philadelphia: University of Pennsylvania Press.

Wild, C. P. (2012) 'The Exposome: From Concept to Utility', *International Journal of Epidemiology* 41(1): 24–32.

Wild, C. P., Scalbert, A., and Herceg, Z. (2013) 'Measuring the Exposome: A Powerful Basis for Evaluating Environmental Exposures and Cancer Risk', *Environmental and Molecular Mutagenesis* 54(7): 480–499.

Williams, R. (1969) 'Foreword', in A. Fried and R. M. Elman (eds.) *Charles Booth's London: A Portrait of the Poor at the Turn of the Century, Drawn from His 'Life and Labour of the People in London'*, London: Hutchinson.

Williams, R. J. (2004) *The Anxious City: British Urbanism in the Late 20th Century*, London: Routledge.

Wing, J. K. (1980) 'Social Psychiatry in the United Kingdom: The Approach to Schizophrenia', *Schizophrenia Bulletin* 6(4): 556–565.

Winz, M. and Söderström, O. (2021) 'How Environments Get to the Skin: Biosensory Ethnography as a Method for Investigating the Relation between Psychosis and the City', *BioSocieties* 16: 157–176.

Wirth, L. (1938) 'Urbanism as a Way of Life', *American Journal of Sociology* 44(1): 1–24.

Woese, C. R. (2004) 'A New Biology for a New Century', *Microbiology and Molecular Biology Review* 68(2): 173–186.

Wolfe, C. T. and Wong, A. (2014) 'The Return of Vitalism: Canguilhem, Bergson and the Project of Biophilosophy', in M. de Beistegui, G. Bianco, and M. Gracieuse (eds.) *The Care of Life: Transdisciplinary Perspectives in Bioethics and Biopolitics*, London: Rowman & Littlefield.

Wolff, H., Wolf, S., and Hare, C. (1950) *Life Stress and Bodily Disease: Proceedings of the Association of Research in Nervous and Mental Disease*, Vol. 29. New York: Hafner Publishing.

Wolff, H. G. (1953) 'Life Stress and Bodily Disease', in A. Weider (ed.) *Contributions toward Medical Psychology: Theory and Psychodiagnostic Methods Vol. 1*, New York: Ronald Press.

Wolff, J. and de-Shalit, A. (2013) *Disadvantage*, Oxford: Oxford University Press.

World Health Organization (2014) *Social Determinants of Mental Health*, Geneva: World Health Organization.

Wright, N. and Stickley, T. (2013) 'Concepts of Social Inclusion, Exclusion and Mental Health: A Review of the International Literature', *Journal of Psychiatric and Mental Health Nursing* 20(1): 71–81.

Xiang, B. (2004) *Transcending Boundaries: Zhejiangcun: The Story of a Migrant Village in Beijing*, Leiden-Boston: Brill.

Yam, K.-Y., Naninck, E. F. G., Schmidt, M. V., Lucassen, P. J., et al. (2015) 'Early-Life Adversity Programs Emotional Functions and the Neuroendocrine Stress System: The Contribution of Nutrition, Metabolic Hormones and Epigenetic Mechanisms', *Stress* 18(3): 328–342.

Yang, G., Wang, Y., Zeng, Y., Gao, G. F., et al. (2013) 'Rapid Health Transition in China, 1990–2010: Findings from the Global Burden of Disease Study 2010', *The Lancet* 381(9882): 1987–2015.

Yang, J. (2015) *Unknotting the Heart: Unemployment and Therapeutic Governance in China*, Ithaca, NY: Cornell University Press.

Yang, J. (2017) *Mental Health in China: Change, Tradition, and Therapeutic Governance*, New York: John Wiley.

Yang, T., Guo, Y., Ma, M., Li, Y., et al. (2017) 'Job Stress and Presenteeism among Chinese Healthcare Workers: The Mediating Effects of Affective Commitment', *International Journal of Environmental Research and Public Health* 14(9): 978.

Yang, W., Wu, B., Tan, S. Y., Li, B., et al. (2020) 'Understanding Health and Social Challenges for Aging and Long-Term Care in China', *Research on Aging*. doi:10.1177/0164027520938764

Youdell, D. (2017) 'Bioscience and the Sociology of Education: The Case for Biosocial Education', *British Journal of Sociology of Education* 38(8): 1273–1287.

Young, A. (2008) 'A Time to Change Our Minds: Anthropology and Psychiatry in the 21st Century', *Culture, Medicine, and Psychiatry* 32(2): 298–300.

Yu, C., Lou, C., Cheng, Y., Cui, Y., et al. (2019) 'Young Internal Migrants' Major Health Issues and Health Seeking Barriers in Shanghai, China: A Qualitative Study', *BMC Public Health* 19(1): 336.

Yuan, Y. (2014) *A Different Place in the Making: The Everyday Life Practices of Chinese Rural Migrants in Urban Villages*, Bern: Peter Lang AG.

Zacharias, J. and Tang, Y. (2010) 'Restructuring and Repositioning Shenzhen, China's New Mega City', *Progress in Planning* 73(4): 209–249.

Zeiderman, A. (2013) 'Living Dangerously: Biopolitics and Urban Citizenship in Bogotá, Colombia', *American Ethnologist* 40(1): 71–87.

Zhang, L. (2017) 'The Rise of Therapeutic Governing in Postsocialist China', *Medical Anthropology* 36(1): 6–18.

Zhang, L. (2018) 'Cultivating the Therapeutic Self in China', *Medical Anthropology* 37(1): 45–58.

Zhong, B.-L., Liu, T.-B., Huang, J.-X., Fung, H. H., et al. (2016) 'Acculturative Stress of Chinese Rural-to-Urban Migrant Workers: A Qualitative Study', *PLoS One* 11(6).

Zhou, H. (2002) 'A Review, Summary and Discussion of Population Migration Study in China', *Population & Economics* 1.

Zhu, Y., Gao, J., Nie, X., Dai, J., et al. (2019) 'Associations of Individual Social Capital with Subjective Well-Being and Mental Health among Migrants: A Survey from Five Cities in China', *International Health* 11(Supplement_1): S64–S71.

Zhu, Y., Hu, X., Yang, B., Wu, G., et al. (2018) 'Association between Migrant Worker Experience, Limitations on Insurance Coverage, and Hospitalization for Schizophrenia in Hunan Province, China', *Schizophrenia Research* 197: 93–97.

INDEX

Abbot, Alison, 152–53
Abbot, Andrew, 33, 36, 38
acculturation, 76–77. *See also* assimilation
Adams, John, 129–30, 222n17
Adli, Mazda, 140, 223n1
affordances, 188–91
African Americans, 40, 44, 54. *See also* race
Age of Stress, The (Jackson), 120–23, 221n5, 222n8
agriculture, 22, 24, 69. *See also* food production
Alaimo, Stacey, 184
Allbutt, Clifford, 120
allostasis, 156. *See also* homeostasis
Alzheimer's disease, 196
American Journal of Psychiatry, 69, 71
American Psychiatric Association, 103
Amin, Ash, 63, 98, 101–2, 114–16, 192, 214nn13–14, 219n18
Anatomy of Courage, The (Moran), 222n10
Anderson, Bridget, 12
Anderson, Elijah, 42
Andrade, Laura, 80
Anthropocene, 9
antidepressants, 59, 220n34. *See also* depression
anti-racism, 43. *See also* racism
anxiety, 76, 80, 145
Architects Journal, 228n1
Ash, Alec, 218–19n5
Ashby, William Ross, 134
assemblages, 8–9, 214n15
assimilation, 55. *See also* acculturation; migration
asylums, 3, 67–68, 104, 216n9. *See also* mental illness
Atwater, Wilbur, 52
authoritarianism, 177

Bach-y-Rita, Paul, 225n32
Baltimore, 128–29
Bangladesh, 81

Baoji, 111
Barker, David, 159
Baudelaire, Charles, 26–27, 120
Bay, Mia, 42, 44
Beard, George, 64
Béhague, Dominique, 81
Belkin, Gary, 208
Bell, Florence, 13
Benjamin, Walter, 13, 26–27, 120, 201
Berlin, 24, 27, 29
Bernard, Claude, 121
Berridge, Virginia, 222n11
Berry, John W., 77
Bhugra, Dinesh, 76
biology, 1–2, 7, 14, 31, 34, 38–39, 136, 182, 200, 203, 205, 213n2
biopolitics, 3, 50, 176–77, 182, 204, 206. *See also* necropolitics
biopsychosocial models, 15, 57, 70, 174
biosensory ethnography, 198
Birk, Rasmus, 227n13
Birmingham, 23
birth control, 67
Bister, Milena, 191–92
Boas, Franz, 43
Booth, Charles, 18, 40, 47–48, 50, 55–56
Booth, Mary, 48
Borrell-Carrió, Francesc, 174
Boughton, John, 211
Bourdieu, Pierre, 143, 158
Bowlby, John, 134, 224n24
Braidwood, Ella, 228n1
brain: as an assemblage, 9; damage to, 168; development of, 141, 167, 169, 183, 196, 225–26n34; embeddedness of, 10; and the environment, 117; and epigenetics, 163–64; inflammation of, 223–24n15; isolation of, 140–41; as a singular organ, 5, 214n10, 225n31; visualization of, 148–49. *See also* humans; neuroimaging; neuroscience; plasticity; urban brain
Brazil, 178, 193

Brenner, Neil, 11
Briggs, Asa, 50, 52
Bristol, 23
Brown, George, 142, 144
Bulmer, Martin, 33–34
Burgess, Ernest, 13, 33–35, 39, 69
Burr, Rollin H., 69

Calhoun, John, 19, 129, 131–32, 134
Canada, 77, 216n12
Canguilhem, Georges, 215n21
Cannon, Walter, 120–21
Cantor-Graae, Elizabeth, 74
capitalism, 15, 30, 96, 219n6
Capon, Anthony, 154
Case, Elizabeth, 214n19
Central Population Registers, 141–42
Chan, Jenny, 93–94, 112
Chang, Lesley, 89, 93, 96, 218–19n5
Chiang, Howard, 104
Chicago, 30–32, 36, 39, 42
Chicago School, 13–14, 30–34, 36–39, 41, 56, 120. *See also* sociology
childhood, 5, 65–66, 157, 159, 168, 193–94, 217n18, 224n17
Chile, 49
China: countryside of, 87; depression in, 106–7; economy of, 88–89, 97, 108–9, 219n6, 219n9; education in, 102; language of mental illness in, 103–4; migration research in, 80; modernization of, 96; psychiatry in, 106–7, 110, 193, 220n27; urban imaginations in, 199
China on the Move (Fan), 90
Chinese Classification of Mental Disorders, 105
Christian, John, 129–30, 222n15
circular migration, 23–24
cities: anxieties of, 19, 21, 69, 142, 181; benefits of, 64, 95, 205; and biopolitics, 161, 176; boundaries of, 11–12; and citizenship, 10, 131; compared to countryside, 87–88; emptiness of, 132; governance of, 177–78, 182; growth of, 35, 201; as habitats, 204, 214n12; hygiene in, 180; and inhabitation, 10; knowledge of, 187; as machines, 214n14; and migration, 4–5, 25, 56; and modernity, 23, 26–28; and mortality rates, 125; as a natural area, 34; as noisy, 171; organization of, 18, 24, 29, 39, 186–87, 226n1; perceptions of, 10, 19, 126, 150, 198; and population growth, 46, 131; and race, 42, 160; and schizophrenia, 142; smell of, 172; as a social laboratory, 34; and social relations, 86; and touch, 172;

as unique spaces, 11, 26, 30, 170–71. *See also* megacities; right to the city; suburbs; urban life; *specific cities*
citizenship, 10, 27, 79, 109, 182
City, The (Park, Burgess, et al.), 34
civilization, 29
class, 10, 35, 40, 64, 81, 165–66, 181, 224n19. *See also* poverty; social mobility
cleanliness, 29, 46, 65, 180
cognitive appraisal, 134–35, 138. *See also* stress
Cohen, Mandel, 124
Cohen, Sheldon, 135–36
Coleman, James, 143, 158
College Settlement movement, 40, 43
Collier, Stephen, 191
Collins, Randall, 144
Colombia, 182
Community Mental Health Journal, 73
Comte, Auguste, 47
Conditions of the Working-Class in England (Engels), 29
Confucianism, 113
Covid-19 pandemic, 194, 214n11, 221n3
Coyne, Richard, 154
Cressey, Paul Frederick, 30
Cressy, Paul Goalby, 30
Crile, George, 120
critical theory, 71
Culver, Helen, 31
Current Opinion in Psychiatry, 145
Current Opinion in Psychology, 155
cybernetics, 134

dagong, 94, 219n13
Danish Civil Registration System, 142–43
Danish Psychiatric Register, 142–43
danwei system, 88, 109
Darwin, Charles, 42, 50
Das, Veena, 58
Davis, David E., 128
Davis, Mike, 84–85, 130
Deaton, Angus, 214n19
deep democracy, 84
Defert, Daniel, 227n6
degeneracy theory, 18, 65–66, 216n6
Deleuze, Gilles, 184, 190, 214n15
Deliveroo, 209
dementia, 145, 209
Deng Xiaoping, 219n6
Dennis, Richard, 26
depression, 76, 103, 105–7, 144, 146, 220n24. *See also* antidepressants
de-Shalit, Avner, 166
determinism, 161–62, 202

Detroit, 24
Developmental Origins of Health and Disease (DOHaD), 159, 223n4
Dhaka, 81, 218n19
Diagnostic and Statistical Manual of Mental Disorders, 103
diagnostic categories, 80–81, 103, 105–6, 142–43. *See also* mental illness; *specific systems*
Dickens, Charles, 47–48
disabilities, 49, 57, 106, 191
DNA, 2, 15, 162–63, 196. *See also* genetics
Dokumaci, Arseli, 191
Dongguan, 89, 93–94
Downey, Greg, 193
DSM-IV, 80, 103, 105
Du Bois, W.E.B., 13–14, 18, 39–43, 55, 60
Duhl, Leonard, 132
Dunham, H. Warren, 69–73
Dunlop, J. C., 52

Ecological Momentary Assessments, 148, 197
ecological urbanism, 214n13
economic stressors, 146
Ecuador, 178
EEG devices, 148–51, 154
enclaves, 56
Engel, George, 57, 174
Engels, Friedrich, 29, 48
epigenetics, 15–16, 161–65, 175, 196, 213n9. *See also* genetics
ethnology, 43
eugenics, 43, 53, 67
Euro-American thought, 104–6
European Union, 223n2
"Experience of Living in Cities, The" (Milgram), 188

Factory Girls (Chang), 89
factory housing, 87, 93, 97
factory labor, 89, 93, 126
family, 97, 181
Fan, Cindy, 90, 218n2
Faris, Ellsworth, 32
Faris, Robert E. Lee, 32, 36–37, 69–73
Fett, Anne-Kathrin, 146
fight or flight response, 155–56
financial insecurity, 4, 194
Firdaus, Gunchar, 79, 82
flâneur, 23, 26–27. *See also* modernity
food production, 23–24, 51–52. *See also* agriculture; nutrition
Foucault, Michel, 19, 180, 190, 204, 220n28, 226n3, 226n5, 227nn8–9

Foxconn, 92–93, 219n9, 219n12
France, 66
Freedman, Jonathan, 131
Freud, Sigmund, 29, 215n3
Frisby, David, 26
Fritz, Angela, 30
functional MRI (fMRI), 148–50, 152
Fund for Race Psychology, 31

Galea, Sandro, 164–66
Gallup, 118–19
Galton, Francis, 42, 50
garden city movement, 199, 204
Gaskell, Elizabeth, 48
gender, 36, 68, 80, 89, 94, 100, 171
general adaptation syndrome, 120–24, 130, 137, 223n19. *See also* stress
General Health Questionnaire-12 (GHQ), 83
genetics, 2, 8, 183. *See also* DNA; epigenetics
gentrification, 204
geographical drift hypothesis, 141–42
geosocial, 213n3
Germany, 23, 29, 53, 68, 104
Gibson, James, 188–91
Giddings, Franklin, 36
GIS mapping, 148
Glasgow, 23
Glass, David, 134
globalization, 21, 96
Global North, 14
Global South, 75, 79, 81, 85, 87, 206, 212
Goffman, Erving, 144, 190
Gomer, Nina, 39
Goodman, Nelson, 186
Gou, Terry, 93
Gould, Elizabeth, 168
GPS trackers, 197
Great Depression, 53
Greece, 118
green spaces, 154, 160, 198
Greenwood, 54
Grinker, Roy R., 134
Grob, Gerald, 69
Grosz, Elizabeth, 183
"Growth of the City, The" (Burgess), 34–35
Gruebner, Oliver, 81
Guangdong Province, 89
Guangzhou, 87

habitats, 9–10, 205–6. *See also* niches
Haerle, Rudolf, 31
Han, Clara, 58–59
Hanssen, Beatrice, 27
Hardie, Keir, 47

Harrington, Anne, 215n2
Harris, Tirril, 142, 144
Harvey, David, 179, 198, 226n3
healthcare access, 57, 63, 77, 79, 92, 113–14, 181, 194, 208
health-seeking behavior, 113–14
healthy immigrant effect, 77
Healthy New Towns initiative, 20, 205
Hebb, Donald, 167
hereditary principle, 66
heterotopias, 19, 180
Hill, Octavia, 13, 47
Hinde, Robert A., 134
Hinkle, Lawrence, 124
HIV, 57
Hochstadt, Steve, 29
Hoffman, Daniel, 159
homeostasis, 121. *See also* allostasis
hormonal feedback, 130
Horwitz, Allan V., 69
House We Live In, The, 130
housing, 44, 47, 87, 92–93, 98–99, 101, 194, 198
hukou system, 89–90, 92, 94, 98, 100, 110, 192–93, 218n1
Hull House, 31, 40
humans: as animals, 2, 10; bodies of, 16, 121, 173, 183; habitats of, 9–10, 34, 214n12; as increasingly urban, 8; models for, 127, 131–32, 138–39, 159, 168–69; relation to the environment, 15–16, 183–85, 195, 200, 202; senses of, 171–72; as social, 8, 144, 213n2. *See also* brain; microbiomes

ICD-10 categories, 59, 103
Image of the City, The (Lynch), 186
income inequality, 88, 158, 210
Independent Labour Party, 47
Indigeneity, 215n1
individualism, 15, 203
inhabitation, 6, 10, 20, 180
inheritance, 8, 65–67, 181
interdisciplinarity, 13, 16, 148
Irish migration, 24, 44, 50, 67–68

Jackson, Mark, 120–23, 221n5, 222n8
Jacobs, Jane, 131
Japan, 104, 109, 149
Jiao, 218n2
Johnson, Peter, 180, 226n5, 227n6
Jones, Peter, 78
Journal of Abnormal and Social Psychology, 71
Journal of Human Stress, 120
Journal of Mammology, 130

Kasinitz, Philip, 55
Katz, Michael, 39, 42
Keiner, Christine, 128
Keith, Michael, 218n2, 219n16
Keswick, Maggie, 228n2
Keyes, Katherine, 166
Kirk, Robert, 133, 223n19
Kirkbride, James, 78
Klausner, Martina, 191–92
Kleinman, Arthur, 104
Knowles, Caroline, 55, 57
Kondo, Michele, 151
Korean War, 124
Krabbendam, Lydia, 142, 146–48
Krieger, Nancy, 175

labor: conditions of, 50–51, 125–26, 194, 219n11; divisions of, 34, 36, 219n13; economics of, 47, 96; forms of, 89, 92–101; and gender, 89, 94, 100; markets of, 110, 214n19; and power, 52; precarity of, 91, 100, 209; and resistance, 95; and rights, 93; as a source of stress, 125; workspaces, 209
Labour and Life of the People in London (Booth), 46
Lakoff, Andrew, 191
Lancet, 63, 125, 145, 223n19
Landecker, Hannah, 51
Lazarus, Richard, 134–35, 158, 195
Lee, Sing, 103
Lefebvre, Henri, 19, 176, 178–79, 185, 199, 210
Lemmers-Jansen, Imke, 146
Lewis, Aubrey, 134
Lewis, David Levering, 40, 43
Liddell, Howard S., 134
Life Stress and Bodily Disease (Wolff, Wolf, and Hare), 123
Lindemann, Eric, 222n18
Lindert, Jutta, 75
Link, Bruce, 165–66
Lipowski, Zbigniew, 136–37
Lipton, Michael, 4
Liu, Yuting, 90
Liverpool, 46
Lock, Margaret, 203
Logan, Alan, 159–60
London, 45–46, 188, 207
London Labour and the London Poor (Mayhew), 47
Lowe, Monica Ellwood, 224n19
Lynch, Kevin, 185, 188, 197, 227n11
Lynch, Richard A., 227n8

managerial revolution, 126. *See also* Taylorism
Manchester, 23, 29–30
Manning, Nick, 227n13
Mao Zedong, 87
Marcuse, Peter, 178
marriage, 67
Marx, Karl, 52, 219n14
Mason, John, 120, 138, 222n8
Mayhew, Henry, 47–48
Mbembe, Achille, 45
McCray, Chirlane, 208
McEwen, Bruce, 19, 156, 158, 224n18
McEwen, Craig, 158
McHarg, Ian, 130
McKenzie, Roderick, 36, 78
Meaney, Michael, 15, 163, 225n28
megacities, 4, 12, 64, 81, 85, 87, 92, 212.
    See also cities; urban villages
Melosi, Martin, 10
Menken, H. L., 127
Mental Disorders in Urban Areas (Faris and
    Dunham), 69–71
mental health: measurement of, 81, 105,
    110–12, 142, 207; perceptions of, 3, 7, 102,
    114; research on, 75; and risk factors, 83;
    terminology of, 3, 107, 112, 116
Mental Health Research Fund, 133–34
mental illness: categorization of, 59, 80–81,
    83, 103, 110–11; as hereditary, 105, 161;
    measurement of, 49, 70, 109, 119; percep-
    tions of, 58; rates of, 4, 8, 69, 75, 210; risk
    factors, 13, 142, 165. *See also* asylums;
    diagnostic categories; *specific conditions*
metaphysics, 16
Meyer, Adolf, 127, 217n12
Meyer-Lindenberg, Andreas, 152–53, 155
miasmatic theory, 174
microbiomes, 145, 173–74, 210. *See also*
    humans
migrants: aspirations of, 18, 78; in asylums, 67,
    216–17n9; as entrepreneurial, 85, 100–102;
    health of, 47, 57, 75, 113; housing for,
    97–98; relationship to home, 88, 91, 96,
    112, 115; socioeconomic status of, 78; stud-
    ies of, 64; terminology of, 74, 214n17
migration: and adversity, 143; definitions
    of, 76–77, 218n2; focus on international
    migration, 12; and health risks, 113–14;
    and labor supply, 91, 110; limits on, 53–54,
    101, 216n12; and modernity, 23; motiva-
    tions for, 23, 47, 54, 75, 82, 88, 218–19n5;
    and opportunity, 99; patterns of, 12–13,
    22–23, 29, 39–41, 80, 96, 111, 214n16,
    218n2; perceptions of, 21, 55, 99; and

population growth, 4–5, 29–31, 46; stud-
    ies of, 8, 25, 32, 39, 53–55, 60, 110, 201;
    and urbanization, 23. *See also* assimila-
    tion; rural-to-urban migration
Milgram, Stanley, 13, 187–88, 197
milieu interior, 121
Milwaukee, 24
modernity, 22–23, 26–28, 30, 172. *See also*
    flâneur
Moore, Robert, 56
morals, 25, 64–65
Moran, John, 222n10
Morel, Benedict, 65–67, 216n6
Morgan, Craig, 75
Morris, Aldon, 40, 42–43
Morris, Jerry, 125
Mortensen, Preben Bo, 142
Mumbai, 82, 84

National Health Service, 20, 205, 228n3
National Institute of Mental Health, 129
National Origins Act of 1924, 54
Nature, 152, 163
Near Infrared Spectroscopy (NIRS), 149
necropolitics, 45. *See also* biopolitics
neoliberalism, 15
neo-Marxist sociology, 71
neurasthenia, 64, 105
neurecosocial approaches, 141, 161, 203,
    206, 209
neurobiology, 5, 19, 223n2
neuroimaging, 147–50, 154, 197, 224n19.
    See also brain; *specific technologies*
neuroscience, 8, 175, 203, 213n6. *See also*
    brain
neurosocial knowledge, 119, 177
New Towns, 199
new urban sociology, 71
New York, 188, 207, 222n13
New York Times, 40, 118
Ng, Emily, 220n33
niches, 10, 185, 189, 191, 193–94, 196, 200,
    208–9. *See also* habitats
niching, 192–98
Niewöhner, Jörg, 191–92
90/10 gap, 79–80
NIRS caps, 197
noise, 171
nostalgia, 178
nutrition, 51–53, 159, 216n9. *See also* food
    production

Oakley, Ann, 222n11
Ødegård, Ørnulv, 73–74, 217n12

one child policy, 218n4
Ong, Aihwa, 219n12
operationalization, 79, 144
Os, Jim van, 142
Osborne, Thomas, 215n21
Osler, William, 120

Paris, 23–24, 26–27, 188
Park, Robert, 13, 34, 36, 69
Pasquino, Pasquale, 227n9
Patient Health Questionnaire-9 (PHQ-9),
    220n31–220n32
Pedersen, Carsten Bøcker, 142
Perfume (Süskind), 172
Persian Letters (Montesquieu), 7
Personal Well-Being Index scale (PWI),
    220n33
Phelan, Jo, 165–66
phenomenology, 202
Philadelphia, 39–40. *See also* Seventh Ward
Philadelphia Negro, The (Du Bois), 39–45
Philadelphia Settlement, 40
Phillips, Michael, 105
Pile, Steve, 28
Pisarevskaya, Asya, 57
Planet of Slums (Davis), 84
plasticity, 156, 167–70, 225n33. *See also* brain
Plumber, Norman, 124
policing, 181, 227n9
policymakers, 7–8, 21
Polish Peasant in Europe and America, The
    (Thomas and Znaniecki), 31–32, 54, 215n4
Pollock, Horatio M., 69
Pollock, Kristian, 138
population: birth rates, 49; density, 54, 90,
    129, 131–32; distribution, 4, 62; growth
    of, 23, 29, 46, 50, 62, 175; limits of, 130;
    measurement of, 89, 141; mortality rates,
    49, 181
Portes, Alejandro, 55–56
Positron Emission Tomography (PET), 148–49
poverty, 24, 47–48, 51, 53, 63, 157, 194, 196.
    See also class
Poverty and Population, 222n11
Poverty: A Study of Town Life (Rowntree), 50
Povinelli, Elizabeth, 98
Power, D'Arcy, 120
Power/Knowledge (Gordon), 227n8
Prague, 24
precarity, 4, 91, 98, 112, 116, 161, 191, 194, 201
Prescott, Susan, 159–60
psychiatric epidemiology, 13, 73
psychiatry: and diagnoses, 70; discourse
    of, 106; and genetics, 162; goals of, 69;

growth of, 127; professionalization of,
    64–65, 104, 161; and sociology, 71–73;
    as somatic, 69
psychoanalysis, 95
psychobiology, 127
psychology, 13, 107–8, 138
psychosomatic medicine, 136–37
psychotherapy, 59, 108
psy complex, 25, 107, 193, 220n27
Pun, Ngai, 83, 94, 98, 112

race, 7, 31, 41–42, 44–45, 55–56, 73, 79.
    See also African Americans
racism, 4, 14, 43, 55–57, 74, 210. *See also*
    anti-racism
Ramsden, Ed, 127, 129–30, 222n12,
    222n17–222n18
Ranney, M. H., 68
Rapoport, Amos, 137
rat cities, 19, 129, 131, 134, 137
rat poison, 128
rats: economic burden of, 128; emergent
    behaviors in, 129; as model for humans,
    127, 131–32, 134, 138–39, 159, 163–64,
    224n24; neurogenesis in, 168–69;
    as pests, 222n13; in slums, 83; stress
    response in, 126–27
Reardon, Jenny, 213n7
Redfield, Robert, 76–77
reductionism, 6–7, 14, 38, 203
Rees, W. Linford, 134
refugees, 57, 75–76
regime of living, 191
Reichert, Markus, 155
religion, 68–69
remittances, 88, 98
Research Memorandum on Migration Differ-
    entials (Thomas), 53
Rex, John, 56
Richaud, Lisa, 98, 101–2, 114–16, 182, 219n18
Richter, Curt, 126, 128
Rietveld, Erik, 189–91
right to the city, 19, 176–78, 183, 199, 203.
    See also cities
Roberts, Ffrangcon, 123
Rodent Ecology Project, 128
Rosen, George, 227n9
Roth, Martin, 134
Rowntree, Seebohm, 18, 50–51, 55, 60
Royal Statistical Society, 47, 49
Rude, George, 24
rural-to-urban migration, 4, 8, 18–25, 47,
    63–64, 87–88, 94, 115, 192–93, 201,
    218nn1–3. *See also* migration

Russell Sage Foundation, 52
Rutter, Michael, 207
Ryle, John, 222n11

Sadler, William, 120
Sampson, Laura, 146
Sampson, Robert, 33, 36
Santiago, 59
São Paulo, 80, 201
São Salvador de Bahia, 193
Saunders, Doug, 85
Savage, Mike, 28, 32, 38
scent marketing, 172
schizophrenia, 72, 74–75, 142
Schofield, Peter, 143
Schopler, John, 135
Schore, Allan, 224n24
Science, 152
Selten, Jean-Paul, 74
Selye, Hans, 119, 121–24, 126, 130, 134, 137
Seventh Ward, 40–41, 44. *See also* Philadelphia
sex, 44, 58, 94, 121, 123, 129–30
Shanghai, 18, 80–81, 86–87, 91, 101–2, 111, 157, 192, 201, 218n1. *See also* Tongli Road
sharecropping, 40
Shenzhen, 87, 89, 94, 219n6
Shonkoff, Jack P., 158–59, 224n17
Simmel, Georg, 8, 13, 18, 27–29, 34, 60, 86, 120, 201, 215n2
Simone, Abdoumaliq, 12
Singer, Jerome, 134
Siu, Kaxton, 97
Slum Adversity Index (SAI), 83
slums, 47, 63, 79, 81, 83–84, 87, 216n3, 216n5, 217n18
smartphones, 113
Smith, Barry, 189
Smith, Dennis, 33
Smith, Hubert Llewellyn, 46
Smith, Michael Peter, 29
Snow, Herbert, 120
Snyder, Jason, 225n34
social capital, 143–44, 154–55
Social Darwinism, 36, 43
social defeat paradigm, 75, 217n13
Social Democratic Federation, 48
Social Determinants of Mental Health, 157
social epidemiology, 166
Social Forces (Schatzman and Strauss), 71
Social Justice and the City (Harvey), 179, 198
social mobility, 76, 85. *See also* class
Social Science Research Council, 54
social suffering, 57–58

social ties, 33, 42, 99, 158
social workers, 36
Society for Neuroscience, 223n2
sociodevelopmental model, 75
sociology, 1–2, 5, 8, 11, 38, 55, 60, 69, 71–73, 200, 213n2. *See also* Chicago School
sociology of inhabitation, 203
Söderström, Ole, 197, 223n9
Solinger, Dorothy, 88, 218n3
soundscapes, 171
Space Cadets, 132–33
spatial justice, 8, 203
Spencer, Herbert, 42
statistics, 42, 47–51, 54, 57, 112, 213n5
St. Louis, 24
Stockdale, Janet, 135
St. Petersburg, 24
stress: causes of, 122–25, 151–53, 155; and disease, 120; effects of, 120, 137, 147, 154, 156, 165, 195–96, 221n3, 223n19; language of, 119, 123, 132; as a linking mechanism, 133, 137–38; measurement of, 102, 119, 135, 148, 152; and the microbiome, 173; and migration, 102–3, 112–13; mitigation of, 158, 161, 206; perceptions of, 19, 107, 133–34, 145, 175, 202; prevalence of, 116–18, 221n4; as subjective, 121, 134–35, 138, 157, 195, 210; terminology of, 107, 120–21, 131; as toxic, 157. *See also* cognitive appraisal; general adaptation syndrome
Subbaraman, Ramnath, 82, 84
suburbs, 23, 35. *See also* cities
Sugrue, Thomas, 39, 42
suicide, 92, 217n18, 219n9
Sullivan, Robert, 222n15
Süskind, Patrick, 172
Swider, Sarah, 92, 98–99

Taub, Edward, 225n33
Taxi-Dance Hall, The (Cressy), 30
Taylorism, 96, 219n14. *See also* managerial revolution
Thaxton, Ralph, 220n22
Thomas, Dorothy Swaine, 32, 53–54, 215n4
Thomas, W. I., 31–32, 54, 215n4
Thompson, E. P., 96
Thrift, Nigel, 214nn13–14
Thrive movement, 198–99, 207, 228n10
Thurston, Anne, 220n22
Tillot, P. M., 50
Tilly, Charley, 22
Times, 120
Titmuss, Richard, 125, 222n11
toilet access, 83

Tongli Road, 101, 104, 114–15, 192–93. *See also* Shanghai
Toronto, 207
touch, 172
toxic stress, 157–58
Toynbee Hall, 40
transcultural psychiatry, 104

UK Economic and Social Research Council, 213n1
Umwelt, 170–71, 185–86, 206, 227n16
"Uncanny, The" (Freud), 29
United Kingdom, 23, 53, 55, 72, 118, 133
United Nations, 62, 214n16
United Nations Habitat, 79
United Nations Human Development Report, 63
United States, 24, 30, 53, 56, 68–69, 103–4, 118, 124, 127–28, 214n19, 216n12
United States Census, 53
United States Department of Agriculture, 52
urban bias theory, 4, 63–64, 216n2
urban brain, 7–9, 141, 154, 161, 175. *See also* brain
Urban Brain workshops, 223n1
urban drift, 72, 142
Urban Ecology, 137
urbanicity, 141–42, 145–46
urbanism, 29
"Urbanism as a Way of Life" (Wirth), 37
urbanization, 62, 82, 91, 142
urban life, 4, 6, 11–12, 15, 18, 21, 28, 37, 126, 129, 178, 182. *See also* cities
urban planning, 24, 154, 160, 198, 205–6, 209–10
urban-rural distinctions, 145, 150
urban villages, 87, 90, 97, 100. *See also* megacities
Urry, John, 172
Uses of Epidemiology (Morris), 125

Vienna, 24
vitalism, 5–6, 9, 16–17, 22, 31, 55–56, 59–60, 69, 203, 205
von Uexküll, Jakob, 170, 185

Wahlberg, Ayo, 191
Walker, Francis Amasa, 53, 216n11
walking interview, 187, 197
Walter, W. Grey, 134
Walter Reed Army Medical Centre, 124
Wang, Wen-ji, 104
Warde, Alan, 28, 32, 38

Warsaw, 24
Watson, John B., 126
Webb, Beatrice, 46, 50
Wheaton, Blair, 195
White, Paul, 124
white supremacy, 45
Whyte, William H., 13, 131–32, 189
Williams, Raymond, 48
Williams, Richard, 29
Wilson, E. O., 147
Windelband, Wilhelm, 34
Wing, John, 72
Winz, Marc, 197
Wired, 152
Wirth, Louis, 29, 33, 37
Wittgenstein, Ludwig, 191
Woese, Carl, 213n1
Wolf, Steward G., 123
Wolff, Harold, 123–24
Wolff, Jonathan, 166
World Health Organization, 103, 157–58
World Health Organization Composite International Diagnostic Interview (CIDI), 80, 103
World Health Organization Disability Assessment Schedule 2.0 (WHO DAS), 83
World Health Organization Well-Being Index (WHO-5), 81–82, 218n20, 220n31
World Psychiatric Association, 217n15
World Urbanization Prospects, 62
World War I, 54
World War II, 55, 125, 128, 134–35, 177
Wuhan, 81, 220n27

Xiang, Biao, 219n8
Xingyang, 111
Xinzheng, 111

Yang, Jie, 106–7
Yan Yuan, 91
York, 50
Yu, Chunyan, 114

Zangwill, Oliver L., 134
Zeiderman, Austin, 182
Zhang, Li, 108
Zheijiancun, 219n8
Zhengzhou, 111
Zhong, Bao-Liang, 112
Zhou, Min, 55
Ziqui, Li, 219n7
Znaniecki, Florian, 31–32

A NOTE ON THE TYPE

This book has been composed in Adobe Text and Gotham.
Adobe Text, designed by Robert Slimbach for Adobe,
bridges the gap between fifteenth- and sixteenth-century
calligraphic and eighteenth-century Modern styles.
Gotham, inspired by New York street signs, was designed
by Tobias Frere-Jones for Hoefler & Co.